ENDORSEMENTS

I grew up reading weight-loss books and have written a few myself, but I have never come upon one that encapsulates the food-and-weight conundrum as effectively as this one. Dr. Sabatino delves brilliantly into the physical, emotional, social, ethical, and spiritual aspects of the problem, addressing all of them in his practical, workable lifestyle solution. Like that solution, this book is based on a great deal of science and even more love.

Victoria Moran,
author of *The Love-Powered Diet,*
Main Street Vegan, and *Age Like a Yog*i

This superb book is needed now, more than ever, as Dr. Sabatino provides a truly compassionate solution for the most pressing health issue that is causing misery and distress to billions of people worldwide. Obesity is a hugely complex topic and while there is no "quick fix," in this book Dr. Sabatino lays out lifestyle adjustments that genuinely work, as evidenced by the many thousands of patients who have benefited from his recommendations and have shed excess weight and actually kept it off long-term. There is no doubt that this book, based on a bedrock of the most up-to-date science, will become an indispensable guide to people suffering with obesity who are looking for lasting, sustainable health and a classic among healthcare professionals as it provides the most brilliant insight into how best to support patients.

Jayney Goddard MSc FCMA FRSM
President, The Complementary Medical Association,
author of *Rewind Your Body Clock*

PRAISE FOR DR. SABATINO AND HIS PROGRAM

From medication to freedom, from morbid obesity to normal, healthy weight and body fat, I lost 140 pounds on Dr. Sabatino's program and have kept it off for several decades. From depression to happiness, I eliminated cravings to refined sugars and sodas and broke lifelong addictions to processed foods. Through Dr. Sabatino's program and his compassionate support, I was able to resolve my compulsive eating behavior, start and maintain a healthy exercise program, start really loving myself more, and get on a good path to wellness. Without any question, Dr. Sabatino's program changed my life!

MB
Brooklyn, New York

Dr. Frank Sabatino has helped many people live more fulfilling lives and lose substantial amounts of weight by making adjustments to their diet, exercise, sleep, and stress management programs. He has been instrumental in my own self-care. Through Dr. Sabatino, I have learned and now practice a lifestyle that is free from toxic food and habits. He has helped me resolve major addictions and food cravings in my life. His lectures resonate with profound truth. He knows just what I need to recalibrate my health. I have been one of his followers for 25+ years.

CL
Memphis, Tennessee

My journey to health began 30 years ago when I had the pleasure of first meeting Dr. Frank Sabatino at The Regency Health Spa he was supervising in Hollywood, FL. His knowledge and expertise about health and wellness changed my life. I attended his remarkable lectures daily and realized that the vegan lifestyle was the best approach to a new and healthy way of life. Under Dr. Sabatino's care I lost 25 pounds and kept it off. That dramatically increased my energy and improved my health. I have been a vegan ever since, maintaining his whole plant food approach without added salt, oil or sugar, and at almost 80 years of age, I can't thank Dr. Sabatino enough for putting me on the path to a healthy lifestyle.

I have also attended many personal health retreats that Dr. Sabatino has supervised in Florida and Chicago and have always been impressed with his compassion and knowledge and how he has shared and spread this knowledge to all my friends and family.

BP
Hollywood, FL

Thanks to Dr. Frank Sabatino I am no longer an asthmatic, was able to correct my vitamin D deficiency within three months' time, and learned how I could prevent repeating my family's history of diabetes. Dr. Sabatino impacted me with his outstanding lectures and helped me through his teaching and care. Following his whole-food, plant-exclusive approach without processed food, I was able to reduce my dangerous blood sugar levels and won my lifelong battle with weight, losing more than 50 pounds and keeping it off for more than 25 years. At age 70, I look and feel better than ever, which is also evident in my health exams.

Dr. Sabatino goes beyond providing educated nutritional and exercise suggestions to facilitating lasting lifestyle changes that always help me connect to what is realistic and healthy for me. He assists me in being more aware of my body and mind connection and helps me prevent health problems from arising. I am a firm believer that Dr. Sabatino has saved my life through his tremendous support.

MT
New York, NY

I have known and been under the care of Dr. Frank Sabatino for almost 30 years. He is the best health lecturer I have ever heard and the most compassionate doctor I have ever met. His teaching and counsel helped me understand the important role of plant-based nutrition for maintaining high-level health, and his program of organic vegetable juices and raw and cooked whole-plant vegan foods without added salt, oil and sugar, together with exercise and stress management, helped me lose a substantial amount of weight and detoxify and recover from cancer and life-threatening blood clots. He has also played an important role in promoting and maintaining the health of my children. I have worked with him in a private office setting and shared his counsel in a spa/retreat setting as well as in personal retreats he has organized and directed. He is unequivocally the most inspirational, knowledgeable doctor I have ever known, and he has the ability to dramatically transform people's lives.

FBV
West Palm Beach, FL

My life changed the very first time I spent one week with Dr. Frank Sabatino. After 22 years of going to the spa that Dr. Sabatino directed, I can honestly say he has improved so many difficult health issues for me. Talk about a change of life! Even that was easier to face with the knowledge that Dr. Sabatino provided me. My blood sugar levels are more under control, and my need for insulin is so much less when I follow his program. With the help of Dr. Sabatino, I am a happier and healthier 76-year-young lady who enjoys life. Thank you, Dr. Sabatino, and I want to say I look forward to spending more time with you and learning more of what life can offer in a healthier world.

RF
Hallandale, FL

Twenty-nine years ago, I was in a terrible car accident. I checked into the Regency Health Spa where Dr. Sabatino was the health director and chiropractor, and he took me under his wing. He guided me with his knowledge and created a plan that changed my life. Twenty-nine years later, I still go to Dr. Frank for adjustments and have him look at my blood work. Besides being in excellent health, I have kept my weight down with his plant-exclusive food program while enjoying healthy recipes Dr. Sabatino has shared with me. He is tops in his field and a wealth of knowledge. Thank you, Dr. Sabatino, for being a positive light in my life!

AM
Aventura, FL

Dr. Frank Sabatino's ability to communicate and explain what can be difficult biochemistry for the layman to understand is brilliant. It is no wonder that since I met him in 1994, I stopped eating meat and poultry and dramatically improved my health immediately. Through the years he was able to guide me on a road to health that took me deeper into the path of being a total vegan and helped me maintain the healthiest weight and body fat of my life. His lectures are life-changing, and his accessibility is like no other. Being under his care is an opportunity that should be taken by anyone who wants to better their health in any way.

EB
Ancramdale, NY

When I was experiencing a great deal of inflammation related to an ongoing health issue, I consulted with Dr. Sabatino, and he suggested that a short fast would be appropriate in my situation. Since I only had a small window of time in which to do the fast and refeeding, I allocated two weeks total to this process, and I undertook a week-long, water-only fast under his care. By the third day of fasting, my pain was significantly less, and the inflammatory marker in my blood, Hs-CRP, dropped 40 points, from a high of 43 down to 3.

Dr. Sabatino supported me every step of the way with wisdom, compassion, and profound kindness. When strange symptoms and discomfort came up, he was able to dispel my worries with keen and accurate observation and sensible explanations. I'm the kind of person who needs to understand the science behind any approach to health care, and Dr. Sabatino patiently gave me all of the information I needed. With decades of experience under his belt and having supervised many thousands of water-only fasts, Dr. Sabatino is an acknowledged world expert in this field. I would not hesitate to fast under Dr. Sabatino's supervision again. In addition, while I was already eating plant-based when I met Dr. Sabatino, his emphasis on eliminating salt, oil, and sugar took my vegan diet to a healthier, higher level and has helped me maintain an optimal weight, very low body fat, and without any further inflammation. He is a physician I would trust with my life.

JG
London, England

Twenty years ago I discovered Dr. Frank Sabatino and his amazing, life-changing way of eating and living. My 70-year-old mother dragged me down to the health spa he was running in Florida, and we never really left again. Dr. Sabatino is the most incredible teacher, and I trust him with my life. His instincts on medical matters are astounding, and his lifestyle changes have been amazing for my whole family.

Dr. Sabatino is not only the best doctor I've ever encountered—and believe me, I've had tons—but also, he is so funny and understanding that all his information can be absorbed in the most delightful way. My mother, my son, and my daughter became "groupies" to the healthy and easy-to-live-by rules for a healthier life that Dr. Sabatino introduced us to. More importantly, Dr. Sabatino changed my mother's life. She so believed in his way of life and tried very hard to live by it, although she was over 70 years old when she met him and into her bad eating habits and lack of exercise her whole life. She never missed his lectures at the spa, never; she even took notes. Dr. Sabatino gave her the best years of her life.

In my years under his care at the spa, I lost over 30 pounds and never gained it back due to the way Dr. Sabatino teaches you about healthy eating. We've spent Thanksgiving at his spa, choosing to spend this wonderful time in Florida with Dr. Sabatino rather than stuffing ourselves with an unhealthy meal at home. I know that my mother lived longer and healthier because of Dr. Sabatino, and I know that my children and I will be now part of his program forever.

LLG
Denver, Colorado

WEIGHTLESS

COMPASSIONATE WEIGHT LOSS FOR LIFE

DR. FRANK SABATINO

Title: Weightless: Compassionate Weight Loss for Life

First published in 2024 by Let's Tell Your Story Publishing

ISBN 978-1-910600-45-0

Cover design: Coral McCloud
Book design: Amit Dey
Editing: Janice Ziegler

This book is written only as a source of information. The information contained in this book should by no means be considered a substitute for the advice of a qualified medical professional. Always consult your primary healthcare provider before beginning any new diet, exercise, or other health program.

All efforts have been made to ensure the accuracy of the information contained in this book as of the date published. The author and the publisher expressly disclaim responsibility for any adverse effects arising from the use or application of the information contained herein.

DEDICATION

To my sons Dante and Rodin, through light and dark you have taught me what love and compassion are all about and filled the world and my life with beautiful music. There are no better gifts.

ACKNOWLEDGMENTS

Writing a book is an arduous introspective journey. It takes a small tribe of supportive people to bring a book to fruition. I am so grateful for the support of the following tribe of friends and professionals and want to thank and acknowledge them for their significant contributions.

Big thanks to Jim Lennon, my true brother from another mother, and his wife Susan Taylor. Their patient readings, impactful comments, initial edits of the early stages of this manuscript, and especially my always entertaining conversations with Jim on natural hygiene, music, art, and life inspired my confidence and motivation to stay the course. A truly special thank you to my main editor, Janice Ziegler. Working with her and having her in my corner was a pleasure beyond words. Her relentless honesty, integrity, insight, expertise, and tireless effort are special gifts that truly honed my voice and vision into a more readable and accessible work. I couldn't have done it without her. A big thank you to my dear friends, Mark and Wanda Huberman, the President and Executive Director, respectively, of the National Health Association, for their constant, unwavering belief in me and my work and especially for the resources and support in getting this book published. I am especially appreciative of Jayney Goddard, my partner in life and love. Jayney's brilliant skills and accomplishments as a writer and editor were indispensable for the organization and layout of the figures and index in this book. More importantly, our conversations about this subject matter, as well as her insightful critiques and criticisms of my work, always colored with unconditional love, provided an honest sanctuary for the nurturing and expression of my voice and vision. A special thanks to my dear family friend of over 30 years, Bethany Vinal, for her remarkable kindness and constant support, and especially for introducing me to my beloved Jayney Goddard. Finally, I am ever so grateful for the professional support and work of Mitali Deypurkaystha and her brilliant team at The Vegan Publisher. I so appreciate their belief in my work and their willingness to publish this book and bring my vision to the public. It is a blessing to have a publisher that embodies the principles of compassionate, vegan living that have been the foundation of my life and thought for the greater part of my personal and professional life.

TABLE OF CONTENTS

FOREWORD

This is a very special book authored by Dr. Frank Sabatino, a highly accomplished professional in the discipline of human health. It addresses the most visible and, for many, the most tormenting health problem of our time, obesity. It is now a vast health problem costing an astounding $150–170 billion per year in the U.S. in addition to the mental anguish that so many individuals and their families experience.

Dr. Sabatino offers an unexcelled combination of patient-centered clinical experience, science-based proficiency, and personal experience with obesity to tell this story. He knows and discusses this issue as well as anyone I know. I especially like his commentary on the causation of a complex disease like obesity. Although many people understandably want simple solutions, that's not the way a health problem like obesity occurs, especially when consumption of foods and their nutritional effects are involved as causes of the disease.

Many behavioral, physiological, nutritional, hormonal, emotional, and biochemical categories of biological responses relate to obesity and related diseases. When investigating and finding ever more mechanisms operating within these complex conditions, however, there is no end to the details that might be encountered. Discovering yet another factor within these processes often leads to development of apparent remedies to correct the whole by treating specific details. As a result, we ignore lifestyle choices that are best described as often acting in unison. It's a process called "nature." Aristotle of ancient Greece knew about this phenomenon when he said that the whole is greater than the sum of its parts.

I don't mean to overlook claims of specific solutions for specific details gone amiss, but this cannot be a substitute for comprehensive solutions. This has long been a difficult concept to describe for the public. But I make the point here because Dr. Sabatino does this in a way that, in my experience, is unexcelled. His book is encyclopedic, practical, and exceedingly well written.

I am hopeful and confident that this is *the* most important book on obesity that has ever been written. It is urgently needed to counter our endless and ugly race to control obesity only by developing yet another lucrative business opportunity. Worse, the greedy, short-sighted approaches to control this problem are often based on the vulgar argument that obesity is primarily genetic, which then requires the development of anti-obesity drugs. Ample evidence has now shown that genes perform their tasks best when they are expressed by modifiable lifestyle practices, especially nutrition, that make the real difference in disease causation.

It's an honor for me to endorse this book.

T. Colin Campbell, PhD
Jacob Gould Schurman Professor Emeritus of Nutritional Biochemistry, Cornell University
Coauthor of *The China Study* (2005, 2016), *Whole* (2014), and *The Future of Nutrition* (2020)

INTRODUCTION

The earth is groaning under the collective weight of the people standing on it. Globally, in 2022, overweight people topped the three billion mark.[1] Growing up as a child on the streets of New York City, I'll always remember the Statue of Liberty standing on Liberty Island in New York Harbor as a looming monument to hope and freedom. But there's a new statue of American liberty. She's exhausted, overweight, slumping, wheezing, and puffing, barely able to carry the torch that's supposed to light our way. She's sporting a new inscription: We are your fatter-than-evers, your tired, your depressed, your swollen-limbed, your bloated-bellied, your fatty-livered, your diabetic blind, your broken-hearted, your disabled and diseased. She no longer stands alone looking out on the island of Manhattan. She's the reflection in many mirrors of the fattest people in the history of the world from Asia to the Americas, mirroring the most dangerous pandemic that has ever threatened the bodies and minds of humankind—a pandemic that crosses all countries, colors, genders, and ages.

Obesity has become *the* modern-day global scourge of humanity. Currently, obesity costs the U.S. healthcare system a startling $170-175 billion annually, including $14 billion for pediatric obesity, which is $470 million daily and $19.6 million per hour. However, none of the developed countries of the world have escaped the spread of this devastation. The Office of Health Economics in England has indicated that while the U.S. has the largest rate of obesity of any developed nation, the United Kingdom (U.K.) is fifth, right behind the U.S., Mexico, New Zealand, and Australia.[2] In 2008, a quarter of the population of the U.K. was obese compared with less than 20% ten years earlier. These shocking realities are associated with extremely dire consequences and burdens on both health and socioeconomic levels. According to the Tony Blair Institute, the cost of being overweight in the U.K. has recently approached 100 billion pounds annually. The cost of being overweight, including disease, disability, lost productivity of the work force, etc. rose from 58 billion pounds annually in 2020 to 98 billion pounds in 2023. This represents an annual increase in direct healthcare costs to the National Health Service of the U.K. from 10.8 to 19.2 billion pounds for obesity-related health problems.[3] That is a shocking 50 million pounds (63 million dollars) per day and approximately 2.1 million pounds (2.6 million dollars) per hour! Unless obesity is dealt with, the government of the U.K. predicts that 75 percent of men, 67 percent of women, and more than 30 percent of children will be obese by 2040.

Yet as much as overweight and obesity impact people from the Americas to the U.K., other countries of western Europe, and distant parts of Asia, the United States is the most glaring example of these pervasive problems. More than 70% of Americans are overweight, and more than 40% are obese.[4] What makes this even more devastating and unsettling is that since 1980, one of the most rapidly growing overweight and overfat segments of our population has been children under the age of 18.[5] The U.S. has achieved the frightening distinction of having the fattest children in the history of the world! In fact, the deplorable truth is that the current generation of children may be the first children who do not live as long as their parents. As a doctor, a scientist, and especially as a father, this fills me with grave concern.

Excessive weight and body fat is clearly associated with an increased risk of heart disease, diabetes, stroke, and cancer, arguably the four most devastating diseases of the modern world. In fact, since fat cells promote the production and release of reproductive growth hormones and inflammatory factors, an increase in fatness can exaggerate the levels of these factors and promote hormone-induced cancers of the breast, uterus, ovaries, and prostate. As a result, obesity has become one of the leading causes of cancer in our culture today.[6]

Yet as pervasive as this problem is, the approaches to solving it have been incredibly shortsighted. Too many people just adopt fad diets that can reinforce disease and weight gain, or they resort to off-label pharmaceutical approaches or mutilating surgical and liposuction procedures that are fraught with the potential risks and complications of anesthesia and infection. Unfortunately, reducing weight and fat often seem to be the focus of a narrow-minded debate of calories in vs. calories out, which places the burden of responsibility for weight gain solely on individual people's dieting and exercise habits. As a result, a panorama of quick-fix diet plans and exercise programs are held out as the only answer to the prayers of the overweight, even as millions of people who religiously adopt these approaches meet with failure and, even worse, reactive long-term weight gain. It should be no mystery, then, to discover that the dieting industry in the U.S., which preys on the false hope of people trying desperately to lose weight, is a mega-billion-dollar industry[7] with as much as a 95% failure rate.

There is no question that more discipline in our eating and exercise habits is necessary to reduce weight. However, an extensive body of clinical and research evidence strongly suggests that it is imperative to consider the importance, and even synergistic interaction, of several key factors to solve the problem of obesity. These factors include the quantity, quality, and type of food we eat; the exercise and activity we maintain; how we handle daily and chronic stress; the psycho-emotional context of our food use; the sleep we need and get; the drugs and stimulants we overuse; how we balance our immune and hormonal systems; and the impact of industrial and environmental pollution and toxicity. As a result, excessive weight and body fat must be more accurately viewed as consequences of a lifestyle that has either neglected or is in direct conflict with the biological, psychological, and even spiritual requirements of life and health.

Long before the current growing field of lifestyle medicine took root, profound health pioneers in the U.S. codified and described a system of healthful living called Natural Hygiene. The principles of this system are the very foundation of this book and the deep roots of my personal practice and understanding. In this context, health and healing is the natural outcome of the normal functions of all living organisms, recognized as a ceaseless biological process that is as constant as the earth turning on its axis. In addition, the body is a masterpiece of wisdom and order. It is constantly using energy to maintain order, stability, and renewal of all cells and systems to resist the relentless environmental forces that eventually lead to overwhelming damage and death.

Yet all living things require a constellation of biological factors for health and survival, including healthy food, fresh air, fresh water, activity, rest, and emotional balance. To the extent that these requirements are appropriated and maintained, health and ease will follow like water flows downhill. However, when the needs of life are neglected, energy is dissipated, toxic conditions accrue, the body is threatened, and a lack of ease, "dis-ease," ensues. In early stages of dis-ease, the body will manifest acute actions and responses like headache, fever, and diarrhea to eliminate threatening conditions and restore a state of ease, wholeness, and health. Unfortunately, within the typical medical system, we have all been conditioned to fear our own vitality and medicate these remedial, supportive symptoms out of existence. This interference coupled with ongoing choices and conditions of abuse can eventually lead to chronic cell and organ damage and the panorama of chronic diseases that plague our entire population.

In this context, obesity is a unique flavor of chronic disease. Its consequences influence many other comorbid outcomes throughout diverse organs and systems of the body, reducing quality of life and decreasing optimal healthspan and performance. Obesity can't be medicated and treated out of existence. Both immediate and long-term success can only be effectively resolved by addressing the lifestyle choices and factors that contribute to its outcome, as addressed in this book. Remember, you are free to make personal choices, but you are not free to choose the consequences. It is only through whole-plant nutrition and supportive lifestyle choices that you can achieve the successful consequences of healthy weight and body fat while respecting the life of all species and the environment that nurtures you.

Do not underestimate the widespread impact of these personal and lifestyle factors. All too often genetics is used to explain, and even justify, dysfunction and disease, including the outcomes of excessive weight and body fat. So many people buy into the concept that since their parents were overweight or had high blood pressure, diabetes, or heart disease, they will have no choice but to develop and express these same problems. This could not be further from the truth.

Health problems and the genes that may be associated with them can be significantly affected by a plethora of lifestyle choices outside the genetic environment that are referred to as epigenetic factors. If you have a family history of high blood pressure, there may be an underlying genetic environment that makes it easier for you to develop this problem. However, even with a genetic predisposition, you still have to create and maintain the poor nutrition, inactivity, and stress choices that promote any genetic tendency to express itself. It is true that some health issues may be unavoidable. There may be predetermined genetic problems that you will express regardless of the personal choices you make in your life. A person born with the inability to produce insulin or compromised function of insulin due to autoimmune disease, which results in the type 1 form of diabetes, is a classic example of an unavoidable, genetically determined condition that requires hormone treatment for life.

However, the majority of genetically affected health conditions are more recessive genetic problems associated with an increased tendency or predisposition to developing a particular dysfunction. It is imperative to realize that these tendencies and predispositions can be minimized or eliminated by adopting routine healthy lifestyle choices grounded in whole-plant-exclusive nutrition. These lifestyle choices can modify, inhibit, or promote the expression of genes that directly affect the outcome of health or disease. Very often, the genetic argument is used to shirk responsibility for the poor lifestyle choices that are truly causing disability and disease. Consistent with the epigenetic argument, there is extensive evidence from diverse populations and cultures across the globe that clearly shows that when people eat similar poor diets, become less active, and maintain relentless stress in their lives, they develop the same chronic conditions of obesity, premature aging, heart disease, diabetes, and cancer, regardless of their distinct personal or ethnically inherited genetic differences.

Obesity is a major health problem with devastating consequences of disability, disease, and potentially death. Yet it is a problem that can be prevented, reversed and solved—but only if we are willing as individuals to address the constellation of causative lifestyle factors that contribute to its outcome. There is no simple, quick-fix solution, but understanding and adopting whole-plant nutrition and other important lifestyle factors discussed in this book is the quickest and most direct path to eliminating debilitating food addictions while promoting permanent, healthy weight and body-fat levels. That is the truth, and it is the truth that I offer you in the pages that follow. In the process, I will be challenging and debunking popular approaches that, while they may produce ephemeral, short-term weight loss, only reinforce failure and misery over time. By applying the ideas and strategies in this book, you can embody the byline of Dr. Herbert Shelton, one of my most influential mentors and a major icon of the Hygiene movement: "Let us have truth though the Heavens fall." Therefore, this book will not be about political correctness. Biased conventional approaches with hidden agendas need to be vehemently exposed, challenged, and rejected so that we can intelligently embrace an unbiased program grounded in the best that science has to offer.

With this in mind, it also is important to realize that there are people and forces in business, science, politics, and government that seek their own profit while promoting food and lifestyle choices that compromise life and health. Their subsidies of the animal and junk-food industries establish economic pressures and social injustice that coerce people to buy foods that foster disease and weight gain. Their advertising dollars are spent and hell-bent on spreading the insidious notion that the only way to promote health and beneficial weight is by the consumption of animal and dairy products. This unconscionable mind control has no real scientific foundation, is motivated by pure greed, and continues to destroy the health and well-being of our planet and people.

As someone who has lived and taught a vegan lifestyle for almost 50 years, I have helped myself and thousands of others maintain superb health and beneficial weight with the strategies and practices presented in this book, exclusively with whole plant food. For clarification and personal preference, I have chosen to describe my nutritional approach throughout this book as a low-fat, whole-food, plant-exclusive (WFPE) diet or vegan, whole-food, plant-exclusive diet, without added salt, oil, and sugar (SOS-free) in lieu of just vegan or the more popular term, plant-based. My emphasis is always on whole, unprocessed plant foods. The term "plant-based" can include food choices that are not strictly of plant origin and the general term "vegan" can include highly processed vegan products and junk foods that are not of animal origin but are not optimal for successful weight and fat loss.

There are populations of people that have promoted health and weight loss with diets that are predominantly plant-based and contain very small amounts of animal products. Unfortunately, this approach still supports industries of death and destruction that are unnecessary, are untenable, and wantonly destroy other helpless, sentient creatures along with our atmosphere and environment. Make no mistake, my approach embraces the vegan philosophy of harmlessness and compassion for all creatures and the earth, always in the context of whole plant foods.

The plant-exclusive approach that I will share with you is time-tested and remarkably successful. In addition, as much as I vehemently challenge the quick-fix fad approaches to this complex problem that truly requires a long-term solution, if you are in love with quick results, there is nothing quicker and healthier than a vegan, whole-plant-exclusive approach. It has been shown consistently, over many years, to promote a comfortable, healthy three to five pounds per week of fat/weight loss in the first few weeks, with steady one- to two-pound weight losses per week over extended periods of time. However, I have had people, depending on initial weight and gender, lose as much as 20-plus pounds in a single month! From a wealth of clinical experience and my heart, I can honestly tell you without a doubt in my mind: if you embrace the principles, ideas, and practices espoused in this book, you will NEVER have to diet again.

You must understand that this program is not about deprivation. No one likes to be deprived. This program is about eating well, not eating less. You will be exposed to remarkably tasty food options, recipes, meal plans, and even jump-start strategies. I will also share my years of experience exploring the incredibly delicious and diverse options available in ethnic cuisine, and the viable and healthy substitutions you can make in ethnic restaurants in your community for takeouts or dining out, while still promoting a WFPE, SOS-free diet. My goal is to inspire you with the incredible diversity and options available in whole-plant nutrition by providing strategies that enhance your ability to function socially as you adopt more of these choices, while also increasing your fun and joy as you eat and live in your "real" world.

I urge you to recognize, abhor, and avoid the violence and devastation involved in animal food production from the soulless industries of commercial fishing and animal agriculture. I implore you to remember that there is no need for any animal to be tortured or killed to promote weight loss. There is no need to damage the earth or ravage its land and water resources to promote healthy weight. Nothing and no one needs to suffer for any of us to create healthy weight and body image. In fact, routinely eating animal foods only fosters potential inflammation, disability, disease, and long-term problems with weight regulation.

This compassionate, mindful approach to weight loss is grounded in a life-above-all-else philosophy—a way of living and thinking that promotes more respect for ourselves and others and better balance and connection in our relationships with the world, animals, and people around us. As a result, it also nurtures a strong sense and experience of self-love and a greater desire to make choices that are in our best interest. It is so important to realize that obesity is often a symptom of a deeper craving and hunger—a hunger to find peace, balance, and well-being in our lives and within ourselves. Especially since we live in a culture that all too often does not honor our core value and constantly pulls us outside of ourselves, disconnecting us from the deeper inner truth of who and what we really are, thereby disengaging and dissuading us from the life-affirming expression and realization of our own deep sense of purpose, passion, and creativity.

Does the world really need another diet and weight-loss book? I don't think so. That's why this is not a diet book. It is a road map. In fact, it's more like a combination GPS and map. A map is only good when it accurately represents the territory it attempts to describe. The information in this book will serve as the most accurate map for the territory of health, well-being, and weight control. For that purpose, I have presented the book in five parts that start with the essentials and importance of whole plant nutrition, move on to important lifestyle factors that are essential for long-term success, and finally progress toward the psychological and emotional factors that can eliminate self-sabotage and insure your best opportunity for success. It will truly help you get to where you want to go with your weight and body-image goals, and it will continue to help you navigate the territory of health and weight regulation so you can stay there. With that in mind, I also believe that knowledge is power, and this is a book of empowerment. I hope and I truly believe that it will empower you to take charge of your own health and weight-loss story.

Just know that I am not writing this book from some isolated ivory tower. I was an overweight, overfat kid raised in the Bronx on the streets of New York City. I come from an Italian family that had some of the fattest people I have ever known. I have experienced problems with compulsive food use, food addiction, and obesity up close and personal for a long time. I have lived through the stress of raising five children, a painful broken marriage and divorce, debilitating emotional and physical traumas, and crippling financial burdens. There were so many times I felt like nothing I did ever seemed good enough. I know what it's like to feel helpless and hopeless. I have compulsively used my fair share of food, drugs, and sex to feed and placate the demons of my own personal dark night.

However, I'm here to tell you that there is light at the end of the tunnel if you are willing to open your mind and heart and let it in. I offer you this manual of hope. So, no matter how many failed diets or weight-loss approaches you may have tried in the past, I urge you to embrace the unique opportunity presented in this book. The holistic vision, ideas, strategies, and practices shared in this book can truly help you satisfy your hunger on many levels, promote remarkable health and well-being, and result in the healthy weight and body image you would love to have, not only for the next few days, weeks, or months, but permanently, for years to come.

PART
1

ESSENTIAL FACTS AND FUNDAMENTALS

CHAPTER 1

WHY WEIGHT? THE NEED FOR CHANGING FOCUS

Have you ever found it difficult to lose weight or had the experience of successfully taking weight off but having a difficult time keeping it off? Unfortunately, too many of us have. If you are one of the desperate millions who have taken, or continue to take, the seemingly endless ride on the typical roller coaster of weight gain and weight loss fueled by the false hopes of quick-fix diet scams, you are not alone. While we continue to grow fatter and fatter, with over 40% of our population obese and more than 70% overweight or obese, the dieting industry in the United States alone is an approximately $70 billion industry with a 95% failure rate.[1] So, it is critical to explore the bigger picture of weight and obesity that has been obscured by shortsighted approaches and limited perceptions. I offer you an oasis, a sanctuary, in a desert of falsehoods and failures. I am going to present a cornucopia of ideas and remarkably successful strategies that I have put together over 46 years of teaching and practice, in both my own life and family and in the lives of thousands of others. My goal, my hope, is to help you flesh out the truth and develop the skills and consciousness to promote long-term, successful weight loss and contribute to the resolution of this devastating pandemic, both personally and globally.

Excessive weight is not just a cosmetic issue. Just being overweight and overfat are significant risk factors in the four most profound causes of death in the Western world: heart disease, cancer, stroke, and type 2 diabetes.[2-4] Obesity and these chronic diseases account for an alarming 70% of all deaths annually worldwide. The good news is that obesity and excessive weight gain is by far the most preventable cause of death in the world today. The bad news is that obesity costs the U.S. healthcare system approximately $147-210 billion annually ($400-575 million daily). The most significant contribution to this exorbitant healthcare cost has come from weight-related increases in heart disease, high blood pressure, and type 2 diabetes.[5,6] Type 2 diabetes is the most prevalent form of diabetes, affecting more than 90% of diabetics, and typically occurs as people get older and fatter as a direct by-product of poor food and lifestyle choices. According to The Centers for Disease Control, type 2 diabetes has more than doubled in the U.S. over the past 20 years as the American population has become more overweight and obese. However, a large, significant number of these new cases of "older person" diabetes have occurred in teenagers and young adults. That frightening fact should not be a great mystery when you realize that in the past 30 years, arguably one of the most rapidly growing groups of overweight and overfat people in America has been children under the age of 19. Our children are marching toward premature aging, chronic disease, and economic strangulation from the burden of these potential healthcare costs at a rate never before seen in history.

Much Ado About Body Fat: Activity and Function

Fat cells (adipocytes) are a unique type of cell in the human body. For the longest time, fat cells were portrayed as rather inert, just hanging out, making us look somewhat less physically attractive, burdening our hearts, and compromising our physical fitness. However, we now know that fat cells are among the more dynamic cells of the body. They function like an additional organ of our endocrine system, releasing a variety of hormones and proteins involved in regulating appetite, food intake, immune system response, and metabolism. The hormones and proteins they release establish important signals and communication with other endocrine organs as well as with the brain and nervous system. This helps ensure a balance of the creation, accumulation, and movement of fat (lipids) in fat cells (adipose tissue) in response to changes in nutrient intake and calorie demands.[7]

Fat cells are also capable of producing and releasing a variety of proteins and hormones that promote inflammation and cancer. Similar to the immune system itself, fat cells synthesize a class of proteins called cytokines, unique chemical messengers that influence and modulate the function of the immune system. Several of these fat-generated cytokines (also referred to as adipokines, including adiponectin, resistin, tumor necrosis factor-alpha, and interleukins, along with macrophage colony-stimulation factor) can stimulate the immune system and increase inflammation.[8] Why is that important? The inflammatory process is a natural protective response of a healthy immune system. However, when this natural process is exaggerated and prolonged by chronic, irritating lifestyle and dietary choices (especially refined and animal-based foods high in added salt, oil, and sugar) and by the increase in body fat, it can be a significant causative factor for pandemic chronic diseases such as heart disease and cancer. The impact of obesity on inflammation and the immune system has also been a significant factor in the recent pandemic of viral infection; obese people infected with COVID-19 were six times more likely to be hospitalized and end up on respirators due to lung complications.

As you gain weight, fat cells are involved in the production and release of chemicals that can increase blood pressure and cholesterol, damage blood vessels, and significantly increase the risk of heart and brain disease. The hormone estrogen is typically involved in regulating sexuality and reproduction. However, when the level of this hormone rises due to the accumulation of excess body fat and the exaggerated release from fat cells, it can increase the abnormal growth of cells in the reproductive system, promoting tumor and cancer growth. Similarly, when obesity and body fat levels increase in people anywhere in the world, the number of cancers of the breast, ovaries, and uterus also increase. This led an international group of cancer research physicians and scientists who studied people in the U.S., Canada, the United Kingdom, and other parts of western Europe over the 30-year period from 1966-1996 to conclude that even modest weight gain was a significant factor for increased cancer incidence.[9]

Another major investigation has clearly shown the relationship between obesity and other cancer outcomes.[10] The relationship of weight and obesity to cancer was evaluated in this study using body mass index (essentially a ratio function of the weight and height of an individual) to measure obesity.[i] People with BMIs below 24.9 are considered to be normal weight, people between 25-29.9 are considered overweight, and those above 30 are considered obese.

Interestingly, while cancers of the colon and blood (leukemia) in this study showed some of the most significant weight-related increases, all cancers significantly increased as BMI increased. The heaviest people observed had death rates from all cancers combined that were 52% higher in men and 62% higher in women than people of normal weight. While you might expect that reproductive cancers of the breast, ovaries, uterus, and prostate would be increased by weight and body fat because of the increased reproductive hormones in fat cells, it was startling to see the high impact of weight on death rates from cancers of the esophagus, colon, rectum, liver, gallbladder, pancreas, and kidney. Remarkably, the results of this study suggested that the extent of overweight and obesity

---

[i] BMI = weight (kg)/height (m)^2

in the U.S. could account for 14% of all deaths from cancer in men and as much as 20% in women.

Body Weight and Body Fat: The Whole Story

Height and weight considerations alone are dangerously shortsighted and not enough to accurately assess obesity because body fat, with all its implications for disease risk, also must be considered to understand the complete picture and significance of body weight. For example, if BMI alone were used to evaluate the impact of weight gain, athletes with high body weight and low body fat would all be classified as obese, even though they are obviously lean and sculpted. You can also have a normal weight, as measured by BMI, but be dangerously overfat. A health study done in Finland in 2007, the National FINRISK Study, identified a new syndrome called normal-weight obesity.[11] A significant number of men and women with normal weight (BMIs less than 25) were found to be overfat. Consistent with the story that I will unfold throughout this book, this condition of normal-weight obesity was promoted by lifestyle factors including decreased physical activity, increased meat and refined sugar consumption, increased alcohol intake, and a lack of plant foods. In addition, information from the 1999-2004 National Health and Nutrition Examination Surveys (NHANES) showed that a significant number of average American men and women in lower BMI categories had body-fat percentages associated with obesity.[12]

However, body weight is still an important consideration, and as the pandemic of overweight and obesity continues to grow, there are fewer and fewer people in lower weight and BMI categories. Statistics from a survey conducted from 2007-2010 by the U.S. Department of Health and Human Services and the Centers for Disease Control and Prevention (CDC) paint a picture that is difficult to believe, suggesting that the prevalence of overweight and obesity is even worse than you and I could have ever imagined.[13] In this survey of thousands of American men and women 20 years and older from different racial and ethnic groups, the average weight of women was 166 pounds, with an average BMI of 28.7 and average waist size of 37.5 inches. Unfortunately, while the average height of black women was similar to other racial/ethnic groups, their average weight of 187.9 pounds and average BMI of 32 were significantly higher, suggesting even greater danger in the African American population. In addition, while the height, weight, and BMIs of men did not vary much among racial and ethnic groups, their measurements indicated significant health risk. On average, men were approximately 69 inches tall with an average weight of 195.5 pounds, an average waist size of 39.7 inches, and an average BMI of 28.6. This tendency toward increased waist size in both men and women is an important consideration, because increased abdominal weight gain is associated with a higher risk of heart disease, stroke, and type 2 diabetes. Therefore, due to the importance and relationship of these various factors to the bigger picture of obesity and weight gain, I recommend using the combination of weight, BMI, body-fat percentage, and waist size/abdominal belly fat to get the most accurate and meaningful picture of obesity. (Body-fat percentages should be 9-17% for men and 14-25% for women; the waist-to-hip ratio should be less than one.)

This has even greater implications when you consider that the typical American is gaining a pound and a half of body fat per year after the age of 25.[14] This means that in the 30 years between the ages of 25-55, one can put on as much as 45 pounds of body fat. Also consider that for every additional pound of fat, the body adds five miles of extra blood vessels to feed this increase in body mass. Since the heart beats about 100,000 times a day, the heart has to pump blood through an extra 500,000 miles a day for every added pound of body fat, or an extra 22.5 million miles for the 45-pound fat gain described above. Think of the burden this can put on the heart as it is compelled to exert energy to pump blood through all these added blood vessels and fat to just sustain normal function! Therefore, when we talk about weight gain, it is essential that the discussion includes the reality and risk of body fat.

Don't Let Gravity Get You Down

When we talk about body fat, that includes the fat that you can visibly see, that stuff we can pinch, jiggle, and shake. This brings to mind my own sweet, heartwarming memory of my Italian grandmother, my bubbie, loving and embracing me with her plentiful arms, squeezing a deep smile of comfort from my little-boy face and soul. When we parted, she would wave goodbye from her windowsill perch in our Bronx tenement apartment building, arms undulating like a hammock of fat that, even when she stopped waving, continued a goodbye wave that never seemed to stop.

However, body fat also includes fat that you can't see, the fat lurking underneath the skin (subcutaneous fat), around our internal organs (visceral fat, the most harmful of all), in the growing apron of belly fat (omentum), and weaving through the striations of muscles. If you were to look at a piece of steak, you would see fat marbling the muscle meat. If you were to cut open a human body, you would similarly see fat streaking within a palette of red muscle meat. That intramuscular fat directly affects our individual metabolism and metabolic efficiency, i.e., how effectively we utilize the glucose and calories we consume.

So, while it is necessary to acknowledge that obesity is truly both a weight- and fat-related problem, our attention is unfortunately focused all too often just on the numbers on the scale. Weight is certainly not the best, or only, criterion for health, since it does not provide the information necessary to effectively evaluate the risky components of fat mass and body-fat percentage. This shortcoming is further exemplified by studies of high-performance athletes who, in their training programs, can gain significant amounts of weight but lose body fat in the process, an outcome of leanness that is truly a healthy circumstance, even at a high body weight. Yet, since it is more convenient to accurately measure scale weight rather than routinely calculating BMI or measuring body-fat percentage, our attention continues to be pulled in the wrong direction, even as the obsession with scale weight often promotes undo psychological upset and harm for so many.[ii] The great news is that by following the diet and lifestyle recommendations of this program you will successfully reduce weight, BMI, and body fat in the healthiest way possible.

The following scenario will emphasize how this misdirection can affect our quality of life and our ability to appreciate and truly live the precious moments that we have. For many years, I directed a health retreat where people came to improve their health and lose weight. At the center where the retreat was held, there was a scale tucked away in the side shadows of the lobby of the main building. The guests of the retreat used this scale, often obsessively, to chart their own progress during their stay. One early morning as I was passing through the lobby, I encountered a female guest walking through the lobby getting ready to weigh herself on the lobby scale. I said, "Good morning! How are you doing?" With her oh-so-serious, edgy, pensive face in play, and without any hesitation, she replied, "I'll let you know in a second." Sadly, her fortune, the quality and potential of that day for her, would rise or fall with the result on the scale at that one moment. There was a time when I made the lobby scale disappear. I removed it from the lobby and put it in the storage room. Guests went to bed in the safety and security of the center at night, and when they got up in the morning to take the solitary journey in their underwear to the hidden recesses of the lobby to weigh themselves, the scale was gone. As you can imagine, this caused a minor revolt that came close to having images of me burned in effigy on the retreat grounds.

Near where I live in Florida, there is a science museum that has scales where you can get your weight on the moon and all the planets in the solar system. On the moon scale, nobody weighs more than 20 pounds or less than 15 pounds. I recommend getting a moon scale for

---

[ii] For this reason, I pair references to weight and fat throughout this book to acknowledge their related, but also separate, roles in health.

your home. Then you can banish the scale issues from your mind and focus on the real work at hand: addressing the integrated lifestyle factors that are critical to promoting high-level health in addition to long-term weight regulation. Yes, excessive weight should be a concern and should motivate your desire for improvement, weight loss, and change. But in this process of change, it is vital to remember (and continue to remind yourself) that you are so much more than your weight and body image. The abnormal preoccupation and upsets that come with the fluctuating ounces and pounds on the scale only interfere with your ability to appreciate the magnificent being that you truly are and to be mindful and open to the experiences and precious moments of your life. These moments are precious. Live them, don't lose them. As a Buddhist monk once said to me, "May you live every moment of your life."

Beware the Starvation Response

As you may know, because of the pervasive preoccupation with weight and fat, many quick-fix dietary approaches have been created to help people take weight off as quickly as possible. If we polled people throughout the U.S., Canada, the U.K., Western Europe, and Asia, we would come up with all the strange and sundry ways that have been tried in an effort to take weight off rapidly (and, I might add, mindlessly) through the years. Yet as different as these approaches may be, they have one thing in common—they are basically failures.

As I already mentioned, 95% or more of all people who take weight off with quick-fix diet programs not only put the weight back on, but typically put it back on with a vengeance. For example, researchers subjected rats to two rounds of rapid weight loss on short-term, extreme calorie restriction. By the third round, the animals lost weight two times slower and gained weight back three times faster on the same number of calories that they originally were able to eat while maintaining their weight.[11] These problems with dieting and weight control are seen not only in animal studies, but also in all the people who fail on

extreme diets and weight-loss programs. Extreme dieting and deprivation typically promote a response that inevitably leads to reactive
weight gain. Why?

As human primates, we are built to eat primarily a plant-exclusive
diet. Historical evidence suggests that the original food supply of our
species was the fruits and plants that grew around us and were readily
available for the taking. However, there were times in our past when
these original food supplies became scarce as a result of harsh environmental pressures and changes. Therefore, we were driven to hunt and
kill for food in a very arduous and threatening environment. In this scenario, food was no longer easy to come by, and there would likely be long
gaps between times when we could eat.

As a result, a "starvation response" developed in response to these
periods of deprivation. Hormonal and chemical changes were established that could program an intensification of hunger signals and
override satiety signals when food was available again, to encourage
overeating and the storage of calories for a future time of need. This
same ancient starvation response still exists within each of us today and
is often triggered by the recurring use of extreme calorie-restricted or
fragmented fad diets loaded with the provocative agents salt, oil, and
sugar. In modern times, however, this becomes very problematic: there
are no longer big gaps between the "kills" or even big gaps between trips
to fast-food convenient stores. Instead, we are constantly overexposed
to all the calorie-dense meat and dairy products and processed, refined
"junk foods" that are so readily available today, while our calorie output is decreased by the remarkable reduction of physical activity in our
modern society and school systems. This is an obvious recipe for disaster
and a sure path to dangerous weight gain. Due to the hormonal and
biochemical changes of the inborn survival response, fad diets based
on calorie restriction and focused on certain categories of food (e.g.,
low-carbohydrate, high-protein, or high-fat animal-based diets) without
regard for the quantity and synergy of key nutrients or other ancillary

lifestyle factors that I will discuss in depth typically promote long-term reactive weight gain.

There are many programs that promote initial weight loss, but, unfortunately, they urge you to mortgage your health future in the process. I will continue to expose and challenge these approaches, because the last thing anyone needs is fleeting, short-term weight loss that simultaneously increases health risk. It is essential that we embrace the best information that science has to offer to promote long-term weight and fat loss along with a healthy body image. Plant-exclusive diet and nutrition choices are essential lifestyle factors that enhance the opportunity for healthy, compassionate weight loss. Let's journey through the remarkable world of plant-exclusive nutrition for optimum results and long-term success.

CHAPTER 2

DIET AND NUTRITION: THE VEGAN, PLANT-EXCLUSIVE SOLUTION

There has been such a long history in our culture focused on the abnormal preoccupation, even obsession, with risky diets and dieting. It is undeniable that the quality and composition of your diet is one of the most significant and important parts of any long-term weight-loss program. Unfortunately, however, people who are trying to secure some small piece of weight-loss success are left to choose from a wide range of questionable approaches, many of which lead to damaging results. To add to the confusion, these programs often make no distinction between the concepts of diet and nutrition, lumping them together and speaking about them as if they were the same thing. While diet and nutrition are intimately connected, they are not the same thing, and it is important to appreciate and understand the fundamental difference between and relationship of these concepts.

Diet refers specifically to what you decide to put into your mouth and eat on a regular basis. Nutrition, on the other hand, is not just about what you consume; it also embraces the bigger picture of digestibility and nutrient availability. It involves not only what you eat, but also all the relationships and reactions that your body has with those things, including considerations of how you digest your food, how you absorb the available nutrients, and how you circulate those nutrients within the bloodstream. It includes how these nutrients are incorporated into the cells of the body to nurture all of the body's tissues, organs, and systems and to promote new growth and life of the entire living ecosystem we call the human body. All of these steps come under the umbrella of nutrition, affecting the bioavailability of nutrients to promote life and health.

Any aspect of your life and lifestyle choices that enhances or compromises any of these steps will influence the quality of your nutrition. For example, improved, consistent sleep and exercise habits promote better digestion, circulation, and absorption that enhance the quality of nutrition. By contrast, chronic stress can compromise effective nutrition. Your natural stress response to threatening or traumatic events in your environment is an arousal response that diverts energy and blood away from the digestive system and toward skeletal muscles in order to help us face the threat or run away from it. Historically, these strategies have been referred to as the fight-or-flight response. (See Chapter 18.)

Under chronic stress, the digestive system is basically shut down and, therefore, less able to digest anything. But when do so many of us eat the most? Under stress. And what do we tend to eat the most under stress? Typically, the most refined, processed foods high in animal protein, fat, sugar, and salt that are often low in fiber, require more time and acid production in the stomach, and are the most difficult to digest and the most weight-promoting. Is it really any wonder then why there are so many digestive- and bowel-related difficulties, distresses, and diseases in our culture, including relentless acid reflux, gas, and bloating? Is it really any wonder why anti-reflux drugs are some of the most overused and abused drugs in our stressed-out culture?

It is important to view the variety of your synergistic lifestyle factors as important factors of nutrition that are critical for improving both the quality of nutrition and your opportunity for long-term, successful weight loss.

Nutritional Keys for Long-Term Weight Loss

Calorie and Nutrient Density

For any diet or eating plan to promote successful weight loss over time, it must satisfy some very specific needs and meet some basic requirements. Perhaps the most basic requirement of any successful weight-control diet is that it must have the lowest calorie density, i.e., calories per weight of food, typically measured as calories per pound. The concept of calorie density was developed by Barbara Rolls, PhD, a veteran nutrition scientist and professor of nutritional sciences at Pennsylvania State University, and is detailed in her bestselling book, *Volumetrics*.

The beautiful, important takeaway of this concept is this: the eating plan that provides the greatest opportunity for weight regulation is the one with the lowest calorie density, which is a low-fat, whole-food, plant-exclusive diet without any added salt, oil, or sugar (WFPE, SOS-free). That means a diet devoid of all animal products, dairy products, and processed junk food, and loaded with raw and cooked organic, unrefined, unprocessed plant foods. As rigorous and different as this diet is compared with the standard Western fare currently consumed by most people, it is unequivocally the most powerful and provocative weight and fat-loss approach. Here's why.

Research has shown that people tend to consume a consistent amount of food from day to day, typically between three and five pounds.[1] If those three to five pounds are of high-calorie-density foods—as is typical of the standard American diet—daily intake can easily range from 2,700 to 10,000 calories. Since the average woman needs 1,800-2,200 calories per day and the average man needs 2,000-2,500 calories per day, it's clear that weight gain will result. However, if those three to five pounds are from foods averaging 600 calories per pound, the resulting daily intake will range between 1,800 and 3,000 calories, and weight will remain stable.

Consider the following table, which presents the calorie densities of different categories of foods.[2]

The Calorie Density Scale	
Foods	**Calories per pound**
Non-starchy vegetables	65 – 195
Fresh fruit	140 - 420
Potatoes, pasta, rice, barley, yams, corn, hot cereals	320 - 630
Beans, peas, lentils (cooked)	310 – 780
Avocados	725
Breads, bagels, fat-free muffins, tortillas, dried fruit	920 – 1,360
Sugars (i.e., sugar, molasses, agave, corn syrup, etc.)	1,200 -1,800
Dry cereals, baked chips, fat-free crackers, pretzels	1480 – 1,760
Nuts/seeds	2,400 – 3,200
Oils	4,000

Table 1. The calorie density of whole-plant and processed food items measured in total calories per pound.

As you can see, the calorie content of the cornucopia of fruits and non-starchy vegetables—the variety of leafy greens, leafy herbs, cucumbers, celery, peppers, etc.—is the lowest of all foods, in the approximate range of 100-400 calories per pound. These foods have a high fiber and water content (non-caloric components accounting for a significant amount of their weight) and can be eaten freely and plentifully to support healthy weight loss and weight control, with the added benefit that their fiber and water content provide a stabilizing sense of fullness and satiety.

Starchy vegetables, such as potatoes and yams, whole grains and cereals, and legumes (including beans, peas, and lentils), are in the range of 300-780 calories per pound and also promote the calorie-density levels, nutritional values, and satiety essential for the long-term maintenance of healthy body weight and body fat.

Furthermore, the American Cancer Institute and the World Cancer Research Fund have suggested that a diet containing foods with an average calorie density of approximately 600 calories or less per pound is ideal for reducing cancer risk and promoting long-term weight regulation. Therefore, the fruits, vegetables, and starches listed on the first four lines of the chart should comprise 90-95% of everything you eat.

Concentrated, processed foods, including many bread products (bagels, crackers, breads, pastas, and dry cereals), dried fruits, and especially refined-sugar products, are 920-1,800 calories per pound, and the most calorie-dense, high-fat foods (nuts, seeds, and oils) have a calorie density in the range of 2,400-4,000 calories per pound. In general, these should be used only very sparingly on any weight-loss program. These foods are best used as a garnish or small addition to meals replete with fruits and non-starchy and starchy vegetables. For example, you may decide to use some bread and pasta in your diet, and that's okay.

However, it is best to avoid all refined breads and pastas, as well as all refined sugar products. If you decide to use some bread products and pasta in your diet, make certain that these foods are made from whole, unrefined grains. Keep in mind that the closer a food is to the way it grows in nature, the lower is its calorie density and the more ideal it is for weight loss. So, for example, if you want brown rice, it is more advantageous to eat whole, cooked brown rice rather than brown rice bread or brown rice pasta. So while whole-grain bread and pasta products can be used, they should be used more sparingly than unprocessed, whole grains on any weight-loss program. As a rule, you can consume a very limited amount of dried fruit, including the use of dates as a sweetener in smoothies and salad dressings, but it is best to eat fruit primarily in its natural, juicy form that is significantly lower in calorie density. Nuts, seeds, and avocados provide significant essential nutrients and health benefits. However, because of their high fat and calorie density, I recommend a limited consumption of these foods, usually no more than one to two ounces of nuts or a few slices of avocado in any day, as part of a healthy diet and weight-regulation program. These foods are best used as a garnish or small addition to meals replete with fruits and non-starchy and starchy vegetables.

Food should also be eaten primarily in whole-food form, chewed thoroughly, and eaten slowly. While consuming your calories in lique-fied form in juices and smoothies may provide concentrated nutrients following periods of dietary deficiency, and some benefits during times of disease, detoxification, or recovery, it can increase calorie density, and, in the case of juice, reduce fiber content and interfere with comfortable satiety.

To summarize, the most effective diet for long-term weight loss should be abundant in whole fruits and non-starchy vegetables and contain large amounts of starchy vegetables, whole grains, and legumes without added refined sugar, oil, or salt. These additives offer no nutritional value to your diet; instead, they add unnecessary calorie density, interfere with your experience of satiety, provoke toxic and inflammatory by-products, and provoke craving and overeating.

Another significant feature of the WFPE, SOS-free diet I recommend is that the foods with the lowest calorie density also have the greatest nutrient density (nutrient availability), or the greatest nutrient to calorie ratio (N/C). When you eat a diet that is primarily fruits and vegetables, it provides the greatest amount of nutrients, especially vitamins, minerals, phytonutrients, and antioxidants, for the fewest number of calories.

However, if you look at the refined, processed diet consumed by most Americans, the N/C ratio is dangerously reversed and nutrient availability is poor. The typical eating plan for many Americans contains 60% processed and ultra-processed food, 30% cooked animal products, and only 1% to 5% greens and multicolored fruits and vegetables. Too many people are eating a diet like this that is nutrient-poor and calorie-dense, leading to some of the fattest starving people in the world. And while they're out there getting bigger than the houses in which they live, they're walking around in a constant state of craving, because they are never nutritionally satisfied. ·

Macronutrients and Micronutrients

It is important to understand the difference between macronutrients and micronutrients. All diets contain macronutrients (protein, fat, and carbohydrates). They are called macronutrients because they are the largest compounds of nutrition typically measured and are consumed in greater amounts, i.e., grams, ounces, and, unfortunately for too many of us, pounds. They also provide the calorie-containing part of any diet. On the other hand, micronutrients (vitamins, minerals, phytonutrients, and antioxidants) are the non-caloric parts of the diet, and are measured and needed in extremely small amounts, often in milligrams or micrograms (1,000 to 1,000,000 times smaller than a gram, respectively). Understand, however, that even though micronutrients are needed in very small quantities, they are absolutely critical for the proper balance and expression of life and health.

With few exceptions, micronutrients are found in their greatest concentrations in plant-exclusive foods. In addition to vitamins and minerals, plant foods contain a wide variety of specific phytonutrients, antioxidants, and anti-aging factors: isothiocyanates in broccoli, cabbage, and Brussels sprouts; isoflavones in soybeans; curcuminoids in turmeric; tannins in berries, pomegranates, walnuts, and almonds; fisetin in strawberries, onions, and grapes; and quercetin in apples, onions, parsley, and dark berries. When a diet becomes deficient in micronutrients, imbalances and craving can be significantly increased. When you eat a plant-exclusive diet and the micronutrient needs of the body are met, however, you can experience a degree of well-being and satisfaction that even helps to overcome compulsive overeating and food addiction.

When you look at the standard processed American diet, however, it is the combination of risky excesses of macronutrients combined with deficiencies of key micronutrients that is the problem. These excesses fall into three categories: the excess of animal protein; the excess of saturated, oxidized, and trans fats; and the excess of refined sugar/carbohydrates.

There are several problems associated with these excesses. Via the building blocks of fats and proteins (fatty acids and amino acids, respectively) and the capacity of refined sugar to promote a major inflammatory pathway in the body involving linolenic acid (omega-6) prostaglandin production, these excesses promote a condition of metabolic acidosis, potential irritation, and inflammation. There also are a number of other chemical agents that are increased by the excessive consumption of cooked animal and processed foods (e.g., heterocyclic amines, saturated and trans fats, oxysterols/oxidized cholesterol, advanced glycation end-products (AGEs), heme iron, N-glycolylneuraminic acid (NeuG5c), trimethylamine N-oxide (TMAO), methionine, and arachidonic acid) that contribute to toxicity, cell damage, chronic inflammation, and the risk of heart disease and a variety of cancers. The key word is "acid"; by virtue of their basic structures, these foods are acid-forming. However, the body strives to be more alkaline or soothing. The fluid in your joints and lymphatic system, your blood, saliva, and urine are slightly alkaline under optimal health conditions. When the body is exposed to eating habits that routinely and consistently increase acidity and promote a plethora of chronic inflammatory agents, there can be increased wear and tear, irritation, and potential damage to blood vessels, vital organs, and tissues.

The body responds to tissue damage by mobilizing the immune system to initiate the process of acute inflammation. This natural acute inflammatory response promotes healing and survival. But if wear and tear and irritation continue day in and day out, meal in and meal out, exacerbated by the dangerous excesses of processed oils, animal protein, refined sugar, and irritating agents, inflammation can become more chronic and can even become a contributing factor for further tissue damage. These excesses (especially when foods are subjected to frying and high-heat cooking) also lead to excesses of the reactive oxygen scavengers called free radicals or oxidants. When free-radical damage overwhelms the body's antioxidant defenses, the condition of oxidative stress occurs, working hand in hand with chronic inflammation to provoke dysfunction and disease.

How important is this? There are many physicians and scientists, armed with a significant evidence base, who believe that the combination of chronic relentless inflammation and oxidative stress are the foundation for most of the major pandemics of our culture: heart disease, cancer, diabetes, stroke, obesity, and unhealthy aging. For example, ongoing irritation, oxidative stress, and chronic inflammation can damage the inner wall (endothelium) of blood vessels in the heart, brain, and genitals, which can lead to plaque formation, vascular blockage, and the reduction of oxygen and blood supply to these vital organs. This can lead to all the symptoms and pathology of cardiovascular disease, brain disease, dementia, and the loss of sexual function. Therefore, it should be no mystery in our inflammatory, meat-eating culture that heart disease is the number-one killer of men and women, killing approximately 25% of all people who die each year in America. The sad commentary is that since the late 1980s and early '90s we have known enough about nutritional science to never have this happen to another human being again.

In addition, as many as one-third to one-half of all men over the age of 45 in the U.S. deal with some aspect of sexual dysfunction. Erectile dysfunction is stimulated to a significant degree by reactive plaque formation and blockage of blood vessels to the genitals, leading to what we can call heart disease of the penis and an endless stream of ads for conventional drugs and so-called natural treatments for erectile dysfunction. Perhaps you are as tired and upset as I am by the blatant manipulation of drug companies and various health professionals that prey on people with this disturbing health problem. Unfortunately, bushels of the drugs Cialis and Viagra, which block an enzyme (phosphodiesterase) that promotes impotence and erectile dysfunction, are sold as a solution for a basic lifestyle problem truly generated by poor food choices, stress, inflammation, vascular blockage, and oxygen deprivation. And the warnings for these drugs are not warnings to most men. They are advertisements. Why? Because for many men having difficulty maintaining an erection, if they can take a magic blue pill to have one, they would tend to overlook any risk as an adverse event, especially the commonly stated risk of having an unabated four-hour erection! In fact, it's probably not that far-fetched to state that if a man has a four-hour erection, he would probably knock on every door in the neighborhood and proudly show it to anyone that he can.

In addition to these major pathological concerns, it is most important to keep in mind that inflammation and oxidative stress can compromise metabolism and are major contributing factors for dangerous, increased weight and body fat.

Our bodies routinely generate metabolic waste and toxins from the normal activity of our trillions of body cells in addition to the onslaught of environmental and dietary toxins entering the body from the outside. The body is always on the job, using energy to eliminate these internal and external toxins or to at least maintain them within an acceptable level that poses minimal threat to the integrity of the body. When we maintain stressful, exhausting lifestyles beyond our energy reserves, there is an energy crisis in the body (enervation) that interferes with the elimination of this internal and external toxicity. This can lead to a buildup of toxins beyond healthy, acceptable levels in the blood (toxemia) and in fat cells, requiring protective elimination by the body that manifests as the acute symptoms of disease, such as fever, discharge, etc. If these conditions of enervation and toxemia are not addressed and reduced by lifestyle factors including rest, sleep, stress reduction, and whole-plant-food nutrition, toxemia can become prolonged over time, promoting chronic degenerative changes associated with long-term damage to the cells and organs of the body, eventually producing cancer and death.

Therefore, to a great extent, the myriad symptoms and diseases that are so prevalent in our culture often occur as a result of chronic enervation/toxemia, chronic inflammation, and oxidative stress that damage body cells and compromise oxygen and blood supply to the vital tissues and organs of the body. Understand that when you developed in your mother's womb, you underwent a process of differentiation. The individual identities of the various cells and organs began to express themselves, as heart became different from liver, which became different from kidney, and so on. The way these different organs respond to similar conditions of irritation, oxidative stress, and inflammation can be quite different and are the direct result of their specific natures, accounting for the unique set of responses and symptoms that are observed in a wide range of pathological conditions. However, the underlying process of a panorama of diseases and dysfunctions is exactly the same: toxicity, irritation, oxidative stress/inflammation, vascular blockage, diminished blood flow, oxygen deprivation, and loss of function. The only thing that's different is location, location, location. The location that any pathology manifests in your body may be determined by prior insults and damage, and your own genetically affected predisposition that the hygienic pioneer/physician, Dr. Herbert Shelton, referred to as your personal diathesis.

So, if you want to decrease heart disease, memory loss, and sexual dysfunction, you've got to minimize factors of enervation and toxemia so as to prevent, reverse, and eliminate the inflammation/oxidative stress and vascular blockage that are dangerously decreasing your oxygen and blood supply, compromising energy, metabolism, and vitality. Anything that reduces toxicity, irritation, and chronic inflammation can reduce the risk of disease, and, as a result of the impact of inflammation on appetite and fat metabolism that is discussed throughout this book, can also decrease potential problems with weight control.

Here's where I give you the Willy Wonka Golden Ticket: a whole-food, plant-exclusive diet, free of added salt, oil, and sugar, is an alkaline-forming diet that eliminates debilitating excesses and provides key macronutrient and micronutrient needs to reduce toxicity, prevent and reverse acidic inflammatory change, prevent free-radical damage, and reduce the risk of major diseases while remarkably enhancing energy and function.

With this in mind, let's take a look at the three major macronutrients: protein, fat, and carbohydrates.

CHAPTER 3

THE BASIC TRUTH ABOUT PROTEIN

Basic Building Blocks

We need protein. It is a significant and crucial macronutrient of any healthy diet. There are thousands of proteins in the body, and they are important for a variety of life-supporting functions, including growth, repair, and the production of hormones and enzymes. All proteins are constructed from 20 amino acids, basic building blocks that are strung together to make up the variety of proteins in the human body, much like chains of letters that make up individual words. Nine of these amino acids are considered essential because we can't make them ourselves; they must be provided by our diet. The remaining 11 non-essential amino acids can either be provided by your diet or produced by the body itself. Keep in mind that when you eat any protein, whether it's from animals or plants, the proteins are broken down first via the process of digestion into their component amino acids which then, following the blueprint of DNA in your genes, can be reorganized and combined to create the full panorama of proteins that you need. From just these 20 amino acids, this mysterious and magical dance of protein synthesis constructs such diverse proteins as the hormone insulin, containing 51 amino acids, and titin, a muscle protein that is the largest protein in the body containing 27,000 amino acids!

All amino acids have an amino portion that contains the element nitrogen. The air you breathe is 70% nitrogen, but this nitrogen cannot be used directly by animal cells and bodies. Only plants, in combination with certain bacteria, can capture atmospheric nitrogen and convert it into a usable form that is then available for animals. Therefore, all amino acids and all proteins are initially made by plants, and all animal protein is actually just recycled plant protein. Contrary to the fear and misunderstanding that many people have about their protein needs, consuming a variety of plant foods provides all the protein you will ever need as well as all the essential amino acids that you are incapable of making yourself.

Unfortunately, because of the importance of protein, we all have been sold the outrageous idea that protein is the holy grail of nutrition, and for us to be healthy, for us to control our weight, it is necessary to eat huge amounts of protein—especially animal protein. Not only is this a glaring lie with no scientific validity, but it also is a myth that defies the science that clearly and unequivocally demonstrates that plants are the fundamental source of all protein, that humans are not meat-eaters, and that by eating animal foods you participate in an unnecessary ritual of wanton violence and killing that lays the insidious foundations for the most devastating diseases affecting our culture today, including widespread fat and weight gain.

Structure and Function

The anatomy and physiology of the body and the digestive system of humans is consistent with true fruit- and plant-eating animals, and completely different from that of true carnivores. Similar to true herbivores, humans have an extremely long digestive tract (10–12 times the length of the trunk); reduced flesh-tearing canine teeth; extensive flattened molars and a unique location of the jaw joint and angle of the jaw for grinding fibrous plants; a small stomach of limited capacity and moderate acidity that requires more frequent feeding to meet daily energy needs; unlimited capacity for digesting plant carbohydrates; an appendix that is part of the immune system; an inability to manufacture vitamin C; and the ability to make vitamin A from beta-carotene. Humans also have a narrow esophagus that only can handle a small bolus of fibrous, watery food as it travels from the mouth to the stomach.

True carnivores have much shorter digestive tracts (just 3–4 times the length of the trunk); well-developed canine teeth for tearing apart flesh and body parts; primarily protein- and fat-digesting enzymes; and a huge stomach of extreme acidity to digest the flesh, hide, bones, and even hooves of their prey. They also have a gut capacity that allows them to eat 20–30% of their entire body weight at one meal, allowing for long gaps between meals. In addition, true carnivores do not develop heart disease, no matter how much fat or cholesterol they eat, and do not develop gallstones because of special emulsifying properties of their bile.

Additional support for our frugivorous/herbivorous nature comes from our mentors in the primate world. Our closest primate relatives on the evolutionary scale are gorillas, chimpanzees, and bonobos, who have a similar anatomy and 97–99+% of the same DNA as humans. Their diets are primarily and consistently fruit, greens, roots, and shoots, with the bonobo, arguably our closest relative, being primarily a fruit eater. It is intriguing that bonobos are also referred to as the "hippies" of the primate world because of their empathetic, compassionate nature. In fact, there has never been any evidence or observation of any bonobo ever killing another bonobo. It would behoove our entire species to pay close attention to these amazing relatives, just eat fruit and plants, and let out our inner bonobo!

Therefore, as much as it may sound like heresy in our culture, I want to emphasize that the diet for health and weight loss needs to be moderate in protein overall—and totally devoid of animal protein. In studies going back to the 1970s and '80s, animals that were exposed to known cancer-causing agents (carcinogens) and then fed on high-protein diets, especially casein (found in milk and dairy products), were more prone to the initiation and promotion of cancers than were animals on low-protein diets.[1] In addition, excessive protein also stimulates pro-aging pathways and premature aging in a wide range of species, including mammals.

Remember, as protein becomes an excessive part of your diet—especially protein from animal food sources—the metabolic acidosis and exaggerated inflammatory agents generated can promote irritation, damage, wear and tear, and debilitating chronic inflammation. Unfortunately, most Americans are getting nearly 70% of their protein from animal sources.[2] Yes, you need protein, but only within a well-defined window of need. Unfortunately, the prevailing philosophy of nutrition in the United States is that if something is good, more must be better, and a lot more must be a lot better. The fact is that all too often, when it comes to nutrition, more may be dangerous, and a lot more may be downright toxic. If you go appreciably beyond a basic window of protein need, you may promote myriad problems and dysfunctions, including damage to the heart, brain, liver, kidney, and colon.

What is the window of need, and what are the best sources of protein? As is natural for many people and cultures on planet Earth, as well as all animals including our primate relatives, it is not necessary to count calories or weigh out grams or ounces of protein or other nutrients for your health and weight goals. Whole plant foods naturally provide all the protein you need. What is most important is to eat a diversity of whole plant foods with 90–95% of your food coming from fresh fruits, cooked and raw starchy and non-starchy vegetables, whole grains, and legumes, and 5–10% from more calorie-dense, higher-fat foods like seeds, nuts, and avocados.

Protein Requirements and Plant Sources

Daily protein needs can be evaluated based on individual body weight or as a percentage of the daily calories you consume (Table 2). On close examination of long-term population studies involving meat-eaters, partial meat-eaters, and plant-exclusive vegans (the Epic-Oxford Study in the U.K. and the Adventist Health Study (AHS-2) in the U.S. and Canada, involving over 102,000 participants), the amount of protein typically consumed by healthier people on vegan, plant-exclusive diets is about 12–14% of total calories, not the 30–50% usually promoted in most high-protein and paleo diets. Since most people are unaware of their total daily calorie intake, this measurement may seem confusing and inaccessible. However, I am presenting it here because it has been used to study human populations. To simplify and clarify the numbers in the human studies and in Table 2, just keep in mind that protein provides 4 calories per gram. So, if you are consuming 2,000 calories per day, 10% of your calories are 200 calories from protein, which divided by 4 calories per gram, is equal to 50 grams per day.

The recommended dietary allowance (RDA) of protein, which is considered to be the average daily dietary intake deemed sufficient to meet the protein needs of more than 97% of the population, is 0.36 grams per pound of body weight (or 0.8 grams of protein per kilogram of body weight). The high-fiber content of whole plant food can cause a small amount of protein (less than 10%) to pass through the intestine, so to ensure adequate availability, it makes sense to slightly increase the daily protein requirement to approximately 0.4 grams per pound of body weight.

The first part of Table 2 below establishes the amount of protein needed to meet the RDA and the adjusted RDA for various body weights; the second part demonstrates that my recommendation that protein be 10-15% of total calories consumed easily provides and even exceeds the RDA amount needed. Note that even for a 200-pound person, since 1 ounce equals 28.3 grams, just 2.5 to 3 ounces of protein per day more than meets the recommended daily allowance! It is important to recognize how different our actual need for protein is compared to the exaggerated amounts typically promoted in our society today.

Protein Requirements by Body Weight

0.36 grams per pound of body weight (or 0.4 grams per pound, adjusted for WPF diets) equates to:

Weight	RDA (0.36g/lb.)	Adjusted RDA (0.4g/lb.)
100 pounds	36 grams	40 grams
150 pounds	54 grams	60 grams
200 pounds	72 grams	80 grams

Protein Requirements as a Percentage of Total Daily Calorie Intake

The recommendation to obtain 10–15% of total daily calories from protein equates to:

1,500 calories	40–56 grams, or 1.4 to 2 ounces
2,000 calories	50–75 grams, or 1.8 to 2.6 ounces
2,500 calories	60–90 grams, or 2.1 to 3.2 ounces

Table 2. Daily protein requirements measured in grams of protein per pound of body weight and amount of protein needed to provide 10–15% of daily calorie intake.

Other factors, including age, activity levels, and pregnancy, can increase protein needs. For older people, approximately 0.55–0.68 grams of protein per pound of body weight are recommended to compensate for some of the contingencies that can occur with aging, including decreased protein metabolism, loss of muscle mass, increased cell damage, declining repair responses to ingested protein, inefficient digestion, and reduced absorption of nutrients.[3] In one study, older men and women (ages 70–79) consuming 91 grams of protein daily lost 40% less lean mass than those eating 50–60 grams a day.[4] Increasing protein intake as you get older may also lower disease risk and help you decrease risky belly fat and body weight. In a national nutritional survey of over 24,000 older adults, the highest protein intake was associated with the lowest body mass index and waist circumference, significant risk factors for obesity, diabetes, and heart disease.[5] Additional increases are also suggested for certain athletes, including weight-training bodybuilders (0.5–0.9 grams per pound), for growing children (0.4 grams per pound), and for pregnant and lactating women (0.5–0.6 grams per pound).

Most people make the mistake of thinking that protein exists only in concentrated foods such as meat, eggs, dairy products, nuts, seeds, soy foods, and beans. In fact, protein exists in every food. Nature doesn't make a piece of fruit or a leaf of lettuce without protein, so even foods that are not typically considered to be high-protein foods provide a meaningful amount of protein. Whole grains are examples of this; although they are not considered to be protein-providing foods, whole grains are between 8% and 20% protein.

In the 1970s, a popular vegetarian cookbook, *Diet for a Small Planet*, made a distinction between foods containing complete protein (having all nine of the essential amino acids) vs. incomplete proteins (having some, but not all, of them). While a variety of plant foods (including quinoa, soybeans, chia seeds, buckwheat, and even broccoli and kale) contain all the essential amino acids, many plant foods are incomplete, so it was thought that vegetarians and vegans had to carefully pair various plant-food categories at each meal to ensure intake of enough high-quality protein to meet the body's needs. Since then, science has proven conclusively that this is not necessary at all. By eating a variety and diversity of plant foods throughout the day, you will consume all the amino acids you need and provide an ongoing pool of amino acids that will support healthy protein production and satisfy the protein requirements of the body.

The following information from the United States Department of Agriculture (USDA) makes this more clear. The USDA National Nutrient Database for Standard Reference[6] lists the following:

Protein Content in Whole Plant Foods

Beans/lentils (180 cal., 14–18 grams/cup)

Nuts and seeds (160 cal., 4–12 grams/ounce)

Oatmeal and quinoa (300 cal., 8 grams/cup)

Broccoli (79 cal., 5.4 grams/8 ounces)

Kale (64 cal., 4.3 grams/8 ounces)

Spinach (52 cal., 6 grams/8 ounces)

Remember, you typically only need 36–90 grams of protein per day. So, for example, if you ate a cup of oatmeal for breakfast with some fruit and 1–2 tablespoons of ground flax seeds, a couple of pounds of greens and vegetables in salads and steamed vegetables throughout the day, 1–2 ounces of nuts, a baked sweet potato with your salad for lunch, and a cup of beans with a half cup of quinoa for dinner, you would consume 70–80 grams of protein, satisfying your protein needs while also providing your daily needs for fiber, micronutrients, and essential fatty acids—which animal foods can't do.

Of course, protein is only one part of the food you eat. The fat content of protein-containing foods must especially be considered because of its high calorie load and some potential detrimental effects that can occur in the body when fat is cooked and processed (discussed in Chapter 4). When you evaluate the amount of fat that comes with the protein in plant foods vs. animal foods, a startling picture emerges that has important implications for health and weight loss. As we have seen, vegetables have extremely low calorie densities (65–195 calories/pound); between 7–33% of their calories are from protein and only

6–19% of their calories are from fat. Fruits, with a calorie density of 140–420 calories/pound, are 2–9% protein and just 3–7% fat, although the highest protein-containing fruits, including guava, apricots, blackberries, and raspberries, are 8–14% protein. Lentils and beans are also low-density (310–780 calories/pound) and have substantial protein content, with 25–30% of their calories from protein but only 3–5% from fat. In contrast, beef, chicken, salmon, and cheddar cheese have high calorie densities (1,100–2,400 calories/pound), with 23–50% of their calories from protein but a whopping 50–74% of their calories from fat![7,iii]

So even though meat and dairy provide substantial protein content, their high calorie density; excessive concentrations of fat calories, cholesterol, and inflammatory and cancer-causing agents; deficient micronutrient content; and complete absence of fiber strongly indicate that these foods should be avoided on any health or weight-regulation program. Since, in comparison to animal products, a wide variety of plant foods provide more than adequate amounts of protein, are extremely low in calorie density, have no cholesterol, have a low fat content (especially of risky saturated fats), and are extremely high in micronutrients, fiber, and water, a large volume of greens and veggies is the best choice for your health and weight-loss program. Therefore, the abundant use of plant foods on a healthy, diverse WFPE diet provides critical but misunderstood sources of abundant quality protein and should be the nutritional focus for long-term, successful weight loss.

To reinforce the idea that eating a diverse plant-exclusive diet easily provides all your protein needs, keep in mind that the largest, strongest mammals on planet earth (elephants, rhinos, hippos, and other large

---

[iii] As discussed earlier, including a variety of nuts in a WFPE diet promotes major benefits, providing much-needed quality protein, essential fatty acids, fiber, vitamins, and minerals. However, since 54–88% of their calories come from fat,[7] their high calorie density dictates that only a very limited quantity (1–2 ounces) should ever be consumed in any day to maintain long-term, successful weight loss.

primates, including our close primate relatives, gorillas and bonobos), with the largest muscle mass, are all strict vegan plant-eaters. An animal like an elephant can weigh more than ten thousand pounds and maintain the largest muscle mass of any animal that walks the earth. Now, it is true that elephants may eat several hundred pounds of salad per day, but they're maintaining all that mass with pure plant protein from leaves, grass, and the bark of trees. Do you think the elephant, this massive, muscular, raw-food vegan, gets up one day, looks out over the savannah, and with a worried look asks, "Where can I get my chicken nuggets, a steak, or some fish?" It's absurd. So, don't worry about your protein needs on a plant-exclusive diet. If the elephant can maintain a 10,000-pound mass on the protein in plants, there's no doubt that you can maintain a 100- to 300-pound mass on the proteins in diverse plant foods.

Most of the animal and dairy products eaten in the U.S. come from cows, sheep, pigs, and goats. Even these animals are strict herbivores who satisfy all of their energy and protein needs from plants. All I'm recommending is to cut out the "middle man"— the middle sheep, pig, cow, and goat—and stop the ritual of pain, torture, and death inherent in animal-food production by eating plants directly and connecting to the primary source of available energy, the sun.

The Roles of Protein and Ecology of Food Choices

As stated earlier, proteins play a major role in growth, repair, and the production of hormones and enzymes. However, protein is not the body's primary energy source as so many people mistakenly think it is. Plants are the only life form capable of transforming the direct energy of the sun into the food that feeds all human and non-human animals on our planet. So, there are only two choices: you either eat plants directly or you eat the body of some animal that ate plants directly. Yet, we have already seen that the calorie density, fat content, and the increase in inflammation and oxidative stress associated with animal food intake increases disease risk and fat/weight gain.

Furthermore, the science of ecology strongly suggests the need for WFPE nutrition to maximize your energy and minimize toxicity. As you go up the food chain from plants to grazing animals or human, to carnivorous predators, there is a natural, logarithmic loss of available energy due to the energy use and dissipation that occurs in the normal metabolism of all animals.

In addition, there is also logarithmic magnification and concentration of toxins that accumulate in the bodies of animals as you go up the food chain. In their fat cells and tissues, animals retain, concentrate, and magnify toxic chemicals from the environment, including harmful elements in plants, pesticides that may be sprayed on the plants they eat, and the toxic by-products of their own metabolisms. If you eat the animals that eat plants rather than eating the plants directly, you will be exposed to a 10-fold increase of the original toxicity. If someone came along and ate you, who ate the animal that ate the plant, they would be exposed to one hundred times the toxicity of the plant. So, as you shorten the food chain and get back to eating plants directly, you are maximizing your energy intake, reducing fatigue, decreasing toxicity, and promoting weight and fat loss.[iv]

Special Animal-Protein Concerns

It is also important to realize that consuming "lean" meat and processed animal foods are definitely not good protein choices for health and weight loss. Cholesterol is concentrated in the membranes of muscle cells—in the lean meat, not the fat—of animals. Processed foods containing milk, cheese, and eggs provide dangerous oxidized forms of cholesterol called oxysterols that can cause inflammation and damage

---

[iv] As you will see clearly in Chapter 20, the exposure to environmental toxicity can promote the accumulation of weight and body fat. This becomes even more shocking when you consider that Americans and people in other industrialized nations are consuming 30–40% of their total calories from animal products and almost 85% of their protein from the flesh, blood, and fluids of animals.

blood vessels. As a result, lean meat and low-fat dairy products are not a solution. Yet this misunderstanding continues to persist, leading people to believe that these are healthy foods when they are not. Between 1960 and 2005, there was a three-fold rise in chicken consumption.[7] Besides the already discussed dangers caused by animal foods, this also may provide a troublesome increase in arsenic contamination and biochemical stress because arsenic has been a government-approved additive in chicken feed for decades. It has been used to kill parasites and promote chicken growth in the animal food industry.[8] Besides this direct effect on chickens, soil can be contaminated by the use of chicken manure, which can affect the quality of commercial produce grown in this soil. Some concern about arsenic toxicity in rice is an example of this. However, boiling trice in large amounts of water and draining the water after cooking can remove a substantial amount of arsenic. Arsenic toxicity may affect hormonal balance, metabolic efficiency, and your ability to achieve long-term weight loss.

Diversify Your Food Choices

Remember that I recommend a *diversity* of plant-based foods. Too often, when people change over to a vegan, plant-exclusive diet, they have very limited imaginations. They sometimes act like a WFPE diet means eating just romaine lettuce and a baked potato. This would not work long-term for anyone. Your health and life would likely be compromised by deficiency and boredom. You will see as we go along that the WFPE diet gives you some of the most varied, exciting, and tasty food options, and also satisfies all of your nutrient needs in the process. I recommend avoiding all animal protein, ideally.

I have lived as a vegan for over 45 years. The last beef, fish, or chicken I had was in the early 1970s. Now in my 70s, I am approximately 6'2" tall, 185 pounds, with low body fat and high muscle mass similar to when I was in my 40s, no belly fat or love handles, completely drug- and pain-free with flexibility, balance, and endurance better than many people half my age. Does that sound like I'm faltering or fading away from the lack of animal protein and animal-based food in my diet? Hardly, and these results are not unique to me. A huge number of people, including well-known entrepreneurs, vegan teachers, activists, chefs, physicians, etc. became ardent promoters of vegan, WFPE living because they were able to overcome major health risks while overcoming addictions and losing hundreds of pounds of weight/body fat, which they have kept off for decades. I have counseled and known countless numbers of people who, after eating conventionally for most of their lives, have switched to eating WFPE and done so for many years. They have dramatically maintained an incredible quality of life, enjoyed high-level performance in all their activities of normal living, and maintained optimal weight and body fat into their 60s, 70s, 80s, and even 90s. There is no need to eat any animal products at any time at all.

You may be aware that the people in many of the lean, long-lived, low-disease-risk cultures termed Blue Zones (populations in Japan, Greece, Italy, and Costa Rica, and Seventh Day Adventists in the U.S.) have been shown to take in a very small amount of their protein from animal sources, usually less than 10% of all the protein consumed. In *The China Study*, that translated to just a few ounces per week.[9] The *Weightless* approach is not about making your life difficult and uncomfortable. It is about making empathetic, compassionate choices that reduce health risk and give you the best opportunity for long-term weight-loss success.

As much as I feel it is imperative to live WFPE, I respect where you are on your own path of life, growth, and change. So, while in transition, if you really can't live without it, limit animal foods to at most a few ounces of animal protein per week. That said, I really believe that once you see that you can live on a few ounces of animal protein per week, you will realize that you can live on no ounces per week. And I hope you can, because there are several additional factors that need to be considered in unveiling the full health impact and physiological stress associated with excessive protein intake from animal sources.

Risks of High-Protein Diets
Uric Acid Toxicity

Increased animal-meat protein intake, in conjunction with the other aspects of our so-called modern diet of affluence (high intakes of other animal products, saturated fat, refined sugar, and alcohol), can lead to a buildup and excess of uric acid. Uric acid is a highly inflammatory agent derived primarily from the purine content of the organs of the dead animal bodies that you're eating, with lesser amounts in dried beans. It can increase irritation and inflammation of anything it contacts as it circulates in the bloodstream.

True carnivores in nature, like lions and tigers, eat virtually nothing but the flesh of all the herbivore/vegan animals that roam the savannah, including gazelles and antelopes. These carnivores generate exorbitant amounts of uric acid via the breakdown of tissues of the animals they are eating. So why don't we see lions and tigers suffering with chronic inflammation, getting hip and knee replacements, and walking with walkers? Simply because these animals have an enzyme called uricase which enables them to metabolize and oxidize uric acid. Uricase converts uric acid into allantoin, which is more soluble than uric acid and can pass more easily and harmlessly from their bodies. If you think about it, it makes sense that if certain animals evolved the capability to eat nothing but huge amounts of flesh, they also would develop the physiological equipment that allows them to comfortably eat that way. Guess what? Human primates like us, primarily equipped for eating a plant-exclusive diet, do not have this enzyme. It is thought that during evolution, humans lost the ability to produce uricase.[10]

Most of the uric acid produced by the body is filtered out by the kidneys. However, when uric acid builds up to an excessive degree from the overconsumption of meat, dairy, and alcohol, the kidneys can become overwhelmed, and elimination will be impeded. As a result, there is no other option but for it to go into the bloodstream, irritating everything it touches, increasing acid wear and tear, precipitating as crystals under the pull of gravity into the joints of the lower legs and feet, and contributing to a form of arthritis called gout. The chemical stress and inflammation inspired by uric acid toxicity can compromise hormonal and neurological function, promoting problems with toxic stress and weight regulation.

You may recall seeing images of an older Henry VIII, the King of England, with his legs up, bandaged, swollen with gout. For this reason, gout has been called the disease of kings. Actually, it is the disease of overweight, carnivorous, alcoholic kings. Henry VIII was on an original modified high-animal-protein/keto-type diet high in fat and meat, with nary a salad in sight. Yet, at least he was eating clean meat killed in small, controlled numbers from the pristine forests of England. Trust me, the meat you're eating today is the furthest thing from pristine, and it's associated with the most brutal killing methods employed by corporate animal agriculture and the commercial fishing industry. It is the most growth-hormone tarnished, genetically modified, antibiotic-poisoned, contaminated crap in history.

Liver Activity: Detoxification and Urea Production

The liver in the human body is like a sentinel on guard, screening and evaluating everything that comes into the body and circulates in the bloodstream. Whether it's the food you eat, the drugs you take, or the pollution and pesticides you are exposed to, the liver, through a separate portal circulation, gets the first look at everything that comes into the body. For those eating the standard American diet, it bears the heavy burden of dealing with the toxicity arising from excessive protein, processed oils, and refined-sugar intake.

To support and protect this first line of defense, then, there is great value in starting a new eating plan or weight-loss regimen with a detoxification process using juices, smoothies, or even water fasting. (See Chapters 10 and 13.) While there may be significant weight loss during a detoxification program, it is important to consider that the detox process is not a weight-loss program per se, but only a means of unburdening the body so it is more efficient metabolically and capable of promoting successful weight and fat loss. If you have been eating large amounts of animal products, refined sugar, fat, and processed food, when you try to get a fresh start, the body's existing chemical stress may impede your progress. Detox programs can provide a valuable jump-start and help you achieve the best results possible.

The liver also plays a major role in protein production and metabolism. For example, albumin is a major blood protein that is produced by the liver. Low levels of albumin on typical blood tests may indicate protein deficiency. In addition, due to the nitrogen content of the amino acids that make up proteins, the metabolism of proteins produces the toxic compound ammonia. The liver converts this ammonia into urea which can be measured in your blood as blood urea nitrogen (BUN) and eliminated in the urine by the kidney. Therefore, abnormally low levels of BUN may also indicate protein deficiency. Conversely, excessively high protein intake from high-protein diets can promote excessive production of urea, burdening the kidneys and compromising their function.

Protein and Transit Time, Intestinal Toxemia, and Weight Regulation

When food is consumed, the time it takes from when it enters your body to when it exits is called transit time. The longer the digestive tract, the longer the transit time. We have one of the longest digestive tracts in nature, which, when paired with the high fiber and water content of plant food, promotes the most optimal transit, digestion, and support of the trillions of life-promoting microorganisms that live in our intestines (the microbiota). Carnivorous animals have much shorter digestive tracts and stomachs that are significantly more acidic than primates like us, so that animal proteins can be processed and digested more efficiently. In humans, however, since animal protein is high in saturated fat and low in fiber and water, it can slow down transit time, decrease the healthy diversity of your gut flora, increase inflammation, and promote blockage, constipation, and incomplete digestion in general. Then, as a result, larger protein fragments can linger longer and break down, decomposing and putrefying rather than being digested in a normal, efficient manner, which can produce debilitating, toxic by-products. These chemicals can create a condition of intestinal toxemia, a toxic condition of the bowel. Bowel toxicity can affect the local environment and cells of the bowel, further damaging your healthy microbiota, and the toxic chemicals can be resorbed into the bloodstream, irritating and even inflaming organs and tissues far removed from the bowel. Headaches, inflammation, damage to the gut lining, leaky gut syndrome, and even autoimmune conditions such as rheumatoid arthritis are to some degree provoked by bowel toxicity.

Anything that helps reduce bowel toxicity provides an opportunity to improve function and efficiency. High-fiber, low-fat plant foods such as fruits, vegetables, lentils, and beans improve overall bowel-transit times, promoting better absorption, circulation, elimination, and utilization of all nutrients. This can dramatically improve your ability to more effectively regulate the use of calories and allow for steady, healthy weight loss. I cannot emphasize strongly enough how important the health of the entire digestive system is for effective weight regulation.

High-Protein Diets, Dehydration, and Electrolyte Balance

To wrap up our protein story, consider the following issues related to high-protein diets. The first few problems center around dehydration and electrolyte imbalance. Carbohydrates, the energy source of our bodies, are hydrophilic, or water-loving. When you abruptly stop eating refined sugars and other carbohydrates, there often is a significant water loss—a dehydration effect—that contributes to significant initial weight loss. However, the body doesn't shed water alone; along with the water, it experiences a loss of critical electrolytes. This loss can have major effects on heart function. Thousands of women between the ages of 35–44 die yearly from cardiac arrest as a result of arrhythmia and electrical dysfunction of the heart due to electrolyte loss.

When carbohydrates are removed from the diet, the body needs an alternative energy source and attempts to create energy from available fat and protein. Since the person is eating lots of protein, the muscle mass is spared, but the body will continue to break down nutritional fat and body-fat reserves to compensate for the lack of sugar as an energy source. However, when fat is broken down, it generates a class of acidic compounds called ketones, resulting in an increased state of ketosis that, if maintained over time, will further acidify the body and lead to more potential inflammation. Chronic ketosis can also have negative effects on kidney and brain function, especially when you are maintaining the high activity and stress of your daily life.

Atherosclerotic plaques in the heart build up quickly on inflammatory high-protein diets. People on an Atkins-type diet for one year had a 40% decrease in blood flow to the heart, dramatically reducing the heart's oxygen supply; a 60% increase in the inflammatory marker C-reactive protein; and a 106% increase in the risky form of cholesterol (LDL), thereby increasing the risk of heart disease and stroke.[11]

In a variety of other studies, low-carbohydrate/high-protein diets were associated with approximately a 60% increase in headaches, a 70% increase in constipation, and a 35% increase in muscle cramping and weakness. In addition, often within six months to a year after periods of rapid short-term weight loss from high-protein dieting, there can be a dramatic rebound weight gain when you go back to eating more normally again.

You may be thinking that this information has been interesting and maybe even beneficial. But since you probably know people who have gone on high-protein and/or high-fat ketogenic diets and lost significant amounts of weight, you may be thinking, "I don't care what you say." What you need to realize is that when someone goes on high-protein/high-fat diets, yes, there can be a significant initial weight loss. But unfortunately, all too often they are mortgaging their health future for some ephemeral, short-term success. There are very important concerns about these extreme diets that can have dire, long-term consequences, and to address these concerns, I have included an entire chapter (Chapter 9) for a more in-depth discussion on the dangers of specific fad diets and other controversial weight-loss approaches.

The high-animal-protein approach is a dangerous attempt for a quick fix that mortgages your health future while interfering with long-term successful fat and weight loss. It is an unconscionable assault on your body, animal life, and the planet itself, and it has no place in a compassionate weight-loss program. The WFPE, SOS-free approach provides the balance of carbohydrates, proteins, fats, and micronutrients that gives you the greatest and healthiest opportunity to create the body you desire now and forever, while respecting the sanctity of life around and within you.

CHAPTER 4

THE PROS AND CONS OF FATS AND OIL

F at is an essential macronutrient of any healthy diet. However, it is the most calorie-dense macronutrient, providing nine calories of energy per gram compared with four calories per gram for protein and carbohydrates. Therefore, it is easy to inflate calorie intake when you are eating high-fat foods, and the optimal diet for long-term weight loss must be low in fat.

I recommend a diet that is approximately 10–15% fat, i.e., no more than 15% of your total daily calories coming from fat. Since fat provides 9 calories per gram, if you are consuming a 1,500-calorie diet, as is typically recommended for many women, that would be approximately 150–225 fat calories or 17–25 grams (approximately 0.6–1.0 ounces) of fat daily. On a 2,000- to 2,500-calorie diet, as is typically recommended for men, that would be approximately 200–375 fat calories or 22–42 grams (0.78–1.5 ounces) of fat per day. Once again, since most people are not aware of their daily calorie intake, do not be overly concerned with by these calculations and numbers. Just by making starchy and non-starchy plants (potatoes, whole grains, whole-grain products, legumes, fresh vegetables, and fruit) 90–95% of your diet with just an ounce or two a day of foods with more concentrated fat content (nuts, seeds and avocados), you will automatically achieve an optimal level of fat intake and optimize your health, weight, and body fat.

Understand that the typical total daily calorie recommendations are somewhat arbitrary. To be more accurate, these recommendations must be considered in relationship to your lifestyle, activity, and calorie output. For example, high-performance athletes can sometimes consume 5,000 to 10,000 calories per day during their intense training and performance schedules just to maintain their weight. However, if you are like most people, living a regular work and family life and maintaining a consistent, moderate exercise program, a good recommendation for daily calorie consumption is about 10 to 12 times your body weight (in pounds). Eating more or less than this amount can translate into weight gain or weight loss.

However, as you will continue to see throughout this book, this program is not about calorie counting; it's about eating a significant quantity of plant food with low calorie density and high nutrient density. Remember my mantra: it's about eating well, not less. It's not just the calories you consume that's important, but rather the quality and type of food that is providing those calories and the impact that lifestyle and environmental factors have on your utilization of them. Why am I suggesting around 15% fat when the average person in the U.S. consumes a diet that is typically between 35–40% fat and when the U.S. government and the American Heart Association recommend a diet containing 30% fat?

In addition to the beneficial low calorie density that a low-fat, WFPE diet offers, my recommendations stem from some of the more profound and provocative studies ever done on health and disease. In *The China Study*, the gold standard for human nutritional research, the leanest Chinese subjects with the lowest outcomes of heart disease, colon cancer, and reproductive cancers consumed under 15% fat.[1] This was also the proportion of fat that was most effective in preventing and reversing heart disease in groundbreaking studies by Dr. Caldwell B. Esselstyn,

Jr., and Dr. Dean Ornish. Dr. Esselstyn's work with some of the most debilitated heart disease patients showed a significant reversal of plaque and vascular blockage in blood vessels feeding the heart, an increase in blood flow to the heart, and a significant decrease in serum cholesterol levels and negative cardiac events over a number of years after adoption of a WFPE diet containing 10% or less fat.[2] The beneficial reversal of heart disease was corroborated by Dr. Dean Ornish in studies utilizing a low-fat vegan diet along with regular exercise and a combination of psychological counseling and the practice of yoga for stress management.[3] Based on these data, it is apparent that limited fat intake, with that fat coming only from plant sources, is most optimal for health and weight loss.

But if you follow the 30% fat guidelines of the U.S. government and American Heart Association, you have a pretty good shot at promoting obesity, strokes, and/or heart disease. At this point you might be saying to yourself, "You mean my government is telling me something that's not in my best interest?" Yes, that's exactly what I'm saying. This shouldn't be that hard to believe. Their recommendations are driven by financial, political, and economic forces, stemming from an unholy marriage of the government with the meat, dairy, and junk-food industries that they subsidize to artificially lower consumer prices on risky animal and junk-food products. As a result, sales and profits are increased, and people are economically coerced to excessively consume meat and dairy products, a situation that is in direct conflict with their best interests and that will only promote obesity and weight gain.

To ensure a healthy lower level of fat intake, I also recommend that you get your fats and oils as close to their natural state as possible, i.e., in the whole plant foods in which they exist. This recommendation includes modest amounts (a few ounces a day) of foods that have higher fat content and calorie density, such as nuts, seeds, and avocados. It is in our best interest to consume fats along with all the other nutrients that exist in food (i.e., proteins, carbohydrates, micronutrients, fiber, and water) rather than in isolation. This promotes a natural balance and protection against excess fat intake, calorie excess, and even compulsive overeating.

Extracted, bottled oils are completely unnecessary and not recommended. There are no animals in nature that isolate the pure fat from their food chain, put it in big bottles of liquid fat, and pour it on everything. Isolation and concentration of one food element to the exclusion of all others is consistent with the definition of junk food. Also, all margarine, animal fats, junk foods, and processed foods need to be eliminated.

When the stomach is full, it distends and activates pressure/stretch receptors in the wall of the stomach, creating a neurochemical satiety response that tells your brain that you've had enough to eat. As we've seen, since fruits, vegetables, legumes, whole grains, and salad greens are very low in calorie density but high in fiber and water, the stomach is more quickly filled and the brain is more effectively satiated so that you feel satisfied with very low calorie intakes. On the other hand, since oils and refined foods are so calorie-dense but lacking in fiber and water, they provide excessive calories without this satisfying "filling-up" effect. As a result, even though you're consuming a large number of calories, eating a high-fat, refined diet leads to a lack of satisfaction and increased hunger, craving, and overeating, making weight loss impossible.

Processing and Cooking of Fat: The Impact on Health and Weight

The impact of fats on health and weight loss is not based on the quantity of dietary fat alone. It also depends on what happens to fat when it is processed, prepared, and cooked. To understand these changes, it is necessary to go deeper into the structure and function of fat.

Fat is made up of building blocks called fatty acids, which, again, implies that an excess of dietary fat can have an acidifying effect on the body and promote more potential irritation and inflammation. Every fatty acid is a chain of carbon atoms (C) attached to each other by chemical bonds, with an acid fragment (-COOH) at one end of the chain, and hydrogen atoms (H) attached to the carbon atoms in the chain (Figure 1).

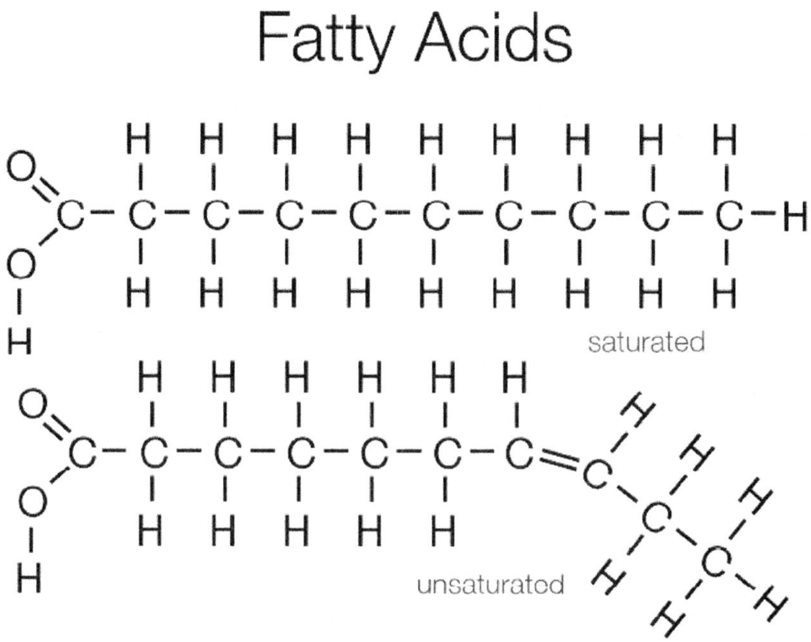

Fatty Acids

Figure 1. The structure of saturated and unsaturated fatty acids. Unsaturated fatty acids have one or more double bonds in the carbon chain. Notice the double bond in the carbon chain of the unsaturated fatty acid in this figure. If the chain has only one double bond it is a monounsaturated fatty acid. If it is unsaturated in multiple places and has multiple double bonds it is a polyunsaturated fatty acid (PUFA). (Image source: Public Domain)

If every carbon atom of the chain has a hydrogen atom attached above and below it, then that fatty acid is called "saturated." When fats are saturated, they have a very high melting point, and are therefore solid at room temperature. That's why, if you were to look at a piece of meat at normal room temperature, you would see solid saturated fat marbling the meat. To some extent, that's also what makes it so dangerous: saturated fat is also somewhat solid at the temperature of the body and may increase the risk of solid fatty plaque accumulating, significantly infiltrating organs and blocking blood vessels throughout the entire body, including the heart and brain.

If hydrogen is removed from any portion of the carbon chain, the chain will be empty at one or more places, or "unsaturated." If they are unsaturated in one place, they are *monounsaturated* fatty acids (such as those contained in olives, avocados, and their oils), and when they are unsaturated at multiple carbons of the chain, they are *polyunsaturated* (like those found in seeds, nuts, and plant oils including corn and safflower oil). When fats are unsaturated, they have a lower melting point, are liquid at room and body temperature, are more unstable chemically, and are more prone to damage from light and (especially) heat.[4] The more unsaturated the fatty acids are, the more fluid they are at room and body temperature. This has important consequences for both the healthy function of the body in general and for weight-loss outcomes in particular.

There are trillions of cells in the human body. Each cell has to be able to live individually and autonomously, taking in nutrients and other important chemicals, eliminating waste, and maintaining its integrity and individuality. Surrounding each individual cell is a cell membrane that acts like a fence defining the boundary of the cell and separating each cell from all the other cells in the neighborhood. Yet, like individuals contributing to a larger society, individual cells come together in a community of cells to make body organs and systems. The cell membrane is a dynamic, fluid structure, made up as a sandwich of protein and fat that serves as memory, protective barrier, and passageway for what the cell needs. Just like you can go through the fence of your property to bring food into your home and to put the trash out on the street for disposal, the cell membrane has to allow nutrients to enter the cell and toxic waste products to leave. However, for things to move in and out of cells efficiently, the fats in the membrane must be as fluid and mobile as possible at body temperature, which would dictate fats that are highly unsaturated. That is exactly the wisdom expressed in the body. The membranes of healthy vital cells are composed primarily of cholesterol and a variety of polyunsaturated fatty acids sandwiched between two layers of proteins that dance and pulse at unique frequencies, similar to the vibrating notes of musical string instruments, to open and close this shimmering biochemical fence so that vital chemicals/nutrients and toxic waste can penetrate, enter, and exit through and around the membrane of the cell.

Both the dietary sources of fat and what we do to it have far-reaching repercussions for weight loss. When fat is processed, prepared, and cooked, there are four major modifications that occur which affect the healthy, dynamic function of all cells and may increase inflammation, biological/oxidative stress, and potential weight gain. These four modifications are: hydrogenation, transformation, oxidation, and production of advanced glycation end-products (AGEs).

Hydrogenation

When unsaturated fatty acids are subjected to even modest heat and pressure in cooking and food processing, hydrogen is added back to the carbon chain, increasing risky saturation. This process of adding hydrogen to the carbon chain is called hydrogenation. It can happen at modest temperatures between 100–200 degrees, yet cooking temperatures are typically in the range of 300–400 degrees or higher. Therefore, sautéing, frying, or cooking with oils in general is never recommended. For weight loss and health considerations, I recommend steaming, boiling, dry sautéing, or sautéing in organic, low-sodium vegetable broth. To provide diverse nutrient availability and exotic flavors that will help you transition to salt- and oil-free food preparation, experiment with cooking with balsamic vinegar or lemon juice and a variety of herbs and spices.

Healthy high-quality, organic, low-sodium vegetable broths, ideal for all cooking/sautéing purposes are readily available in most supermarkets. There are also alternative kosher veggie broths readily available for members of the Jewish faith.

Transformation

When oils are exposed to high heat, not only do they become hydrogenated, but they are also transformed. Transformation of fatty acids can contribute to additional physical stress and cellular dysfunction that promote inflammation and hormonal changes affecting weight gain.

Everything in the world has a certain structure that dictates its function. Similarly, every cell and chemical in the human body has a three-dimensional structure that is critical for optimal function. To visualize the relationship of structure and function, notice that above your waist you have two arms and below your waist you have two legs that allow you to function normally. Imagine that I had a frying pan big enough to lay you in it like a piece of bacon. Now imagine that after I fry you up, one of your arms ends up where one of your legs used to be and vice versa. I think you can appreciate that you might look somewhat the same, but you would function very differently and less optimally.

When fats and oils are subjected to high heat and pressure, the arrangement of hydrogen on the fatty-acid chain of unsaturated fatty acids is altered and transformed. This new structure is the "trans" form of fatty acids, or trans-fatty acids (TFAs), and it's riskier and less functional than its original. Typically, more than 90% of all fatty acids in healthy body cells are in cis form, which is the most fluid and mobile (like a light, thin oil) that allows nutrients, chemicals, and waste products to move, dance, and glide with ease in and out of cells and around cell membranes.[4]

The altered TFAs are more rigid and immobile (like lard) and will not function the way that normal cis fats do. Since they look somewhat the same to the body, they will be used by the body in ways similar to healthy fats. However, the more they are put into the membranes of cells, the more those cells will allow things to enter that they would normally block, and the more they will block things that they would usually allow to exit. As an example, the more trans fats in the diet and in your system, the more prone you are to bacterial and viral infection. When trans fats are put into the walls of blood vessels, these vessels may not handle the pressure of blood moving through them as well and may be more prone to damage, inflammation, and plaque formation, increasing the risk of heart disease. Consistent with this discussion, there is mounting evidence that the increased consumption of TFAs has been associated with increased aggressive behavior,[5] an increased risk of metabolic syndrome (including high blood triglycerides, low HDL cholesterol, and elevated blood sugar), and an increased risk of coronary heart disease.[6,7] In addition, eating more TFAs may trigger systemic inflammation and promote increased body weight, increased abdominal (belly) fat, insulin resistance, and diabetes mellitus.[8]

The impact of trans-fatty acids on inflammation is an important part of the health and weight-loss story. In an extensive study, women who consumed the highest amounts of trans fats in processed junk food had 73% more C-reactive protein and 17% more interleukin 6, well-accepted markers and immune activators of inflammation, than women eating the smallest amounts of trans fats.[9] When inflammation is increased in the body, it creates stress by overworking the adrenal glands, putting undue burden on the hormonal system in general and promoting potential problems with weight regulation. Excessive inflammation also can block the action of a special hormone released from fat cells, leptin, which regulates the brain's experience of satiety. As a result, you can lose the signals that urge you to stop eating when you're full, interfering with your awareness of fullness, and therefore promoting overeating, compulsive food intake, and reactive weight gain. It should be clear, then, that there is no place in the diet for these processed, transformed fats. When you go shopping, read all labels and choose products that contain no trans fats—and make sure that the labels also say no hydrogenated oils, since partially hydrogenated oils can provoke an increase in TFAs.

Oxidation

The third fat modification may be the riskiest of all. When fats are subjected to high heat in processing, not only are they hydrogenated and transformed, but they also are oxidized. Oxidation occurs when the fatty acids are exposed to oxygen. When it comes to fat, "oxidation" is a fancy way of saying that the fat has gone rancid. Rancidity is an oxidation process.

In nature, oxygen is a double-edged sword. In the presence of oxygen, the body converts the carbohydrates in plant foods into energy. As I have mentioned previously, this conversion and energy production occurs in energy factories called mitochondria that exist in all cells. However, oxygen can also create potential harm. Think about oxygen rusting away metal implements in your garage or old buildings being eaten away by exposure to oxygen over time.

In its fundamental structure, oxygen lacks two atomic particles called electrons, making it a relatively unstable element that spends its chemical life seeking electrons to balance and stabilize itself. Oxygen is chemically compelled to find these missing electrons because oxygen, like all of us, is just looking for a stable relationship. However, if it finds those missing electrons in the heart or brain or in cell membranes anywhere in the body, it will attempt to steal them from vital body cells, causing damage and disease wherever in the body it finds them.

Typically, oxygen is coupled with other oxygen atoms in nature to create the stable molecule of oxygen, O_2, or it is combined with hydrogen in a water molecule, H_2O, which allows oxygen to share and secure the electrons it needs. However, since oxygen is being metabolized to such a great extent in the energy factories of our cells, it can be uncoupled to produce single oxygen atoms with free unpaired electrons that are very reactive and threatening. These reactive oxygen species with free unpaired electrons are aptly named "free radicals" or "oxidants." Dangerous free radicals are produced by ionizing radiation from excessive sun exposure, air pollution, tobacco smoke, alcohol consumption, exposure to pesticides and herbicides, and the excessive consumption of animal, dairy, and junk foods that are fried or exposed to high-heat cooking. These highly reactive, free-radical scavengers create a unique form of damage and stress that we previously discssed as oxidative stress and are linked with a panorama of diseases, including premature aging, inflammation, and even cancer.

Excessive reactive oxygen species can extract electrons from the unstable unsaturated fatty acids that exist in all cell membranes. This process of oxidation, or lipid peroxidation of fats, converts unstable unsaturated fatty acids present in all our vital organs into the most dangerous free radical known to man, the lipid peroxyl radical. And since fat is an essential part of all body cells, this oxidation of fat can cause widespread inflammatory and mutagenic (cancer-causing) effects throughout the body. Diets high in animal products subjected to the high heat of cooking (frying, barbecuing, and smoking of meat and cheese) expose the body to dangerous levels of lipid peroxyl radicals, and free radicals trigger excessive inflammation and physical stress which, as we have already discussed, can hinder weight loss and promote abnormal eating habits.

If free radicals (oxidants) are disease-promoting, then antioxidants, whether produced by the body itself or consumed in plant foods we eat, are the micronutrients that counteract and eliminate the destructive action of free radicals and are associated with health promotion, disease reduction, and anti-aging. Since plant-exclusive diets have the greatest amount of antioxidants (more than 50 times more antioxidant activity than any other eating plan!), an exclusively plant diet loaded with fruits and vegetables provides the greatest protection against free-radical damage and the potential inflammation and weight gain that can occur as a result of this oxidative stress.

AGEs (Advanced Glycation End-Products)

Early research on the science of aging revealed that high levels of sugar in the blood can combine with proteins and fats to compromise the vital function of proteins. This chemical combination of sugar and protein creates harmful advanced glycation end-products (AGEs), chemical compounds that are associated with premature aging, inflammation, and a variety of chronic diseases including heart disease, dementia/Alzheimer's disease, and diabetes. The impact of AGEs will be discussed in greater depth in the Chapter 5.

Significant amounts of dangerous AGEs are formed outside the body in foods with high fat and protein content, in processed refined oils, and especially in high-fat and high-protein foods that have been exposed to the high, dry-heat cooking associated with barbecuing, browning, roasting, grilling, frying, and toasting. Foods highest in AGEs include meat (especially red meat), certain cheeses, fried eggs, butter, cream cheese, margarine, mayonnaise, oils, and nuts.

A high-AGE, disease-promoting diet is often considered to be one significantly above 15,000 kilo units daily; anything well below this is considered less risky. Table 3 lists the AGE content per 100 grams (approximately 3½ ounces) of a variety of food items, including whole plant foods, animal products, and refined/processed foods. At a glance, you can see that fruits, vegetables, rice, oatmeal, beans, and potatoes range from 10–200 KU. In dangerous contrast, butter, cheese, steak, and chicken range from 6,000–23,000 KU, with fried bacon checking in at a whopping 91,577 KU. Furthermore, as the fat content of plant foods increases, so does the AGE content. Nuts and olives have a a a higher AGE content, for example, but if you consume these more calorie-dense foods in the recommended smaller amounts of one to two ounces per day, AGE excess is not a problem. Note, however, that when olives are processed into olive oil, the AGE content is increased seven-fold, illustrating why eating the whole foods rather than bottled oils is recommended.

Plant Foods		Animal / Processed Foods	
Carrots	10	Cake	1,113
Apple	13	Fried Egg	1,240
White Potato, boiled	17	Bologna Luncheon Meat	1,640
Oatmeal	18	Pancake	2,263
Cantaloupe	20	Waffle	2,870
Tomato	23	Chips / Crisps	2,883
Rice	30	Salmon, broiled	3,010
Cucumber	31	Cookies / Biscuits	3,228
Celery	43	Tuna - Broiled	5,113
Pita Bread	53	Roasted Chicken	5,828
Sweet Potato, Baked	72	Broiled Steak	7,479
Veggie Burger	100	Big Mac	7,801
Red Kidney Beans, canned	191	Turkey Burger, pan-fried	8,251
Pasta (boiled 12 min)	298	Feta Cheese	8,423
Tofu, steamed	628	BBQ Chicken	8,802
Olives	1,670	Mayonnaise	9,400
Raw Sunflower Seeds	2,510	Cream Cheese	10,063
Tofu fried	4,723	Sausages	10,858
Raw Cashews	6,730	Parmesan Cheese	16,900
Roasted Cashews	9,807	Butter	23,340
Olive Oil	11,900	Fried bacon	91,577

Table 3. The AGE content of foods in kilo units per 100 grams
(3.57 ounces)

Understanding the Impact of Essential Fatty Acids

Looking closer at the fatty acids that make up fat reveals even more ways that refined and animal foods can trigger excessive inflammation. Of all the fatty acids in the body, there are only two that are essential fatty acids (EFAs). In this case, the word "essential" means two things: they are absolutely necessary, and we are incapable of making them. Therefore, they must come into the body in the food we eat. If they are lacking in the diet, deficiency occurs and body function is compromised. The two EFAs are linoleic acid (LA) and alpha-linolenic acid (ALA); due to variations in their structures, they are classified as omega-6 and omega-3 fatty acids, respectively.

EFAs play a major role in balancing the immune system. Our immune system is capable of recognizing everything that we are and everything that we're not (self and non-self). This means if you encounter a bacterial or viral infection, the immune system has to do two things. It has to recognize that these organisms are not you, and then it has to mount some defense to protect you against what's not you. Bacterial and viral organisms do not thrive in elevated temperatures, so the body has evolved the ability to create fevers for its protection. On the other hand, if there is an injury to the body, it can create an essential inflammatory response to clean up tissue damage and promote healing. I think you can appreciate that if fever goes unchecked or inflammation is not controlled, these constructive actions will become detrimental to the body. The immune system must be able to both increase and decrease these responses for healthy function and balance. The chemicals in the body that help the immune system to maintain these inflammatory responses are prostaglandins, eicosanoids, thromboxanes, and leukotrienes, all of which are produced from EFA.[10] The EFAs also balance the function of the brain and nervous system. EFAs are a significant part of the membranes of all nerve cells in the brain and also an important part of the fatty lining around nerve cells called the myelin sheath, which promotes the efficient, rapid conduction of electrical impulses for communication in the brain and nervous system.

The various inflammation-regulating compounds derived from the omega-6 and omega-3 pathways can promote both inflammatory and anti-inflammatory responses to meet the needs of the body and support the healthy function of the immune system. It has been suggested that human beings evolved on a diet with an omega-6/omega-3 ratio of 1:1, but today's highly processed standard American diet has a ratio of 15:1.[11] While a variety of studies have suggested that the optimal ratio of EFAs is different for different diseases, the closer the ratio approaches 4:1 (omega-6:omega-3), the more beneficial it is.

The excessive intake of omega-6 plant-derived oils found in processed foods (notably corn oil, safflower oil, sesame seed oil, and sunflower oil) and arachidonic acid (a dominant fatty acid in all animal cells and animal-food products including all meats, eggs, and dairy products) has led to the dramatically increased levels of omega-6 fatty acids in the American diet, which in turn has increased the ratio of omega-6 to omega-3 fatty acids. The higher ratios have been shown to promote a variety of diseases, including cardiovascular disease, cancer, inflammatory disease, and autoimmune disease.[12] In contrast, omega-3-rich ALA, which is found in walnuts, soybeans, avocados, whole grains, deep greens, cruciferous vegetables, flax, chia, and hemp seeds, promotes the anti-inflammatory omega-3 pathway. The only way this healthy 4:1 ratio can be achieved is by decreasing consumption of all refined foods and all animal foods and increasing the consumption of whole plant foods, especially those rich in omega-3, as listed above.

The body has specific enzymes that can convert anti-inflammatory ALA into longer, more unsaturated members of the omega-3 family, including eicosapentaenoic acid (EPA) and docosahexaenoic acid (DHA), which are important for heart and brain health. The pathway from ALA to DHA only goes in one direction and involves enzymes that convert ALA to the following sequence of products:

ALA ➔ Stearidonic Acid ➔ **ETA** ➔ **EPA** ➔ **DHA**

Since preformed EPA and DHA exist primarily in seaweed and fish (that make it from the seaweed they eat), the amount of EPA and DHA in a plant-exclusive diet can only be provided in one of three ways: by the conversion of ALA, by consuming preformed EPA and DHA in sea vegetation and seaweed, or via supplementation with oil derived from seaweed algae. Since less than 1% of dietary ALA is converted to EPA and DHA, concerns about deficiency typically drive recommendations for additional supplementation. This may be questionable and unwarranted, however. Several studies have shown that even though vegans and vegetarians have lower dietary levels of EPA and DHA than omnivores consuming fish, blood levels in vegans were stable and maintained by the conversion of ALA.[13,14] Maintaining stable lower levels may be advantageous, as some controversial data suggest that higher blood levels may promote a significant increased risk for all grades of prostate cancer.[15]

Furthermore, information from the Adventist Health Study-2, an extensive lifestyle population study done between 2002-2007, indicated that vegans had the highest intake of plant-based ALA and the lowest intake of EPA and DHA compared with vegetarians eating some eggs and dairy and nonvegetarians eating some fish and/or meat. But even though the intake of EPA and DHA was lowest in vegans, they still had high levels of these omega-3 fatty acids in their body fat that was on par with fish-eaters, suggesting that the conversion of ALA to DHA and the potential storage of DHA are significantly greater than previously thought and that the body is quite capable of making all the omega-3s you need from a plant-based diet high in ALA.[12]

When you look at the standard American diet today compared with over 100 years ago, it is apparent that the diet today is much lower in beneficial omega-3 oils. A major reason for this is the hefty increase in refined carbohydrates and animal products in our diets over the last century. These foods have largely replaced whole grains, deep greens, nuts, and seeds, which are significant sources of omega-3s. To better balance omega-3 intake, I recommend routinely consuming walnuts and adding a tablespoon or two of chia, hemp, or ground flaxseed to your diet daily. Flaxseed is not as digestible as these other seeds and needs to be purchased in a ground form or ground up first in a coffee grinder or high-speed blender. These seeds can be added to oatmeal, salads, or even green smoothies for breakfast or as a snack sometime during the day.[v] Additionally, whenever you use grain products, such as rice, breads, and pastas, make sure they are 100% whole-grain.

Prostaglandins, one of the chemicals that increase inflammation, are produced to a great extent from animal products and refined, processed foods. These inflammatory prostaglandins are made from arachidonic acid, which is the long-chain polyunsaturated omega-6 fatty acid that is the most dominant fatty acid found in the membranes of animal cells and in the dairy fluids produced by animals. It is also produced by the enzymatic conversion of the essential omega-6 fatty acid LA in the corn, sunflower, and safflower oils used excessively in processed food production. Consequently, milk and dairy products, chicken, lamb, beef, and pork promote the production of high concentrations of specific inflammatory prostaglandins. This is just one of many reasons why urging people to eat lean meat like chicken and turkey is one of the biggest con jobs of nutrition. It has contributed to a dangerous and false sense of security.

If these animal foods made up only a very small part of our diet, it would not be a big problem. However, as we have emphasized, Americans often get much as 85% of their protein from animal protein sources. As a result, we have skewed our population in the direction of increased inflammation and immune suppression.

---

[v] Recipes for these smoothies will be given in Chapter 13.

It is absolutely critical to adopt a plant-exclusive approach to eating. High-protein and high-fat diets maintain a dangerous illusion: they promote quick-fix, short-term weight loss while reinforcing long-term reactive weight gain. This is not the way to go. Time and time again, it has been shown throughout the world that the leanest, healthiest people are not those who eat a lot of high-protein/animal-protein, but are those who eat an abundance of plant-exclusive carbohydrates. Consistent with this statement, the results of the extensive Adventist Health Study-2 clearly showed that, in more than 70,000 people in the U.S. and Canada, vegans on average had the lowest weight, with average BMIs of 24, compared with fish- and meat-eating nonvegetarians, with average BMIs of almost 29.[12] In addition, vegans in this study also had the lowest levels of inflammation as indicated by the inflammatory blood chemistry marker C-reactive protein.

The conclusion is obvious and compelling: adopting a diverse, whole-plant-exclusive eating plan gives you the greatest protection against all disease and the greatest opportunity for healthy weight loss over weeks, months, and years to come. The vegan, WFPE, SOS-free diet is the best solution for providing the most effective oils and the healthiest ratio of essential fatty acids that reduce rampant inflammation and the associated problems of physiological stress, hormonal imbalance, overeating, and weight gain.

CHAPTER 5

THE CARBOHYDRATE/SUGAR STORY: FUNDAMENTALS AND CONCERNS

The wide variety of whole plant foods contains the greatest concentration of both simple sugar molecules and more complex arrangements of simple sugars called starches that comprise the macronutrient group called carbohydrates.

Carbohydrates are the foundation of all energy production for all animals and are made exclusively by plants. Only plants can take the direct energy of the sun in combination with the carbon dioxide we exhale or produce industrially and, through the process of photosynthesis, produce all the seeds, berries, grains, legumes, fruits, and vegetables that feed the planet. When you eat plants, their carbohydrates, especially the simple sugar glucose, come into the body and, in the presence of the oxygen you breathe in, are converted in the energy factories of all cells (mitochondria) into the energy reserves you need to do all the things that you do.

Carbohydrates are classified into four major groups: monosaccharides (also called simple sugars, the three most important of which are glucose (also known as dextrose), fructose, and galactose); disaccharides (formed of two simple sugars; the three major ones are sucrose, lactose, and maltose); oligosaccharides (formed of three to six simple sugars); and polysaccharides (composed of many molecules of simple sugars; these include cellulose as well as glycogen and starch, which are the storage carbohydrates of animals and plants, respectively).[1]

The simple and complex carbohydrates (starches) in a WFPE diet include a diversity of whole grains, fruits, vegetables, potatoes, and legumes, which provide vitamins, minerals, phytonutrients, and fiber essential to health. Eating a diverse and exclusive diet of whole plant foods, including a small amount of nuts, seeds, and avocados, will provide the 70–80% carbohydrates, as well as the 10–15% protein and 10–15% fat, that are ideal for maintaining optimal health, weight, and body fat. The heavy emphasis on complex carbohydrates reflects the body's need for the fuel and fiber they provide.

Unfortunately, carbohydrates have gotten an unfair reputation, largely thanks to the Paleo/keto approach, which vilifies "carbs" and reveres protein.[vi] The truth is that we need carbohydrates. Why? The short answer is, "For energy." During digestion, unrefined, whole-plant carbohydrates with their high fiber content are broken down, releasing glucose gradually into the bloodstream where it is the primary and preferred source of energy for all the cells and organs in our body—especially the brain, which is just 2% of our body weight but requires 20% of our energy. Unused glucose is also stored as glycogen in the muscles and liver for later use at a time of need. Our bodies need glucose just as our cars need gasoline and our appliances need electricity.

In contrast, refined carbohydrates have little or no nutritional value and are often referred to as "empty calories." These include table sugar, brown sugar, white flour, and high-fructose corn syrup, and they are found in sodas, most baked goods (including breads, pastries, etc.),

---

[vi] See Chapter 9 for more on the dangers of the Paleo/keto approach.

breakfast cereals, and fruit juice concentrates. They are rapidly digested and spike blood sugar levels quickly.[2]

It is the prolonged energy provided by simple and complex whole-plant carbohydrates that supplies the sustained energy needed for all daily activities, from thinking to moving. This is why it's always been interesting to me, even laughable, when people come to me dragging their feet and say, "I'm so tired, I have no energy. I need protein." They, like most people, have been brainwashed to equate protein with the solution for all that ails them. Typically, when your energy is low, you don't need protein. What you need is usually more rest and more whole-plant carbohydrates, including fruits, vegetables, whole grains, and legumes, which will provide you with the glucose needed to fuel your activity.[vii]

The Evils of Refined Sugar

Let me be perfectly clear: there is no place in any effective weight-loss program for any refined sugar products. When I say "refined sugar products," understand what I mean. These products are typically derived from plants like sugar cane, sugar beets, or corn crops. Sugar cane is a bamboo-like stalk that is only about 12% sugar by weight and has a high fiber content (16%); the rest is water (72%). However, when sugar cane is subjected to the sugar-processing industry, the plants are shredded so the pure sugar can be extracted, leaving the fiber and water content behind. The result is a product that can be as much as 99% sugar by weight. It takes three feet of sugar cane to make a teaspoon of sugar, and there are 10 teaspoons of sugar in a 12-ounce can of Coca-Cola. That's thirty feet of sugar cane in a can of soda, and I defy anyone to chew through 30 feet of sugar cane in a month. Yet, how long does it take to inhale a

---

[vii] Although the body can convert and utilize the building blocks of protein, amino acids, for energy production, this is not a direct process. To reiterate what I have stated previously, protein is necessary for growth, repair, and hormonal and enzyme production, not in-the-moment energy availability.

can of Coke? The imbalance of this kind of refined sugar consumption is obvious and dangerous.

Refined flours have been similarly overprocessed to remove the water and healthy, fibrous, nutrient-dense portions of whole grains. Whole grains such as wheat, rice, and millet are milled to strip away the outer bran and germ, and the remaining inner endosperm is ground further into the refined white flours that are used to make products such as breads, cakes, baked goods, and pizza crusts. As mentioned previously, these refined carbohydrates are broken down very quickly during digestion into glucose, rapidly elevating blood sugar levels, promoting food addiction, and reinforcing deficiencies of important micronutrients. This puts an undue burden on the hormonal and neurological systems of the body that control blood sugar levels.

Some of the leanest, healthiest, longest-lived people on our planet— those living in so-called Blue Zone cultures, including Okinawans from Japan, Sardinians off the coast of Italy, Ikarians off the coast of Greece and Turkey, Costa Ricans of the Nicoya Peninsula, and Seventh-Day Adventists in America[3]—consume very few, if any, calories from refined sugar in their diets. Historically, data from the USDA, the U.K., and other countries suggest that in 1815, Americans and other populations were consuming about 15 pounds of refined sugar per person per year, but by 1970, the yearly per capita intake had risen to 122 pounds and now stands at more than 150 pounds per person per year.[4,5] And that 150 pounds doesn't even include all the artificial sweeteners that are used as additives in many refined-food products and so consumed in large amounts today. Unfortunately, refined carbohydrates have replaced whole, unrefined, plant-exclusive carbohydrates for too many of us, bringing with them a number of downsides.

An article published some years ago in the *Wall Street Journal*, entitled "The Supermarket Shopping Basket," clearly showed the nightmare that this has become. The article addressed what Americans are spending their food dollars on when they go shopping, the amount of money spent on these products, and a list of these products in a hierarchy from largest quantity of product and money spent to the least. Do you know what the #1 shopping item of the American public was? It was carbonated soft drinks and sodas loaded with refined sugar, currently costing the public approximately $37 billion per year! Seventh on the list was beer, eighth was cigarettes, and twenty-third was vegetables—right behind dog food, luncheon meat, and toilet paper. Now, toilet paper I can see, but luncheon meat? And fruit didn't even make the top 50 of this list! This clearly contributes to the incredible, reprehensible increase in obesity in our children and teenagers over the past 30 years.

Unfortunately, these disturbing choices are being manipulated and driven by the powers that be. As far back as 2008, a major farm bill in the U.S. provided major subsidies to large farms growing crops that are routinely processed into high-fructose corn syrup, a key ingredient in processed junk food.[viii] These subsidies significantly lowered the cost of processed foods vs. the whole foods that promote health and weight regulation. As a result, junk food is often far less expensive than more nutritious options, and unhealthy calories have become a more affordable option for lower income families and communities. In a study comparing supermarket prices of over 300 food items, high-calorie, nutrient-poor junk foods were significantly less expensive than low-calorie, nutrient-dense fruits and vegetables, so that the healthier choices tended to be made by people of higher socioeconomic status.[6] Over the few years that this study took place, the costs of healthy food increased by almost 20% while junk food prices *dropped* almost 2%. These sinister changes mean that the same amount that can buy thousands of calories of junk food or many hundreds of calories of soda can only buy a few hundred calories of fresh fruits and vegetables.

In contrast, farmers growing fruits and vegetables are only marginally subsidized. The government subsidy policy maintains this huge

---

[viii] A more in-depth discussion of the government subsidy process is presented in Chapter 11.

calories-per-dollar discrepancy between fresh produce and refined junk food and processed animal products, placing financial pressure on many consumers to buy and eat health-damaging, dangerous processed food. It discourages people with low incomes from making healthy choices, especially if they live in poorer, more disenfranchised inner city neighborhoods and communities where healthy food and quality produce is barely available and healthy food choices are virtually impossible. Poor food choices, disturbing declines in physical and mental health, and weight gain are being shaped by economic coercion and greed that sinks its tentacles deep into the foundation of personal and family life.

The disturbing truth of this abuse can sometimes be stranger than fiction. A study was done some years ago on learning behavior in rats. This study involved typical children's breakfast cereals, ones that can contain as much as 60-80% refined sugar. Rats were evaluated for their cognitive ability to learn and perform maze-running behavior. One group of animals was fed the cereals, and another group was fed the box that the cereal came in, ground up to look like shredded wheat. (Rats, like many of us, will nibble on just about anything.) The animals that ate the box performed significantly better on a variety of learning tasks than did those that ate the cereal. So, if you have children or grandchildren who want these processed garbage breakfast cereals, maybe you can get them to eat the boxes instead!

Just recognize that while a compromised diet may seem cheaper initially, you can incur exorbitant long-term financial and personal costs associated with disability and disease if you make these foods a routine part of your life. Trust me, health is always significantly cheaper than disease at any time, and the issue of affordability is actually more within reach than you may think. The good news is that there are many less-expensive whole, natural food options—including grains, legumes, vegetables, and fruit (even including organic choices)—in the supermarkets and health-food stores in your communities. You don't have to be wealthy to be healthy. Consistent with this idea, an analysis from the Physicians Committee for Responsible Medicine (www.pcrm.org) showed that food costs on a low-fat vegan diet decreased by 16 % compared to a diet of meat, dairy, and other animal products, which was a savings of more than $500 per year. With conscious effort and attention to the food items and substitutions recommended in this book, you can provide very healthy options at a very reasonable price for yourself and your family.

Excessive refined sugar affects the body and the weight-loss picture in several critical ways.

- Because refined-sugar products are often devoid of fiber, refined sugar is absorbed rapidly and raises blood sugar levels quickly and dangerously. When sugar goes up even a little bit above a healthy range of normal, it becomes one of the most toxic aging influences known to man. Additionally, when blood sugar levels are abnormally elevated over time, there is a dysfunction and subsequent increased release of the hormone insulin (hyperinsulinemia). This can result in an increased risk of diabetes, an increased conversion of sugar into fat, and the promotion of reactive weight gain. The increase in insulin can also raise cholesterol levels, increasing the risk of heart disease.

- Cancer cells prefer and rely on high levels of sugar for energy production and have a large number of insulin receptors. So, when the body is exposed to exaggerated refined-sugar levels over time, the excessive insulin that is released can bind to receptors on cancer cells, allowing sugar (and amino acids) to enter these cells. This also stimulates the release of insulin-like growth factor (IGF-1), which can trigger genetically produced enzymes and biochemical pathways that promote cancer growth. Notably, this is evident in research that shows breast density, an important precursor to breast cancer, is significantly increased in young girls and women who consume the most refined sugar in sodas and bakery products. Anticancer diets need to be devoid of refined sugar.

- Refined sugar has been shown to exert a cocaine-like effect in the brain. Initially, it can exaggerate the presence of the brain neurotransmitter dopamine that establishes our natural experience of pleasure. However, over time, excessive refined sugar promotes brain changes that eventually deplete the amount of dopamine released as well as the number of dopamine receptors in the brain, diminishing the pleasure response. As a result, you will continue to crave more and more sugar in a hopeless attempt to increase the pleasure response and provide satisfaction.

- If you have had problems with sugar in your life, have you ever had the experience of going back to sugar after staying away from it for a while and finding that you just can't seem to get enough? Refined sugar feeds your addiction to it and your drive to overeat it, thus reinforcing reactive weight gain. (See Chapter 22 for a more in-depth discussion of the impact of sugar on brain reward, compulsive eating, and food addiction.)

- Refined sugar can also promote the release of prostaglandins, which increase inflammation. That increased inflammation can block satiety signals in the brain, urging you to overeat even though you've had enough.

- When blood sugar is maintained at higher levels over time, it can negatively affect the action and function of vital proteins in the body. Proteins are large, complicated molecules made up of multiple strands of amino acids arranged like beads on a string, braided and wound together. For proteins to function properly, these strings of beads must be free to fold and vibrate at particular frequencies, like the strings of a plucked guitar. This electromagnetic dance is crucial to life and health. However, elevated blood sugar levels maintained by the consistent, excessive consumption of refined sugar can react chemically with the amino acids. This chemical reaction cross-links the strands of protein, restricting their movement and ultimately interfering with protein function. This process of sugar and protein interaction is referred to as the glycation of protein, and can result in the formation of chemicals called advanced glycation end-products (AGEs). As was discussed earlier, these products promote premature aging throughout the entire body, e.g., cataract formation in the eye, loss of collagen elasticity in the skin and blood vessels of the body, and even the beta-amyloid plaques seen in the brains of people with Alzheimer's disease. In addition, since all the hormones and enzymes in the body are proteins, the glycation of protein can compromise any hormone or enzyme-related functions, including digestion, nutrition, and metabolism, potentially interfering with your ability to control weight and body fat. Also, it is important to keep in mind that subjecting foods containing sugar, protein, and fat to high-heat dry cooking and processing, especially the toasting, browning, and blackening of foods, increases glycation and the production of AGEs and dangerous acrylamides. To reduce the process of glycation and the production of AGEs, I recommend the following:

- Eliminate the consumption of refined sugar, especially fructose and high-fructose corn syrup, which can promote a glycation effect that is 10 times greater than that of glucose.

- Eat mostly fruits and vegetables—raw, steamed, or boiled.

- Decrease processed and browned, toasted, or blackened foods.

- Decrease animal fat and protein and cook more slowly with low, moist heat; steaming and boiling are ideal.

Many of the perils of refined sugar have been known for quite some time now. Yet, in spite of this knowledge and the insidious effects of sugar on our bodies and brains, I know how difficult it can be to break the stranglehold of refined sugar in your life. It can only be broken with a mindful vigilance that continues to discover and remind you about what may be driving the choice of sugar in your life. What does it mean to you? Is there some deeper issue or conflict that you may be avoiding in the quest for short-term pleasure?

In my opinion, it's imperative to understand that refined sugar is a nutritionally bankrupt, obscene food that provides only empty calories. It is loaded with huge numbers of calories, yet devoid of micronutrients and elements that truly sustain us in body and mind. This bankruptcy, together with the brain changes mentioned above, ensures our inability to be satisfied and drives us to seek more and more. Remember, our brains need sugar. They thrive on it. So, we have a natural drive and taste sensitivity, etched into our gene pool, to seek sugar for energy and survival. But with refined sugar, there just never seems to be enough.

The cornucopia of fresh fruit, with all its fragrances and sweetness, nutrients, fiber, and water, is the most beneficial, natural way to satisfy this basic need. However, just like pornography plays on our inborn drive for reproduction and sexual pleasure, overstimulating refined food is a caricature of our deep-rooted need for sugar, preying on the pleasure process in our brains and sabotaging our natural instincts and needs. Short-term pleasure from hyper-stimulating, pornographic food or other reactive, mindless behaviors/addictions can be an escape to which you may surrender in moments of stress and overwhelming pressure. However, it doesn't help you deal with the deep-rooted issues driving your stress and dysfunction.

Please understand, I don't sit in harsh judgment of occasional attempts to just take a break from the action and discomforts of life. I've done plenty of them in my own life with drugs, sex, and poor choices. However, if the motivations and issues lurking behind our behaviors are not dealt with, an insatiable deep hunger and dissatisfaction will continue to dictate the terms of our lives. Just as a steady diet of porn hijacks our deeper need for intimacy and connection, eliminating obscene refined sugars and bringing natural, succulent, plant-based carbohydrates into your life will imbue you with the whole-food sugars and starches you need to experience balance and reduce craving. The satiety and peace of mind that ensue will help you truly connect with yourself and foster the self-love that ultimately is crucial for health and long-term weight loss.

> *My recommendation is to avoid all refined sugar and refined-grain products. That includes all sodas, bottled juices, high-fructose corn syrup, and refined breads, cereals, and pastas. These foods need to be replaced by fruits and veggies, potatoes, legumes, and whole grains in their natural state (or to a lesser degree in whole-grain breads and pastas).*

CHAPTER 6

HORMONES, GLYCEMIC IMPACT, AND WEIGHT CONTROL

Based on the information I've presented so far, it should be apparent that the excesses of animal protein, fat, and refined sugar in your diet lay the foundation for inflammation, chronic disease, and weight gain. However, the way food directly affects your blood sugar and blood sugar regulation also has a profound impact on your ability to both take weight off and keep it off. With that in mind, the most successful eating plan for long-term weight loss must support optimal hormone function and incorporate whole plant foods with the lowest glycemic impact.

The Hormonal Control of Blood Sugar

To understand the power and significance of the WFPE diet, it is necessary to delve deeper into how the body controls blood sugar. Blood sugar control is one of the most important functions of the body.

The body is always concerned that we have enough glucose in our blood to meet our energy needs. In fact, the body is devoted to the idea of always keeping our blood sugar level within a well-defined, healthy range of normal; if the blood sugar level goes up above this healthy range, it becomes one of the most toxic, aging influences known to man.

Just think about the incredible damage and disease that can occur in diabetics with chronic high blood sugar: devastating heart and kidney damage, loss of eyesight, and amputation of limbs. So, the body is tasked with the challenge of keeping blood sugar within a normal range.

To accomplish the task of keeping blood sugar in a healthy range of normal, the body demonstrates elegant and sophisticated control. In the pancreas, there are small islands of beta cells that release the hormone insulin into the bloodstream. Insulin will circulate in the blood and attach to special proteins (receptors) on the surface of liver and muscle cells (see Figure 2).

The insulin receptors are special proteins designed to exactly match the shape of insulin, like the lock on a door matches its key. When insulin attaches to its receptors, like a key inserting into its lock, there is a signaling pathway inside the cells that opens the door (the glucose transporter, GLUT-4) in the cell membrane and allows the glucose in the blood to enter the cell. So in order for us to control blood sugar, there are really only three important events. The first is the release of insulin, the second is the attachment of insulin to receptors that open doors in the cell membrane, and the third is the entry of sugar into the cells. Effective blood sugar control is driven by insulin release and attachment. This regulation enables blood sugar to be effectively utilized to satisfy current energy needs and be stored for future needs as follows.

First and foremost, blood sugar must satisfy the energy needs of all cells, including brain and red blood cells that are the primary glucose-dependent cells in the body.[1] The importance of supplying blood sugar to the brain is evident when you consider that it requires 20% of our energy but is only 2% of our body weight, as noted earlier. Typically, normal dietary intake of carbohydrates exceeds the needs of these cells, and additional glucose can go into liver and muscle cells where it is stored like a savings account as an energy reserve for a future time of need. In a time of stress or increased activity, when we need additional energy, the glucose stored in the liver and muscle cells can be mobilized back into the bloodstream and made available for energy production.

Effect of Insulin on Glucose Uptake

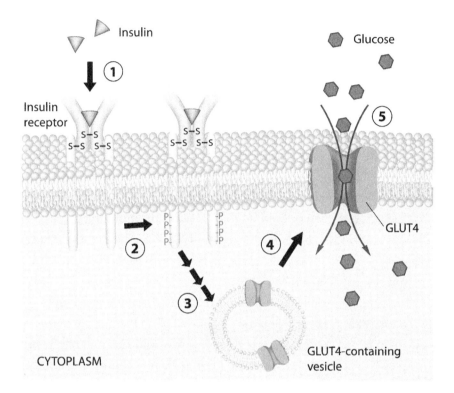

Figure 2. Mechanism of insulin action and function. Insulin attaches to receptors in the cell membrane (1) like a key inserting into a lock in a door and signals a special chemical vehicle called the glucose transporter (GLUT-4) to be inserted into the cell membrane (2)(3) (4), allowing glucose to cross the cell membrane and enter the cell (5). (Image source: Artist; Designua)

The primary destination of excess dietary sugar is the skeletal muscles that move the body.[2] Think about all the activity that the body has to perform on a daily basis and all the energy our muscles have to exert to accomplish this action. In fact, in the fed state when the body is responding to the hormone insulin, skeletal muscle has the greatest impact on the removal of excess sugar from the blood, accounting for as much as 60–70% of glucose removal.[3] The liver accounts for the smallest fraction of excess sugar removal.[4]

Insulin Resistance

Several nutrition and lifestyle factors have a significant impact on insulin function. If you eat the saturated and processed fats in animal and junk foods, their fats are rapidly absorbed into muscle cells, basically taking up space in these cells and making them less available for the needed entry and storage of sugar (glucose). The excessive fat in muscle cells will also alter the receptors for insulin, making insulin less able to attach. This blockage of insulin's ability to effectively promote sugar entry into cells is a condition called insulin resistance. Other factors also promote insulin resistance, including aging, fatness, decreased exercise, chronic stress, and sleep deficiency.

To visualize insulin resistance more clearly, imagine changing a lock on a door, then trying to open the door by sticking the old key in the new lock. It wouldn't work, of course, and you would not be able to open the door. When these nutrition and lifestyle factors change the ability of cells to intake blood sugar (glucose) by altering the cells' "locks," insulin can no longer open the cell "door" and enter the cells. As cells resist the attachment of insulin, the circulating sugar cannot enter muscle and liver cells effectively, and the glucose (sugar) levels in the blood will continue to increase, posing a potentially toxic threat to the body.

Sugar Stress and Weight Gain

This situation leads to a profound example of the wisdom of the body. It's important to note that fat provides us with nine calories of energy per gram compared to protein and carbohydrates which only provide four calories per gram. That's why eating a lot of fat can remarkably increase calorie density and weight gain. However, it also means that fat will provide the most abundant reserve of potential energy for every gram that you store in your fat tissue. So, when the body is confronted with elevated blood sugar, it converts this toxic threat into the most energy-efficient material that it can possibly create—fat—and stores it in your fat cells.[5]

The stored body fat has a purpose: it supplies the body with significant energy reserves that it is able to access and utilize for additional energy, if and when needed. Unfortunately, many of us have stored more of this material than we can ever use in a lifetime. To put a positive spin on it, you can make the case that the pandemic of obesity is fundamentally a direct effect of the body's wise attempt to protect itself against the toxic elevation of blood sugar.

In addition to weight gain, elevated blood sugar is a form of toxic chemical stress on the body that provokes the glands of stress, the adrenal glands, to elicit a fight-or-flight stress response and release the hormone cortisol to mediate this response. (See Chapter 18.) Unfortunately, cortisol has an affinity, a love affair, with fat cells in your abdominal region and can increase abdominal belly fat, the riskiest weight gain of all, significantly increasing the risks of heart disease and diabetes.

Cortisol also has a direct impact on the fat-making enzyme lipoprotein lipase. This enzyme is located in small capillary beds in the vicinity of fat cells; it lures circulating sugar and fatty acids to participate in fat production and storage. Not only does cortisol directly increase the activity of lipoprotein lipase, but cortisol can also directly access and affect the genetic machinery of your cells to stimulate the production of it. This lends credence to the important role of stress management in general, and toxic stress reduction in particular, in fat and weight gain.

This information strongly suggests that ongoing insulin resistance may be the most significant hormonal imbalance of many people with weight problems. Unless insulin resistance is healed over time, it is virtually impossible to handle sugar in a manner that will allow you to keep your weight under control.

Insulin Excess and Burnout

When there is insulin resistance and blood sugar levels rise, the body begins to act as if there's an insulin deficiency. It signals the pancreas to make more and more and more insulin to help push the excess glucose into the cells. In fact, it can produce and release as much as two to three times more insulin than is found in a lean, young, healthy person. It has been known since the 1960s that the excessive release of insulin is a characteristic feature of obesity and weight gain.[1] Elevated levels of insulin in the blood (hyperinsulinemia) increase the risk of heart disease, brain damage, and cancer. Elevated insulin also produces increased hunger, increased food intake, and a heightened perception of the pleasantness of sweet taste and processed foods loaded with refined sugar.[6] When insulin is not working effectively, this cycle continues chronically, and sugar continues to stay elevated despite increasing insulin levels. Type 2 diabetes can develop as a result. To avoid this (and to treat it), what has to be improved is insulin resistance, which is best addressed by lifestyle changes, including a high-fiber, low-fat, high-carbohydrate, plant-exclusive approach to nutrition, consistent activity, better sleep, and stress reduction.

If insulin resistance goes on long enough, the excessive reactive insulin release may overwork the insulin-producing cells in the pancreas, leading to exhaustion and dysfunction of these cells and ultimately an inability to produce insulin. Keep in mind that this potential exhaustion and dysfunction is also promoted by the excessive consumption of processed foods containing refined sugar. When you eat refined sugar products, there is a spike in blood sugar that poses a threat to the system. The body will react by overstimulating the release of insulin, causing a reactive crash of blood sugar (hypoglycemia), which is a major stress to the body. The crash also drives the craving for more sugar. This spiking and crashing can cause wide-swinging fluctuations in your energy as well as major physical and emotional stress and instability. Over time, chronic insulin resistance and/or the consistent nutritional overstimulation of insulin release may promote the development of a type 1-like diabetic state, a more drug-dependent form of diabetes. Typically, type 1 diabetes, previously referred to as juvenile diabetes, is an autoimmune form of diabetes usually found in people who are born with genetic compromised insulin production and/or function. People with this form of diabetes have no choice but to take insulin hormone replacement therapy.

The combination of insulin resistance and refined, sugar-dense, processed foods will maintain high blood sugar levels that can potentially promote reactive fat and weight gain. There's no way around it: to control weight, all processed, refined foods should be eliminated as much as possible. Again, it's the high fat levels in animal products, processed foods, and oils added during cooking that can block insulin attachment and promote insulin resistance and higher blood sugar levels, even if you're also eating healthy plant carbs or modest amounts of refined sugar. That's why, while it's not intuitive, a high-carbohydrate, high-fiber, low-fat, plant-exclusive diet will lower blood sugar levels significantly. I have seen blood sugar levels drop several hundred points within a week or two on an unprocessed, vegan, WFPE diet without added refined sugar or cooked oils. Carbohydrate-rich whole plant foods (low in fat and high in water and fiber) maintain lower sugar levels and promote the best opportunity for weight loss. As a result, it is unequivocal: the eating plan for diabetics must also focus on unrefined, unprocessed, whole, raw and cooked plant-exclusive foods.

So in the big picture, to avoid or remedy excessive weight gain and type 2 diabetes, you must correct the food and lifestyle factors that interfere with insulin attachment, promote insulin resistance, and provoke increases of blood sugar and insulin release. All the factors discussed in this book, along with the strategies I share for integrating these ideas into your daily life, will help you heal the problem of insulin resistance.

Glycemic Impact Defined

To more fully appreciate the effects of whole vs. processed foods on hormone function, blood sugar balance, and weight/fat gain, a consideration of the glycemic impact of food takes on added significance. When you eat any food that has carbohydrate content, whether it's a piece of fruit, some brown rice, a vegetable, or a candy bar, the basic questions that can always be asked are: How rapidly and how high does this food raise blood sugar?

Historically, these questions have been answered by the concepts of glycemic index and glycemic load. The glycemic index (GI) ranks foods on a scale of 0 to 100, with pure glucose (sugar) ranked 100, and assigns a numeric value to foods based on how rapidly they raise your blood sugar compared to that. Typically, the more processed a food is, the higher its GI and the faster it raises blood sugar. Foods with more fiber or fat content, like whole plant foods, tend to have lower GIs.

However, the glycemic index does not go far enough to truly assess the potential impact that any food has on blood sugar and weight gain. To understand a food's complete effect on blood sugar, it is necessary to know both how quickly it makes glucose enter the bloodstream and how much glucose it actually contains and delivers. To address these concerns, a separate measure called glycemic load was created to provide a more accurate picture of the real-life impact of food on your blood sugar. As an example of glycemic index vs. glycemic load, a serving of watermelon has a high GI (80), but since it contains mostly water with very little carbohydrate (sugar), it has a very low glycemic load of 5.

Even including the glycemic load is not enough to clarify the whole picture, though. There are several basic problems when you try to rigidly use glycemic index as the gold standard for measuring the effects of food on blood sugar. First, all of us have different body-fat percentages, different amounts of lean muscle mass, different metabolic and hormonal efficiencies, and different activity and lifestyle patterns, so that the way any one food affects the blood sugars of different people will vary somewhat, regardless of any standard measurement of glycemic index or load. Second, it has now become quite clear that the way any food affects your blood sugar is not determined by its sugar content alone, but also by its fat content, its fiber content, its water content, its micronutrient content, and how refined or processed it is. Encompassing these variables may seem difficult and confusing. So, to simplify healthy food choices and their effects on blood sugar, I have replaced the conventional concept of glycemic index and load with my own empirical, intuitive concept of glycemic impact (GIm).

There are no charts or lists of GIm, but it generally encompasses and simplifies the data of glycemic index and load and includes the consideration of sugar, fat, water, micronutrient, and fiber content in determining blood sugar effects. High-GIm foods are high in refined sugar and fat, and low in micronutrients, fiber, and water, while low-GIm foods are high in whole-plant carbohydrates (with no refined sugar at all), micronutrients (phytonutrients, vitamins, and minerals), water, and fiber and have some slowly absorbable plant fats. As discussed above, when your diet has a higher saturated-fat content from processed junk food and animal products, insulin function and blood sugar regulation will be compromised, promoting elevated blood sugar, and potentially increasing the GIm of even healthy, whole plant foods.

Therefore, by my definition, high-GIm foods are basically all of the refined, processed foods, while low-GIm foods are all of the whole, unrefined, natural fruits, veggies, whole grains, and legumes. This puts an end to all the absurd arguments that people have had in the past over whether they can eat a mango or a baked potato. Trust me, if you are dealing with a weight problem, it's safe to say that mangos are not your problem. In fact, if you are a starch-lover like I am—and I can't emphasize this enough—potatoes and fresh fruit are ideal for both short- and long-term weight control. Remember: whole plant foods not only have the lowest GIm values; with the exception of nuts, seeds, and avocados, they also have the lowest calorie density, magnifying their role in promoting optimal weight and body fat.

Strategies to Reduce Glycemic Impact and Promote Weight Loss

It is important then to keep in mind that all carbohydrates are not created equal. I bring this up because typically you'll hear many people saying the mantra, "My doctor told me I can't eat carbs; I'm carb-sensitive."

The truth is that you can't live without carbohydrates. Carbs are necessary to control weight effectively, but what you need are low-glycemic-impact carbs—and that means all the fresh fruits and vegetables. Yes, yes, yes, I did say fresh fruit. With the resurgence and brainwashing of high-protein animal diets, you would be amazed at how many people in our culture are freaked out about eating a piece of fruit.

All the self-proclaimed gurus of the high-protein persuasion, and even some people promoting raw, plant-based diets, have absolutely terrified people with unfounded, unscientific rhetoric about the dangers of fruit consumption. In fact, as human primates, we are fruit-eaters by nature. Our closest primate relative, the bonobo, takes most of its diet from fresh fruit, and our similar bodies recognize the inborn wisdom of enjoying them, too. It is no mystery, then, why fresh fruit and leafy greens are foods we gravitate toward eating in their natural state without any thought of or need for preparation or cooking; it's ingrained in us to do so because they simply taste so good to us that way. You don't worry about sautéing the mango or cooking it in any way. On the other hand, you have not evolved to jump in full stride on the back of a zebra and rip out a piece of its rump with your front teeth. And if you want to convince me that you should be eating lots of animal protein for weight loss, I have to see you jumping on the back of that zebra and tearing its rump apart.

So, hear me loud and clear: fruit is ideal for weight loss. As an example, if you had a pineapple as big as your chest, it would be just a few hundred calories, high in fiber, more than 95% water, and loaded with antioxidants and phytonutrients. This is exactly what you want in your low-fat, WFPE diet.

I'm going to give you a guarantee right now. There are very few guarantees in life, and I certainly don't promise many of them. But if you are dealing with a weight problem, I will guarantee you one thing: fruit is not your problem. I have counseled people for more than 45 years, and I have yet to have someone come to me and say, "Doc, I got a weight problem. Can you help me with this apple thing?" Let me ask you a question. Were you drawn to this book to try to understand your weight problem because you're at home bingeing uncontrollably on mangos? I have had people come to me weighing over 300 pounds, eating everything but their cars at home, and they will ask, "Do you think I can have a piece of watermelon?" My reply is, "Have a truckload of it!" It's absurd. We have been so brainwashed to barely question our intake of risky animal and processed foods, but even mention eating watermelon or a baked potato to someone with weight concerns, and they will be appalled by the very suggestion. It is apparent that unless your thinking is dramatically re-educated, you will continue to wallow in failure perpetrated by your own and other people's misconceptions.

Finally, it is true that a great deal of modern conventional fruit has been hybridized by compromising agricultural practices that may have intensified its sugar content and diminished some quality and nutritional value. However, there is now so much organic fresh fruit available, even in conventional supermarkets and at farmers markets in your communities, that you can avail yourself of this remarkable, essential food source without worrying about negative hybridization, irradiation, genetic modification, or pesticide poisoning.

With all that in mind, I'm recommending a strategy that you may find very useful.

30-Day Strategy

In the next 30 days, any time you want anything sweet, make it a piece or two of fresh fruit. That means no cookies, no candy, no cake, no refined sugar of any kind, no honey, and no agave. I'm putting you in sugar rehab for 30 days. We will discuss the addictive process in a later chapter, but this period of time will allow you to break your attachment to refined sugar. Furthermore, if you have compromised your endocrine and nervous systems, especially your pancreas, thyroid, and adrenal glands, with excessive refined-sugar products over a long period of time, even the beneficial sugar of fruits may initially elicit a roller coaster of spikes and crashes in your blood sugar levels. Therefore, eating some celery, cucumber, or romaine lettuce leaves with the fruit or blending the fruit in smoothies with greens such as spinach, kale, collards, and bok choy will promote a more measured absorption and utilization of dietary sugar and a stabilizing effect on your blood sugar levels.

Also, understand that the glycemic impact of foods is somewhat affected by how you prepare them. If you compare a raw carrot with a boiled carrot, the cooked carrot will promote a more rapid elevated sugar response. Why? Cooking breaks down and caramelizes the sugar content of the food, whether a carrot or an apple. The breakdown makes the sugars in it more available more quickly, contributing to an increased glycemic impact. Since fruits and vegetables are made up as chains of simple sugars, the more you overripen, cook, or process them, the more the glycemic impact is increased.

Therefore, I recommend that you eat your fruits and vegetables in as close to the raw state as you can or just lightly steam or sauté them—do not embalm them. You don't want them mushy and limp, sliding off your plate. They should still be somewhat crunchy and crispy, maintaining some color and vitality. When you overcook fruits and vegetables, their colors becomes less vibrant and their nutrient content is compromised. These strategies will provide protection against exaggerated sugar responses as well as protect the integrity of their vitamins, phytonutrients, and antioxidants that can be damaged by excessive cooking and heating.

This also becomes an important issue when we consider the consumption of grains and grain products. Every step of the processing of grains leads to products that are higher in calorie density and can raise blood sugar more dramatically and quickly. If you eat brown rice as it comes directly from the field, it will raise your blood sugar to some moderate degree. If you pulverize the rice into flour, expanding the surface area of the grain, and convert it into bread and pasta, the glycemic effect will be raised. If you puff that grain into a puffed rice cereal or puffed rice cake, its GI will rise even higher.

So here is another important strategic approach. During the next 30 days, whenever you want any grain products, choose a 100% whole grain (e.g., brown rice, quinoa, or millet) and avoid all refined starches such as bread and pasta. If you find yourself having difficulty making a full-month commitment, even two weeks would be beneficial, but 30 days will make a much bigger difference. After the 30-day period, if you want bread or pasta, make it 100% gluten-free and whole-grain. Check the packaging and make sure you read the fine print on the ingredient label; it should say "100% whole grain," no matter what the grain is. The great thing is that there is so much variety available now that you can get breads and pastas made from every imaginable whole grain and legume.

Wheat products have been at the center of some controversy in recent years, as there is some concern that the increased consumption of genetically modified, hybridized wheat in the many wheat products developed and sold over the past 70 years has contributed significantly to the epidemic of obesity. Documented effects of wheat consumption include exaggerated glycemic impact, increased glycation of protein, appetite stimulation, and increased inflammation and joint damage.[7] For some, wheat's high gluten content is the focus. Gluten is found in other foods as well, including other wheat varieties and derivatives, such as rye, barley, triticale, malt, and brewer's yeast. But wheat is the most common gluten-containing food we eat, and its gluten content is particularly high. A moderate percentage of people have an allergic gluten sensitivity, and an even smaller number of people have extreme gluten intolerance. About 1% of people suffer from celiac disease, an inflammatory bowel condition caused by a hypersensitivity to gluten in which even tiny amounts can cause severe damage to the small intestine.

While whole-grain wheat products are not a problem for everyone and the gluten issue may seem overhyped at times, the elimination of wheat products and of gluten has helped a substantial number of people lose a significant amount of weight—as much as 20-50 pounds—in a period of several months. My own clinical anecdotal experience is that specific pockets of weight, i.e., abdominal belly fat and love handles, also can be reduced significantly by the removal of wheat and gluten from the diet. So, with this information in mind, I typically recommend only using low-gluten grains (brown rice, quinoa, buckwheat, and millet) for at least the 30-day rehab period, even if you don't have any major reactions to wheat and gluten. Because of the potential problems with hybridized, genetically modified wheat products in our culture, you may want to consider going a step further by avoiding wheat and gluten-containing products for three to six months to better evaluate the potential impact on your energy, pain, inflammation, and weight loss.

There is also a debate in some nutritional circles about the use of grains in general in the human diet. The suggestion is that human and non-human primates are not grain-eaters by nature, but with the development of milling and cooking, we have been able to make grains and grain products more digestible and available for human consumption. I feel that a moderate use of whole grains, in combination with an abundant diversity of potatoes, legumes, leafy green/cruciferous vegetables, onions, mushrooms, fruit, herbs, and spices, provide remarkable benefits for health and weight regulation. Whole grains are abundant in fiber that feeds the healthy bacteria of the gut which in turn support the health of the colon and the immune system and play a major role in satiety signals, food addiction, and weight control.[ix] Remarkably,

---

[ix] The comprehensive impact of a WFPE diet on the integrity, function, and role of the gut microbiota in appetite regulation will be discussed extensively in Chapter 7.

in a study of 4,125 adults 65 years of age or older, a higher intake of fiber from cereals (whole grains) was associated with a significantly greater decrease in inflammation and inflammatory markers, including C-reactive protein, interleukin-6, and TNF-alpha, and in a lower risk of cardiovascular disease as compared with fiber from fruits and vegetables.[8]

A variety of whole-grain starches diversify a plant-exclusive diet, provide fiber and nutrition that enhances the quality of the diet, and make it more interesting and easier to incorporate into your life. Therefore, I recommend a variety of grains (in only whole-grain form) with as little gluten as possible.

Make certain you choose your whole-grain products carefully and consider the ingredients used in breads and pastas. The ingredients in any grain-based product should basically be just grain and water. If a bread and/or pasta has an ingredient list as big as your hand or if there's even one ingredient that you can't pronounce, don't eat it. I call this digestive phonics—if you can't read it, you can't digest it. Just kidding, of course, but it's more truth than not.

It's also important to be sensitive to the amount of bread you consume. Bread consumption is one of those things that can really get away from you, and it can even provoke your craving for more refined carbohydrates. I'm a bread guy. If you are into bread, you are my kind of people. I was born into an Italian household, and when I came out of the womb, I came out on a full moon on a Saturday night with a piece of bread in one hand and a glass of wine in the other, ready to party. And it hasn't changed much since.

Sprouted-grain, flourless breads work well for satisfying your bread hankerings without triggering carb-craving or negative blood sugar changes. I recommend using quality breads like this as a major starch in and of itself. That means eating bread with salad and vegetables by itself, rather than adding other complex foods to it, like other starches, spreads, meat, or dairy products.

This 30-day strategy of a modest use of only gluten-free whole grains when you want something grainy and only fruit when you want something sweet can account for as much as six to eight pounds of weight loss alone over the next month, without your even thinking about it. After that 30-day sugar-rehab period, many people discover that they lose their sugar craving and their taste for fragmented, refined sugar, and that fruit will quite adequately and consistently satisfy their sugar needs and tastes.

Typically, if you crave sweets, your hormonal system, involving the pancreas, thyroid, and adrenal glands, is probably compromised, and you are probably fruit- and complex-carb deficient. Thus, fruit needs to be a bigger part of your diet. I recommend eating fruit that is in season and grown as close to your home as possible. That way, you're not eating fruit that has been picked when still unripened, stored for long periods of time, and shipped over thousands of miles. As a result, nutritional quality will improve while reducing your personal energy demands and carbon footprint.

While fruit availability is more limited in winter (such as apples, pears, some melons, and citrus), the spring and summer are the seasons to be jolly with all the spring and summer fruits, such as peaches, plums, nectarines, berries, and mangos. I never recommend eating conventional berries in the winter. They are usually imported and subjected to extensive pesticide abuse. Again, as you will see in a subsequent chapter, these chemical toxins can promote reactive weight gain. If you want berries in the winter for smoothies or salad dressings, I recommend frozen organic berries, which are readily available. Look for other frozen organic fruits, too. They are often picked at peak ripeness and flash-frozen immediately after harvesting, thereby offering excellent nutritional profiles.

Remember, your body is an intelligent, self-regulating system that is in constant communication with you. This internal dialogue gives us information and feedback about our basic needs for optimal survival.

This innate power and wisdom resides in each of us, and as you improve your health and sensitivity, you will become more mindful, attentive, and responsive to the healthy directives of your own inner voice, making the shift to constructive food choices more successfully. Purely and simply, the vegan, WFPE, SOS-free diet ensures a glycemic impact that will promote the best blood sugar regulation and the best opportunity for long-term, successful weight loss.

CHAPTER 7

FIBER AND WATER AND SALT, OH MY!

Plant-based foods have the highest fiber and water content of any food you can eat. I like to refer to the water content of fruits and vegetables as "living water." As important as it is to drink adequate amounts of water (approximately 100 ounces daily), the water content and quality provided by whole plant foods makes an essential, significant contribution to your daily hydration requirement.

Water content provides a filling-up effect and therefore contributes to a healthy feeling of satiety, even with low calorie intake. However, when you cook (and especially overcook) plant foods using a dry-heat cooking method (broiling, baking, pan frying, roasting, etc.), one of the first things you lose is water content. For example, if you were to weigh a raw potato, bake it, and then weigh it again, the baked potato would weigh less because of water loss. To ensure the best natural hydration in your foods, I definitely recommend eating your fruits and vegetables as close to the raw state as you can. Even if you can't go completely raw, keeping the diet 60–80% raw is in your best interest.

As I mentioned previously, oxygen is an unstable element whose lack of two core electrons drives its unique chemistry. As a result, oxygen promotes the formation of damaging free radicals by appropriating electrons to serve its needs from the chemical compounds it contacts in the cells and tissues of the body. Yet, we have been exposed to oxygen for eons of time, so why haven't we rusted away like some metal tool in a garage? The answer to this question lies in the basic structure of the water molecule. The classic chemical formula of water, H_2O, indicates that every molecule of water is made up of two atoms of hydrogen for each atom of oxygen; so, when oxygen combines with two hydrogen atoms in a water molecule, each hydrogen atom can share an electron with oxygen, thereby providing the two electrons that oxygen lacks and creating the most stable, least reactive state of oxygen.

Therefore, it is no mystery that both the body and planet Earth have similar high water contents (approximately 70%) that support optimal health and life, and foods that have the highest water content—fruits and vegetables—are the most important components of human nutrition. Adequate water intake is essential for health, efficient metabolism, and long-term weight control. The metabolism and breakdown of fat is a water-demanding process, so dehydration interferes with weight loss and promotes fatigue. Furthermore, the water that you drink and that you consume in food may have beneficial antioxidant effects in itself, reducing pain, inflammation, and disease.

It is often suggested that the daily consumption of 8–10 eight-ounce glasses of water per day is optimal for health and well-being. However, your water needs will be dictated to some degree by the way you eat and the lifestyle you lead. If you're eating a refined diet that has very little water content, then your need for water will be much greater, and you would do well to drink 90–100 ounces per day. If you're eating an abundance of fruits and vegetables loaded with water, your thirst and the need for water will be much less, perhaps only 40–60 ounces per day. Try to be more mindful of your own sense of thirst. Your body will let you know, through your thirst, when you need to drink more.

Since a vegan, WFPE diet has the highest water and fiber content (combined with the lowest calorie density) of any weight-loss approach, no other eating plan will promote profound, healthy weight regulation as well as a consistent WFPE diet of raw and lightly steamed/cooked plant foods. As mentioned previously, since we have one of the longest digestive tracts in nature, eating food that is high in water and fiber content fosters the most efficient transit through the digestive system and is necessary for the healthiest digestive and bowel function. A healthy intestinal tract is critical for the efficient absorption and utilization of nutrients and for effective appetite and weight control.

Fantastic Fiber in Plants

In addition to its deficiency of water, a standard Western diet loaded with refined foods is noticeably deficient in fiber. When the diet is deficient in fiber, a litany of stomach- and intestinal-related problems can occur, including reflux, distention, bloating, diverticulitis, and even cancer.

There are trillions of microorganisms that reside in our intestines, referred to as the gut microbiota (GM). In fact, approximately five pounds of your body weight are from the organisms that live within you. The beneficial microorganisms of the GM play an important role in producing vitamins, specific fatty acids, neurotransmitters, and the protective mucous lining of the large intestine that is part of the innate immune system. The GM thrives best on the fiber provided by plants, so when you eat a variety of plant-exclusive foods, you create the greatest and healthiest diversity of GM.

It has been known for some time that high-fiber nutrition reduces the risk of heart disease because the healthy, diverse gut microbiota supported by the fiber in whole plant foods can metabolize all the cholesterol arriving in the large intestine. The cholesterol is converted by the GM into the non-absorbable sterol coprostanol that is eliminated in the feces. This is the most important mechanism for the removal of cholesterol from the body.[1] In addition, the soluble fiber found in plants

binds directly with both dietary cholesterol and any excess biliary cholesterol (produced normally by the liver) to promote its excretion from
the body, pulling that cholesterol into the stool in the normal course
of metabolism. When fiber is too low, or even absent, cholesterol will
not be eliminated effectively; it will be recycled, staying elevated in
the blood and contributing to potential vascular blockage and heart
disease. That's why for a number of years now, you've seen boxes of
cereal and oatmeal with big hearts on them advertising them to be
heart-healthy fare.

In addition, a healthy GM protects you against inflammation and
ferments fiber to produce small, short-chain fatty acids (SCFAs), including butyrate and propionate. These SCFAs maintain the snug fastening
of cells lining the colon that is needed to block the absorption of large by-
products of digestion and toxic molecules, an essential part of our innate
immune response. Excesses of animal protein, saturated fat, low-fiber
junk food, alcohol, pesticides, antibiotics, and chronic stress promote an
unhealthy transformation of the GM and a decrease of GM diversity
referred to as dysbiosis, which can trigger autoimmune responses and
the development of colon cancer. This can increase pathogenic organisms in the gut, decrease the production of SCFAs, damage and break
down the mucous lining, increase inflammation, and interfere with
protective immune activity. The alteration of the GM and overgrowth
of pathogenic organisms, coupled with damage to the mucous lining,
can also cause a leaky gut and the absorption of toxins that can further
increase inflammation, cause food sensitivities/allergies, and potentially
incite the development of autoimmune disease. This toxicity can even
compromise the protective blood vessel barrier of the brain (blood-brain
barrier), allowing toxins to infiltrate the brain and contribute to anxiety,
depression, cognitive deficits, and even Alzheimer's disease.

Importantly, the high fiber and water content of whole plant foods
also have a major impact on a variety of factors that are critical for
maintaining optimal weight and body fat, including appetite, satiety,

compulsive food use, and addiction.[x] When the stomach is filled with food, pressure is exerted on the walls of the stomach, activating nerve cells that let the brain know that you have had enough to eat. Since plant food is so low in calorie density and high in fiber and water, you experience fullness and satiety with a much lower calorie intake than if you ate animal and processed foods that are deficient in fiber and water, take up less space in the stomach, and are significantly more calorie-dense. As a result, animal and processed foods leave you feeling less satiated and lead to overeating despite your having consumed significantly more calories.

Another function of the SCFAs produced by your GM from the fermentation of plant fiber is the production of peptides that slow down the digestion of carbohydrates in the stomach and small intestine, stimulating cells in the distal part of your small intestine that elicit a sense of fullness and satiety. When your diet is heavy in fiber-deficient animal foods and processed foods, your GM is starved for the fiber it needs; is less diverse; contains more risky, toxic organisms; and makes you more prone to inflammation, craving, and overeating. Consistent with this information, obese people eating standard animal-based, processed-food diets have been shown to have a loss of healthy diversity of the GM, an increase of organisms that promote inflammation, and difficulty controlling appetite and achieving healthy satiety.

Excess reproductive hormones, e.g., estrogen and testosterone, are eliminated from the body by attaching to fiber in the colon. A form of dietary fiber (lignin) found in flax seeds, beans, and lentils binds to estrogen and testosterone in the digestive tract to ensure that these hormones are eliminated from the body. Keep in mind that reproductive hormones stimulate the growth of the body and the maturation of sexual organs during puberty. As you get older and growth is no longer necessary, the body naturally decreases the production of these hormones. If these

---

[x] The role of plant foods and fiber on brain chemistry, pleasure/ brain reward, and food addiction will be discussed in Chapter 22.

hormones are increased later in life by excessive hormone replacement therapies or by an increase in body fat that activates the aforementioned enzyme aromatase, they can contribute to abnormal growth of cysts, tumors, and hormone-related cancers. Therefore, when fiber is lacking, these growth-stimulating hormones can elevate in the bloodstream, significantly increasing the risk of developing cancers of the breast, ovaries, uterus, and prostate.

Finally, the increased fiber content of a plant-exclusive diet can reduce and stabilize elevated blood sugar, reduce body weight and obesity, and lower serum levels of the highly sensitive C-reactive protein that is associated with acute and ongoing inflammation, suggesting that high fiber intake may reduce inflammation.[2]

Via these many processes, it's clear that plant foods containing the highest water and fiber content provide the greatest safeguards against a panorama of health problems, including obesity and weight gain.

No Added Salt

Salt is the most ubiquitous, overused, and abused condiment in the human diet. It is the major additive, along with sugar and oil, used by the processed-food industry to produce hyperpalatable junk food that drives compulsive overeating and food addiction and causes major problems with losing weight and keeping it off.[xi]

Salt is a chemical compound made up of just two elements, sodium and chlorine. While excesses of sodium are the villain of this part of the story, I don't want to give sodium totally bad press, because it also is one of the most crucial, essential minerals of the human body.

Every cell in the human body is like a miniature battery, constantly generating electric current. As a result, we are electromagnetic in nature. That's why you can put electrodes on the surface of the chest and measure the electrical discharge of the heart using an electrocardiogram (ECG)

[xi] The addictive quality of these additives and foods is discussed in-depth in Chapter 22.

and why you can put electrodes on the surface of the skull and measure the electrical discharge of the brain using an electroencephalogram (EEG).

The electrical activity produced by the cells of the body is primarily a function of the movement of just two minerals, sodium and potassium. However, the body holds on to sodium like a miser. There is an interplay of hormones and enzymes (the renin-angiotensin-aldosterone system) orchestrated by the kidneys, liver, lungs, brain, and adrenal glands that promotes the balance of sodium and water to ensure adequate blood pressure in the circulatory system. In this process, sodium is rigorously held onto while potassium is more preferentially eliminated. That's why when people are put on a diuretic medication for high blood pressure, they will sometimes be put on a potassium supplement rather than a sodium supplement in order to replenish the more selective loss of potassium.

One of the reasons that a plant-exclusive diet is ideal for human consumption is that, as a rule, fruits and vegetables are high in potassium and low in sodium. Even higher-sodium-containing plants such as Swiss chard, celery, tomato, and zucchini are still loaded with potassium. In contrast, if you look at a diet full of meat, dairy, and processed, refined foods, this ratio is exactly reversed; the conventional, standard American eating plan is low in potassium but off the charts in sodium. It is very important to realize that even if you don't add salt to your food, if you are eating meat and dairy products, your diet is still too high in sodium, because of the sodium naturally retained within the bodies and fluids of animals. Our modest need for sodium is best obtained from whole, natural, plant foods, and there is never a need to add any salt to your food.

The RDA for sodium in the United States is 1,500–2,300 mg per day (depending on certain conditions of disease), or about a 0.6–1 teaspoon of table salt per day. However, the average intake of sodium for adults in the U.S. can be as high as 3,500 mg per day.[3] Because we are a salt-addicted culture, I feel that the recommended daily intake has been set too high. In my opinion, if you are adding salt to your food or eating sodium-containing canned or packaged food, the total you add should never exceed more than 500–800 mg per day. The few hundred milligrams of sodium coming naturally from your WFPE diet will be more than adequate to meet your needs without contributing risky excess.

So, what's the problem with excessive sodium? Increased sodium can foster a loss of calcium from urine that lowers calcium levels in your blood. Since calcium is critical for the contraction of all muscles (including the heart) and the release of transmitters in the brain, a decrease in blood levels of calcium triggers the removal of calcium from bone to replenish the blood supply, increasing the risk of osteoporosis. In fact, sodium's contribution to the current epidemic of bone loss is one of the more overlooked parts of the osteoporosis story. As a result, salt intake should be carefully monitored for the effective management of this problem.

Excess sodium also can trigger the retention of many times its weight in water, so routine excesses of sodium often cause tremendous fluid retention and water-weight gain. Every pint of water you retain adds one pound of body weight. Therefore, low-sodium nutrition is essential for any long-term weight-loss program. This is just one more reason why diets high in animal foods that naturally contain high sodium are a debilitating obstruction to successful weight loss. In addition, the increase of fluid volume caused by excess salt intake is a major contributing factor for high blood pressure, and increased blood pressure is significantly correlated with coronary heart disease, kidney disease, and stroke.[4]

The routine use of excessive salt can also damage the gel-like protective lining (glycocalyx) of the inner endothelial walls of blood vessels. The glycocalyx promotes the conversion of the amino acid L-arginine into nitric oxide in the endothelial cells of blood vessels that dilates blood vessels to increase blood flow to the heart and other vital organs. Salt damage to the glycocalyx and endoothelial cells can compromise nitric oxide production leading to constriction, damage and inflammation of blood vessels, that may restrict blood flow to vital organs as well as promote vascular bleeding and clotting episodes throughout the body. Excess salt can also irritate and stimulate the immune system to increase inflammation throughout the body.

Furthermore, you have taste buds in your mouth that are attached to nerves that inform the brain about the various taste sensations provided by the food you eat (saltiness, sweetness, bitterness, sourness, and savoriness). These taste buds have a threshold of stimulation that must be exceeded by the various taste chemicals before the taste bud can be activated to communicate with your brain. The more salt you use, the more the taste bud will become desensitized over time and require more stimulation before it responds. Think of someone you may know who has a salt shaker going even before they taste their food because they already know that it will probably be tasteless to them. The problem is not that the food is tasteless, it's that the person's habit of oversalting has resulted in their needing much more additional salt stimulation before they can taste anything. The good news is that when you stop adding salt to your food and reduce your dependency on it, you will improve the sensitivity of your taste buds to whole, natural, plant foods, promote a healthy balance in your brain's pleasure system, decrease your craving for processed food, and achieve a healthier level of satiety and quantity of food intake. The WFPE diet provides all the sodium that you need.

PART

2

SPECIAL CONSIDERATIONS, CONCERNS, AND CONSEQUENCES

CHAPTER 8

LIMITED SUPPLEMENTATION, NOT SUBSTITUTION

With very few exceptions, I recommend obtaining the body's nutritional needs with whole, natural, plant-exclusive foods, not supplementation. As I have discussed, harmful excesses of animal and processed foods and deficiencies of the myriad micronutrients found in plants contribute to the most devastating diseases that demand the most healthcare dollars, i.e., cancer, heart disease, stroke, diabetes, and obesity. You cannot solve a problem of excess with supplementation. There's only one way to solve a problem of excess, and that is to reduce it.

When scientists first examined a piece of fruit or a leaf of lettuce, they discovered nutrients that are now well-known, e.g., vitamins, minerals, and other phytonutrients. However, as these foods have been more closely examined over time, an even greater variety of previously unknown nutrients and cofactors have also been discovered. This suggests that whole foods potentially contain an array of important, as-yet-undiscovered factors that will continue to be revealed over time in addition to the myriad of nutrients of which we are currently aware. It is often discovered that newly discovered nutrients are as important, if not more so, than the ones that were known. This suggests, as discussed by

Dr. T. Colin Campbell in his book, *Whole: Rethinking the Science of Nutrition*, that whole foods contain thousands of nutrients that impact thousands of reactions in the body, and calculating the specific influence of individual chemicals and nutrients is not sufficient to explain the effect of any food as a whole.[1]

When you eat the bounty that nature provides, you are eating both the known and unknown micronutrients they provide in combinations and synergies that support their optimal absorption and utilization and are most essential for life and health. Supplements, however, cannot contain the crucial unknown elements contained in whole foods because we don't know what they are yet. Therefore, supplements by their very nature are deficient.

Be very clear: even at its best, supplementation can never be a substitute for a compromised diet. Too many people are spending too much of their food dollar on supplements and not enough on the whole foods that can truly improve the quality of their nutrition. As a result, fragmented nutrition has often replaced the natural, unparalleled integrity of whole-food nutrition. Supplements can create a dangerous false sense of security.

Nutrition is a symphony, an orchestration of known and unknown nutrients directed by the intelligence and wisdom of a body that absorbs, integrates, and transforms them into the substance and expression of creative life. Eating isolated, fragmented nutrients, as many people do, is like trying to appreciate the full brilliance of a Mozart symphony by listening to just the string section. You would get the basic idea, but you would never fully appreciate the splendor of the complete composition. I want you to experience the amazing magnificence of whole-food nutrition.

An argument is often made that because of the compromise of our commercial soils, and even the debilitating hybridization and genetic modification of a variety of plant foods, some form of supplementation is essential. To a certain extent, some of these concerns are warranted, but by eating a diversity of plant foods in an organic form, grown in a variety of different organically nurtured soils, you can eliminate most of these concerns. However, even in a diverse, vegan, WFPE diet, there are a few areas of supplementation that should be considered.

Vitamin B12

Vitamin B12 is essential for the normal maturation of red blood cells and the development and function of the spinal cord, specifically the part that processes sensory information. When B12 is deficient, blood cells are incapable of effectively carrying oxygen, potentially leading to a form of anemia called pernicious anemia. Vitamin B12 is a by-product of bacterial metabolism, so it can be produced by bacteria living naturally in your mouth and certainly on the surface of organic produce that has not been sprayed with pesticides. It is found in greatest concentrations in animal products, however, since these foods are derived from bodies and fluids of animals loaded with bacterial contamination. As a result, vegans can have vitamin B12 levels that are lower than those of meat- and dairy-eaters, but understand that the defined "normal" for vitamin B12 levels on typical blood tests was established in a more typical, meat-eating population. So, the "normal" ranges on blood tests may be typical, but not necessarily accurate for everyone. Therefore, the lower levels seen in vegans may not be unusual for them.

To most accurately assess vitamin B12 levels to determine if there is a problem, I recommend that all vegans have both their B12 and MMA levels checked. MMA (methylmalonic acid) is a chemical in the body that reacts with vitamin B12 to produce a coenzyme (CoA), which is essential for normal cellular function and energy production. MMA is elevated in the urine or blood of more than 90% of people with true B12 deficiency. If your B12 level is lower than normal on a typical blood test and your MMA level is normal or low, it is not likely that you have a true B12 deficiency. However, if your B12 level is low and your MMA level is high, it is likely that you have a true B12 deficiency. Under these circumstances, I recommend 500–1000 micrograms of the cyanocobalamin or methylcobalamin form of B12, taken as sublingual tablets or liquid sprays, three to four times per week.

Vitamin D

Vitamin D levels are linked with bone health, hormonal regulation, and the health of a wide variety of body systems. When sunlight reacts with cholesterol in your skin, it produces vitamin D3 that is transported to your liver and converted into 25-hydroxy vitamin D before it is processed into its final form in the kidney. There is a suggestion that vitamin D deficiency is associated with obesity, but it is not clear whether low levels cause obesity or if a low level is the result of obesity. Interestingly, when the level of 25-hydroxycholecalciferol (the precursor form of vitamin D most commonly used to measure vitamin D levels in the blood) was higher prior to subjects following a calorie-restricted diet over a three-month period, there was a significant increase in the loss of weight and belly fat in adult men and women.[2]

Typically, 10–15 minutes of soft sun exposure (early morning or late afternoon) three to four times per week on as much of the body surface as you can expose should be adequate to meet your vitamin D needs. However, I have had patients in South Florida come to me so tanned and sun-exposed that their skin looked like weathered luggage, and they were vitamin D deficient on typical blood tests. Since vitamin D is fat-soluble, an increase in weight and body fat may sequester it, thereby increasing your vitamin D requirement. People with darker skin color may also require additional vitamin D. Consequently, I recommend measuring vitamin D levels on everyone. Typically, 30–100 nanograms (ng)/milliliter (ml) is considered normal. I like to see the blood levels closer to mid-range (40–50 ng/ml). There are some who feel that 20 ng/ml or greater may still be normal, but many doctors typically supplement people with levels less than 30. For me, sun exposure is the first approach, but if this is not working to maintain normal levels, I recommend supplementing 1,000–2,000 IU of vitamin D3 per day for a period of three months and then doing a follow-up test.

Iodine

Iodine is a mineral that plays a major role in a variety of important body systems and functions, including the growth of the skeletal and central nervous systems in the developing fetus, infants, and children as well as the production of thyroid hormones throughout life. Unfortunately, insufficient iodine intake is a global problem affecting two billion people worldwide, particularly people in South Asia and parts of Africa, with mild iodine deficiency affecting 50% of Europe and declining levels becoming more apparent in the U.S. in recent years. Iodine deficiency interferes with the healthy growth and development of children, promotes an increase in infant mortality, and fosters a decline in thyroid function in people of all ages that can significantly increase weight gain and obesity.[3]

The pituitary hormone called thyroid-stimulating hormone (TSH) increases the entry of iodine into the thyroid gland. There it is combined with thyroglobulin, containing the amino acid tyrosine, to produce the thyroid hormones T3 and T4. Thyroid hormones play a major role in energy metabolism; some of the symptoms of low thyroid function are uncontrollable weight gain, hair thinning, and fatigue. Adequate iodine intake is critical for overall energy production and weight regulation. The RDA recommended by the Food and Nutrition Board of the U.S. is 150 micrograms per day for children and adults, with 220 and 290 micrograms per day for pregnant and lactating women, respectively.

The content of iodine in the food supply is quite variable, depending on the iodine content of different soil conditions and locations. Typically, plant foods are too low in iodine to meet the RDAs, with the exception of sea vegetation (seaweed), which extracts iodine from sea water. Iodine can be obtained from small amounts of iodized salt, but since I am advocating a whole plant diet without added salt, this is not an option. Keep in mind that unless the salt container states that it is iodized, commercial salt, sea salt, and Himalayan salt do not contain iodine.

While eating some seaweed can satisfy your daily need for iodine, the iodine content in seaweed, especially kelp and wakame, is too high and can promote health problems associated with excessive iodine consumption. The seaweed hijiki should also be avoided because of its high arsenic content. Instead, the best seaweed options to satisfy your daily need for iodine are ⅛ to ¼ teaspoon of dried dulse flakes or one teaspoon of vegan, fish-free nori. These options will provide the 150 micrograms of iodine you need and can be sprinkled on salads, used in cooked dishes, or consumed in dishes like veggie sushi. A liquid mineral supplement containing 150 micrograms of iodine can also be used to provide the daily iodine requirement.

Omega-3 Fatty Acids

There has been some confusion and controversy about the sources and requirement for supplementation of the essential omega-3 polyunsaturated fatty acids (EFAs). Various health organizations recommend an omega-3 alpha-linolenic acid (ALA) intake of 1.1 and 1.6 grams a day, respectively, for adult women and men, which is easily provided by a diverse plant-exclusive diet that includes ground flaxseed, chia seeds, and walnuts. A tablespoon of ground flaxseed contains more than 2 grams of ALA while an ounce of walnuts (about seven walnuts) provides 2.5 grams of ALA, significantly exceeding your daily need. Even a variety of deep greens and cruciferous vegetables provides a modest amount of ALA (e.g., half a cup of cooked Brussels sprouts contains about 135 mg of ALA, about 12% of your daily requirement). Therefore, plant foods can provide adequate and high-quality sources of ALA.

As discussed previously, ALA is converted by specific enzymes into additional members of the omega-3 family, EPA (eicosapentaenoic acid) and DHA (docosahexaenoic acid), that have widespread impact on health. It is commonly believed, though, that less than 1% of dietary ALA is converted to EPA and DHA, which is found primarily in seaweeds and fish that eat seaweeds. As a result, there is concern that deficiencies may occur in vegans eating limited amounts of sea vegetation, and an additional minimal supplemental intake for vegans—250–500 mg per day of combined EPA and DHA in algal oil form—is often recommended by many physicians and nutritionists. But this may be questionable and unwarranted. Extensive research has shown that while the dietary intake of preformed DHA and EPA is significantly less in vegans compared with people eating meat and fish, the average blood levels of these essential fatty acids were significantly higher in vegans compared with fish-eaters, and the conversion process from ALA to EPA and DHA and the converting enzymes are significantly more effective and efficient in vegans than in people eating fish.[4]

The production of these critical EFAs is affected by the process of end-product inhibition, which is common to all chemical reactions and pathways in the body. End-product inhibition is when the final product of any chemical reaction or pathway acts to inhibit the reactions and enzymes that create that product. To explain this another way, if your body makes a chemical or hormone naturally and you add that chemical or hormone into the body from the outside, your body will stop making its own. For example, if someone gets diagnosed with a low-functioning thyroid and then takes prescription thyroid hormones, the body will stop the natural production of its own thyroid hormones, ensuring a dependency on the medication for life. If you consistently take preformed EPA and DHA, this will signal the body to interfere with its conversion process and stop making its own. That's why it is more advantageous to consume adequate ALA in plant foods as a precursor for making your own EPA and DHA, which will more effectively support enzyme efficiency and your natural process of production.

Furthermore, since the conversion pathway is a one-way pathway from ALA to DHA, supplementing with preformed DHA does *not* provide essential ALA and EPA, and you can still develop deficiencies of ALA and other omega-3 family members derived from ALA that promote their own significant health benefits. ALA and its direct derivatives in the omega-3 pathway, stearidonic acid and ETA, promote an increase in the volume of grey matter in the frontal parietal cortex of the brain and an enhanced fluid intelligence. Decline of fluid intelligence is one of the most debilitating aspects of cognitive decline with aging.[5]

There is no doubt that adequate DHA and EPA are required for normal brain function throughout life. DHA makes up 60% of all polyunsaturated fatty acids in nerve cell membranes and is essential for neurotransmission and synaptic plasticity in the brain. Along with EPA, the decline of these fatty acids is clearly associated with the pathology of Alzheimer's disease, including inflammation, oxidative stress, and the development of beta-amyloid plaques. Alzheimer's patients have significantly decreased levels of DHA compared with age-matched controls.[6,7]

Unfortunately, since fish contain preformed EPA and DHA, fish and fish oil have gotten much positive airplay as a desirable source of food and supplementation. This is a devastating development, and I never recommend consuming either fish or supplementation derived from fish. The fishing industry has catastrophic effects on the environment and sea creatures. Trillions of fish are killed yearly while countless other creatures are caught in the bykill of this wanton, industrial slaughter and the oxygen-producing algae, flora, and coral beds are decimated. This, along with the appalling amount of plastic pollution being produced worldwide from the commercial fishing industry, is contributing to the destruction of the ocean ecosystem. In addition, as a result of the devastating environmental changes affecting our oceans and water supply, there can be remarkably dangerous levels of mercury contamination in fish. Symptoms of mercury contamination are similar to the symptoms of low thyroid, chronic fatigue, and fibromyalgia. If you have the symptoms of any of these problems and you've been eating a lot of fish, I recommend that you test your urine and/or blood or hair for mercury contamination. Heavy metal toxicity can seriously compromise the integrity of the endocrine and nervous systems and compromise your ability to control your weight.

Consider, too, how much commercially sold fish comes from fish farms that are more brutal than many animal factories. The goal of these fish farms is to grow fish big enough and fast enough to maximize commercial profit. This process often compromises nutritional value and decreases the availability of omega-3 oils in these creatures. Also, to make sure that the farm-raised salmon, for example, have that nice orangey-pink color found in the wild, they are given feed that dyes them that color and contains PCBs (polychlorinated biphenyls), the same stuff that shows up in the feathery insulation in the attics of our homes.[xii] Similar to land animals maintained in factory farms, these fish are also fed large amounts of antibiotics to counter the potential infections present in fish farms' abnormal, crowded conditions while also promoting rapid growth and weight gain to boost commercial profits. These antibiotics foster dysbiosis and weight gain in human consumers. All of these factors underline the importance or realizing that for issues of health, weight control, and compassion, there is no reason at any time to eat fish for your nutrition or omega-3 needs.

There also is some concern that the ALA-converting enzymes can be either less effective with age or even lacking in certain individuals, potentially leading to a deficiency of DHA in those who do not supplement. This has led to some suggestions that, since true vegans are not eating fish, they may be at greater risk for developing a potential deficiency of DHA with age. Under these conditions, which ultimately would be

---

[xii] We will discuss at great length in Chapter 20 how industrial toxins like PCBs feed the epidemic of weight gain and interfere with your individual weight-loss program.

determined by genetic analysis, vegans would be advised to eat sea vegetation and/or take an algal-oil-based supplemental form of DHA.

To measure EPA and DHA more effectively, an easily accessible, finger-prick home blood test to check the omega-3 index was developed to calculate the total amount of EPA and DHA as a percentage of all the fatty acids contained and transported in the membranes of red blood cells.[8] In early studies, an index of 8% or greater was associated with the lowest risk of heart disease while an index less than 4% was associated with the greatest risk. The KORA-Age study evaluated people in the age range of 68–92 and established that an omega index less than 5.7% and greater than 6.8% was associated with the highest and lowest cognitive impairment, respectively.[9] Just keep in mind that this test measures circulating blood levels of EFAs and may not be a true indicator of what actually exists within body organs and tissues. Even though it is widely accepted that a small percentage of ALA is converted into EPA and DHA, there are data suggesting that DHA can be concentrated and synthesized in liver and fat cells over long periods of time and released on demand to satisfy body and brain needs, eliminating concerns about inadequate conversion.

If you are concerned about a potential deficiency, taking algae-derived supplements of DHA is an option. But the better option is to eat whole plant foods with high ALA content and/or take a supplement with higher doses of DHA precursors including ALA, stearidonic acid, and EPA. Always keep in mind that for the most part, a whole-food, plant-exclusive diet with added walnuts, seeds, greens, legumes, and whole grains will provide an amount of ALA that will allow you to produce all the EPA and DHA you need.

CHAPTER 9

FADS, FIXES, AND MAGIC BULLETS: THE DANGERS OF PALEO AND KETO DIETS, SURGERY, AND OFF-LABEL DRUGS

Addressing the full constellation of nutrition and lifestyle factors involved in fat and weight gain is the true path to both short- and long-term success. Unfortunately, we live in a culture of internet hucksters, influencers, and so-called "experts" with very little evidence on which to base their claims, coercing you to sidestep the true causes of your problems and crave their questionable quick fixes and short-cuts. These approaches feed failure, hopelessness, and disease that can distract and deter you from healthy, consistent success and may dangerously mortgage your health future. They center around fad diets, surgical procedures, and drugs that are currently having their heyday of popularity, while promoting myths and choices that are putting you and the entire world at risk.

Diet Fads and Myths: The Paleo Diet

Proponents of the Paleo diet point out that we have bodies genetically tied to the Stone Age while living in a fast-food world. They suggest that, therefore, modern humans should be eating the way that hunter-gatherers ate during the Paleolithic era, which extended from about 2.5 million years ago to the start of the agricultural revolution about 10,000 years ago. This has led to the promotion of a Paleo diet that advocates getting more than half of all your calories from meat (mostly lean meat and fish) and the elimination of dairy products, beans, and cereal grains that were introduced into our modern diets after the advent of cooking and agriculture.

While the Paleo approach may be appealing to many people who are still grossly misinformed, mistakenly carbohydrate-phobic, or lost in high-animal-protein diets, and while it may seem to be the best approach for long-term weight loss, it is based on misconceptions and shortsighted interpretations of the best available information. It is important to realize that we are not just limited to fossil records to try to understand the eating and living habits of hunter-gatherer tribes from the Paleolithic period. There are still a number of nomadic hunter-gatherer tribes scattered on Earth today with short ties to the distant past who provide a modern context for exploration of ancient eating habits. These include the Tsimané in the Bolivian rainforest, the Hadza of Tanzania, the Yanomami Indians of the Amazon, the Kung tribe in Africa, the Bajau of Malaysia, the Kyrgyz in the mountains of Afghanistan, and the Inuit of Greenland.[1]

Promoters of the Paleo diet, which contains close to 50% protein, have tried to make the case that we have evolved as carnivorous creatures that relied on the flesh and blood of animals for our health and the evolution of the human brain. In fact, there are data that clearly challenge these assumptions. The observations of indigenous cultures suggest that today, and probably even more dramatically in the past, hunter-gatherers typically have very little success as hunters with the primitive weapons at their disposal, and unless they are a tribe of people who live in an environment where plants just don't grow effectively, such as the Inuit of Greenland, they often rely on plants for the bulk of their diets. The Hadza get close to 70% of their calories from plants, and other hunter-gatherers incorporate a substantial amount of tubers, yams, and wild nuts into their diets. Furthermore, there is a strong suggestion that when cooking became part of the human lifestyle approximately 500,000 to 1,000,000 years ago, the increased availability of nutrients and energy from cooked food fostered the development of bigger, better functioning brains in early humans even more than did hunting and eating meat.

While early humans may have eaten some meat, the evidence suggests that when plant foods were available, they lived primarily on plant foods. Paleobiologist Amanda Henry found starch granules from plants on fossil teeth and stone tools, suggesting that humans have been eating grains and tubers a lot longer than previously thought and certainly long enough to tolerate and digest them effectively. In fact, the extremely variable environmental conditions and genetic diversity of the different hunter-gatherer groups suggest that there is a huge variation in the types of food that humans have consumed and thrived on in the past and continue to utilize today. Therefore, there is no one Paleo diet. On the contrary, being human does not rely on our consumption of meat but on our ability to adapt to many different habitats and to promote our survival with a variety of potentially healthy food options.

Although the Paleo diet correctly recommends the elimination of processed food, it also erroneously recommends the elimination of whole grains and legumes, which enhance the quality of a healthy plant-exclusive diet. The heavy focus on meat in the Paleo diet clearly does not replicate the diversity of foods that our ancestors ate; worse, it creates an environment favorable to the development of a variety of disease-promoting factors. Aside from the high saturated fat, oxidized cholesterol, heme iron, trimethylamine N-oxide (TMAO), and inflammatory prostaglandins provided by meat, research has shown that the human immune system attacks a sugar in red meat called N-Glycolylneuraminic acid (Neu5Gc), causing inflammation that can eventually cause cancer.

And as revealed in our previous discussion of protein, high-animal-protein diets promote dehydration and electrolyte imbalances, chronic ketosis/inflammation, increased liver production of urea, strain on the kidneys, increased oxidized LDL cholesterol, increased formation of atherosclerotic plaques and heart disease, increased migraine headache risk, dysbiosis of gut flora, chronic constipation, and debilitating, reactive weight gain.

There is no reason or need to consume animal products and processed junk food. The increased consumption of these foods is the foundation for today's pandemics of obesity, heart disease, diabetes, and cancer, and it takes the greatest toll on animal life, land, and water resources. This is also consistent with the observation that when healthy indigenous cultures adopt the excesses of our modern diets, they develop all the same chronic diseases affecting modern civilization.

No one needs another diet that masquerades as truth behind the veneer of questionable science while planting the seeds for more disability and disease. No one should condone or participate in any diet that promotes the disgusting, wanton abuse and killing of other creatures and the devastation of our planet with the absurd argument that it is necessary for weight loss. There is no sane justification for animal product consumption, ever. It is an approach that is untenable and unsupported scientifically, morally, and ethically. Rather than getting lost in one more questionable diet plan, your focus should be on eliminating all animal products and refined processed food from your diet and instead eating a diverse low fat, WFPE, SOS-free diet instead.

In direct contrast to the Paleo diet, an unprocessed WFPE diet gives you the greatest nutrient and energy availability for the smallest number of calories with only positive health consequences, and it does so while respecting the planet and its other sentient beings. For these reasons, it is the ideal eating plan for health and long-term weight regulation, especially when combined with regular physical activity and other crucial lifestyle factors.

Diet Fads and Myths: The Keto Diet

The ketogenic diet is another fad diet that emphasizes processed and cooked animal foods while excluding or limiting a variety of carbohydrate-rich plant foods and refined processed sugar in all forms. It differs from the Paleo approach by typically advocating as much as 70–80% high-fat foods (butter, cheese, milk, bottled oils, avocados, and nuts), 10–25% protein (meat, eggs, fish, and bacon), and only 5–10% carbohydrate foods (specifically low-glycemic vegetables). Its strict limitations on carbohydrate foods requires the exclusion of virtually all refined sugar products and sweeteners.

Because of the extreme constraints the keto diet places on carbohydrate-rich plant foods like fruits, vegetables, whole grains, and legumes, the body has to rely on nutritional and body fat as its energy source. As we mentioned previously, when fat is metabolized for energy, ketones are generated by the liver, creating the physiological condition of ketosis, which provides fuel for the body. The restriction of carbohydrates and the increase in ketones causes a decrease in the hunger/appetite-stimulating hormones insulin and ghrelin, which reduces cravings, and an increased access of body fat for fuel. Since excess protein can be converted into glucose and interfere with ketosis, the amount of protein is also restricted on this plan.

While this approach may trigger some rapid initial fat and weight loss, it promotes a variety of potential health risks over time.

- One of the primary ketones is acetone, commonly found in nail polish remover, so bad acetone breath can result.
- A set of symptoms referred to as "keto flu" often occur early on. These symptoms include body aches, muscle cramps, fatigue, diarrhea or constipation, general weakness, and skin rashes, which are all associated with dehydration related to the loss of water and crucial electrolytes. The restriction of plant foods causes deficiencies of dietary water and potassium content.

- Restriction of plant foods also potentially can lead to deficiencies of crucial micronutrients—vitamins, minerals, antioxidants, and phytonutrients—found in a variety of carbohydrate-rich plant foods.

- Since fat is the most calorie-dense nutrient, you can easily consume too many calories on this high-fat diet, urging the body to use that dietary fat for its energy rather than body fat and interfering with weight loss.

- A high-fat, animal-based diet that is low in fiber can cause a loss of diversity of the gut microbiota, promoting damage to and alteration of the healthy probiotic environment of the colon, resulting in dysbiosis and inflammation.

- The diet's significant amounts of saturated and trans fats can promote insulin resistance and an excessive release of insulin (hyperinsulinemia), resulting in long-term problems with blood sugar, increasing chronic inflammation, and potential fat and weight gain.

- This diet also can lead to long-term losses in muscle mass and energy, decreased performance, and reduced overall metabolic efficiency.

In short, the overall risks of the keto diet far outweigh any short-term benefits. There is no substitute for the low-calorie, high-nutrient-dense, WFPE, SOS-free eating plan for both short- and long-term weight-loss success.

Surgical Fixes

For decades, bariatric surgeries for weight loss have been offered as a bastion of hope for people suffering with chronic morbid obesity who have often failed on an endless array of diets and calorie-restriction programs. A 10-year study of surgical trends discovered that these procedures have increased significantly, with gastric sleeve surgery (in which 80% of the stomach is surgically removed and the remainder sewn into a small, slender, banana-shaped tube) showing the most significant increases.[2] Gastric bypass and gastric band surgeries are the other common bariatric procedures.

In gastric bypass surgery, also called Roux-en-Y gastric bypass, a small stomach pouch is created and attached directly to the small intestine, bypassing the remaining part of the stomach and part of the small intestine, and the normal architecture of the gastrointestinal tract is rerouted to accommodate the newly formed pouch. Gastric band surgery creates a small stomach pouch by placing an inflatable band around a portion of the stomach that can be adjusted to alter the size of the pouch and the size of the opening between the pouch and the rest of the stomach. The goal of these procedures is to reduce the size of the stomach so that it can hold just a few ounces of food, forcing you to eat less.

Keep in mind that these surgical procedures have all the risks associated with surgery, including potential problems with general anesthesia, blood loss, blood clots in your legs and lungs, infection, and possible postoperative complications that include bowel obstruction, the formation of gallstones, "dumping syndrome" (associated with nausea, vomiting, and relentless diarrhea), gastroesophageal reflux (GERD), stomach perforation, and ulcers. Yet, for the morbidly obese person who loses significant weight from these procedures, the advantages can also be substantial, including decreased risks of high blood pressure, stroke, sleep apnea, fatty liver disease, hip and knee inflammation, and pain, and of type 2 diabetes and its complications.

In comparison, the food and lifestyle program recommended in this book will prevent and reverse these conditions even more effectively without the abuse, mutilation, and potential complications of surgery. One of the profound things about the WFPE program I recommend is that it is not about eating less, it is about eating well. When the entire eating plan is focused on foods with the lowest calorie density, lowest glycemic impact, and the highest fiber, water, and nutrient density, you can eat volumes of food; your appetite and satiety will be naturally controlled, and you'll achieve and maintain an optimal weight without surgically mutilating and rerouting your magnificent gastrointestinal tract and digestive system.

The sad commentary is that around 25–30% of people who take weight off with surgical procedures tend to put it all back on within the next decade unless they follow up with a more rigorous lifestyle approach that is more consistent with the program I am proposing. It therefore makes the most sense to embrace the information and approach emphasized in this book as soon as possible, no matter what your starting weight may be, to ensure both short-term and long-term success.

Magic Bullets and Drug Abuse

The hope for quick-fix pills, potions, and drugs for weight loss is a glaring example of the seemingly endless cultural and medical search for the elusive holy grail solution that can rescue a hopeless world suffering the consequences of excessive fat and weight gain. Well, at least for the moment, some think this search has ended. A magic bullet has supposedly been discovered in the arsenal of drugs used to treat type 2 diabetes, and it's being touted and endorsed for melting away excess weight by physicians, influencers, and the image-conscious world of celebrity. That magic bullet is the drug semaglutide.

I have previously described the important role of insulin in blood sugar control and weight gain. To understand the impact of the new drug approach, we need to revisit and expand our understanding of the world of digestive hormones involved in the regulation of blood sugar and food use. When we eat, hormones called incretins are released by your digestive tract that cause the pancreas to release insulin, block your liver from releasing sugar that it has stored as a reserve, and slow down how fast food leaves your stomach. This increases the entry and storage of glucose in your muscles and helps you feel full longer.

Semaglutide, marketed as Ozempic and Wegovy, mimics the incretin glucagon-like peptide 1 (GLP-1) produced by the body. The drug is used to treat type 2 diabetes because of its impact on insulin release and blood sugar control. However, because Ozempic can help you feel less hungry and full for longer so that you eat less, it is now being prescribed off-label as a weight-management drug—even though it is not approved by the FDA for weight loss. The higher-dose form of semaglutide, Wegovy, is intended for long-term use and has been approved for chronic weight management in more morbid obesity. So even with a high out-of-pocket cost of almost $1,000 per month, catchy ads on many social media platforms and Ozempic Facebook groups have influenced massive numbers of regular folks as well as celebrities to jump on the Ozempic bandwagon.

Unfortunately, like all drugs, there is a litany of potential adverse effects that people may choose to overlook in their giddiness about rapid, initial weight loss. Semaglutide is usually given as an injectable drug in weekly doses, with the dose increasing over time to ensure more effective weight loss. As the dose gets higher, a significant number of people experience very disturbing nausea, diarrhea, and vomiting. To deal with some of this, you are recommended to eat smaller meals, avoid high-fat foods, and remain upright after eating. Commonly, there can be fatigue and stomach pain and, in a small number of cases, severe stomach pain indicative of life-threatening pancreatitis. In addition, gallstones and kidney disease may develop in a small number of cases. Another common occurrence is the development referred to as "Ozempic face" in which there is a rapid and extensive loss of facial fat leading to loose, wrinkled skin. An article in *New York Magazine* described women on this drug experiencing overwhelming fatigue, relentless projectile-type vomiting that one woman called "power puking," and heart rate spikes so strong as to disturb sleep.[3] Semaglutide's weight-loss results plateau as the patient's body adapts to the drug, topping out at around 16% of the original body weight. And to top it off, when people stop taking this drug, there is almost an immediate gain of all the weight that was lost.

The recommendation for people taking this drug is that it should be paired with a healthy diet and exercise. My contention is that if you follow the healthy, supportive diet and exercise recommendations and other important lifestyle factors I am sharing with you, there is no reason to take questionable drugs with potentially dangerous adverse effects to achieve some transient, short-lived weight loss. I completely understand the frustration, helplessness, and hopelessness that can follow repeated rounds of failed diets. But there are no magic-bullet drugs or pills without even more frustrating, dangerous consequences. The real magic and hope are in the WFPE, SOS-free eating plan in combination with the constellation of supportive lifestyle factors that I will continue to explain, because nothing can equal this approach for promoting both the healthiest, rapid, significant, short-term health gains with stable long-term results.

CHAPTER 10

WATER-ONLY FASTING: DETOXIFICATION AND WEIGHT LOSS

As I have discussed in previous chapters, lifestyle choices and behaviors that promote decreased inflammation, decreased oxidative stress, and detoxification of the body can provide major support for a successful weight-loss program. Therefore, to improve your chance for effective weight control over time, it may be important to consider implementing one of the most misunderstood but profound approaches in health care: water-only fasting.

The word fasting comes from the old English word, faestan, which means to be strict, to have discipline. By definition, fasting means the abstinence from all food and liquids, except water, for some extended period of time. Now, I can appreciate that in our culture of gluttony and overeating, including my roots in a food-centered Italian family, the idea of voluntarily abstaining from food may seem like a mind-blowing idea teetering on the brink of absurdity. Yet, there is an extensive body of evidence compiled over many decades, including lab studies in a wide variety of species and clinical observations in humans, supporting the use of water-only fasting for a wide range of health problems, including obesity. These data are consistent with the idea that throughout evolution, all life forms, from bacteria to humans, have experienced periods of starvation and food deprivation alternating with periods of abundant food availability. As a result, we have evolved the ability to adapt to long periods without food.[1]

Over the past 46 years, I have personally supervised the fasts of thousands of people for a wide range of health concerns. I also have been part of an association of hygienic physicians who have supervised more than 50,000 fasts over the past 50 years. I was extremely fortunate and grateful to do an apprenticeship at the fasting institute of Dr. David Scott back in the 1970s. Dr. Scott was a pioneer in the monitoring of blood chemistries in the fasting state. His knowledge and experience were an inspiration, a major influence, and the foundation of my own studies and clinical fasting practice.

In addition to the clinical fasting experience with humans, nature presents us with some remarkable examples of fasting in a variety of other species. As part of their reproductive cycle, salmon swim upstream, battling the force of relentless currents to make their way to their original spawning grounds and complete the dance of reproduction. All of that tremendous activity and output of energy is done in the fasting state.

There is a time when large seal bulls migrate to islands in the northern waters to mate and ensure the propagation of their species. During this time, the large male seals have a harem of females with whom they must copulate as many as a dozen times or more each to ensure fertilization. Now it's not all fun and games in the northern waters. These dominant males have to defend their harems and territory from the challenges of all the young bulls in the neighborhood. All this mating and fighting goes on over a period of several months, during which time these seal bulls can lose almost half their body weight—and it is all done in the fasting state. Afterwards, these bulls move to some nearby islands for an unlimited salmon buffet to put their weight back on.[2]

Apart from these unique experiences of the fasting state, the loss of appetite and fasting are natural to all animals, including humans, in response to disease and stress. If you observe animals in the wild, or even your own house pets, you will notice that when they are injured or diseased, they often retire to a quiet and comfortable place and stop the intake of all food. They will drink water but abstain completely from eating. The loss of appetite in disease is also present in humans, but the idea for most people in our culture to stop eating is such an abhorrent notion that they will continue to eat even when all their natural instincts are telling them to stop. As you will see, when less energy is required for eating, digesting, and procuring food, more energy is available for healing and repair.

Fasting and the Dance of Life

To understand some of the intricacies of fasting, it is necessary to have some understanding of the processes of digestion and elimination. The human digestive system is basically a lubricated tube about 30 feet long, open from mouth to anus, segregated into a series of connected organs that comprise this functional system. It has the specific job of taking the complicated stuff from the environment we call food, breaking it down into simple nutrient building blocks that can be absorbed by the cells of the body, and eliminating the fiber and waste that is left over.

There is a profound wisdom and intelligence that manifests and weaves through the dynamic action of the body and ensures its balanced function. Consistent with this tapestry of homeostasis and survival, the body has developed a variety of back-up and fail-safe mechanisms to safeguard life and health. In this case, it is possible that nutrients can make their way to the cells of the body in a form that is still too complicated for the cells to handle. So not only do we have a digestive system at large, but every one of the trillions of body cells has its own back-up digestive system called the lysosome.[3] Lysosomes are microscopic organelles within the cells that have a highly acidic internal environment containing approximately 60 different digestive enzymes and functions to complete the digestive process. Just as the digestive system of the body is lined by a mucous membrane that serves as a protective barrier, lysosomes have a protective membrane around them, a barrier that controls the release of its enzymes, confining and controlling their action to protect the cell from being destroyed.[4]

Lysosomes are also involved in another very important function. Every day, millions of cells are being born while millions of cells are being destroyed and eliminated. When a cell has outlived its usefulness and is slated for death (apoptosis), the membranes of its lysosomes break down, flooding the cell with enzymes that dismantle and destroy it. Under conditions of nutrient deprivation, microscopic vesicles in the cell (autophagosomes) transport and recycle the damaged parts, old proteins, and toxic debris to the lysosomes, where they are metabolized to foster the support of vital tissues and organs. This process of cell "housecleaning" is referred to as autophagy and is one of the more incredible demonstrations of cellular alchemy that occurs in the fasting state. It is a process of self-digestion and is going on in the body every second of every day. However, during fasting, more energy is available for autophagy and elimination since the body is diverted away from the procurement of food, digestion, and cellular growth. In fact, it has been shown that when cells of mammals are completely deprived of essential nutrients in the fasting state, including glucose and other growth factors, the process of autophagy is triggered, regulated by genes that also decrease aging and increase the resistance of cells to environmental and chemical stress.[1] So in fasting, the natural process of autophagy, which modulates the life and death of all cells, is enhanced and allows the body to maintain and protect healthy, functional body cells while digesting, dissolving, and reutilizing worn-out and damaged cells (including nonessential extraneous growths such as tumors, cysts, and stones) for its energy needs.

Interestingly, this has much in common with the formation of the butterfly. If you were a caterpillar, you would have one job: to eat non-stop from sunrise to sunset, sometimes for a period of days and weeks. (I know that there are a few two-legged caterpillars out there thinking this is nice work if you can get it.) However, at the end of eating time, a genetic program jump-starts the autophagic process that dissolves the body of the caterpillar into a chrysalis, eventually shaping and restructuring the chrysalis into the shimmering iridescent butterfly that emerges from the autophagic soup of metamorphosis. I have seen a lot of shimmering human butterflies emerge from the metamorphosis of fasting.

Where Does All the Energy Come From?

As I have mentioned, the body has a deep-rooted need for energy and therefore for the sugar that provides it. The way the body handles food (and the lack of food) to meet this need speaks directly to the role of fasting in fat and weight loss. When food comes into the body, it is digested, and the building blocks of carbohydrates (glucose or fructose), proteins (amino acids), and fats (fatty acids) are absorbed into the bloodstream and circulated to all body cells.

Because sugar (glucose) is needed to produce energy in the body, the food we eat must replenish and maintain adequate blood sugar levels. Since elevated blood sugar levels can be dangerous, it also is critical that blood sugar be maintained in a well-defined range of normal. As previously discussed, if you overeat sugar or maintain lifestyle factors that interfere with sugar metabolism, glucose levels may increase beyond normal blood levels. The body can protect itself and create a savings account of glucose for future energy needs by storing excess glucose in the liver and especially skeletal muscles. In muscle and liver cells, it is stored as a long chain of glucose molecules bonded together called glycogen. If you consume more sugar than what the bloodstream can handle and what the liver/muscles can accept, the surplus will be moved by the body into fat cells for long-term energy storage, contributing to fat and weight gain.

Now, as you can imagine, when you stop eating, the first thing that happens is that blood sugar levels drop. This is a primary stress and threat to the body. As a result, the body begins to access the glycogen that is stored in the liver, pulling it into the bloodstream to replenish the declining blood sugar level. The glycogen reserve in the liver is typically depleted within the first 24–36 hours of fasting, however, and if you continue to fast, the body needs to find some other way to satisfy its blood sugar and energy needs. Therefore, by the second day of fasting, the body begins to use the amino acids of protein in our muscles and glycerol (one of the building blocks of fat) from the fat in our fat cells to create sugar. This process of creating sugar from protein and fat is called gluconeogenesis, gluco (glucose), neo (new), genesis (creation), the creation of new forms of sugar from other existing nutrients. By the third day of fasting, the dominant source of energy becomes the metabolism of the fatty acids from the body's fat, producing a class of compounds called ketone bodies (acetone, acetoacetate, and beta-hydroxybutyrate), which provide the major energy needs of the brain and body, thereby conserving and sparing protein.[5-7] Some estimates suggest that a person between 150–160 pounds can obtain basal caloric requirements from their fat reserves for up to two to three months of fasting.[8]

Unwarranted Concerns

Due to the body's use of proteins and fats in the fasting state, some people have expressed concerns about the efficacy and risks of fasting. However, when fasting is done with professional supervision under proper resting and stress-free conditions, the clinical and research evidence has shown these concerns to be unfounded.[9] In fact, fasting is a remarkably valuable tool for promoting health recovery from a wide range of pathological conditions, in addition to promoting and supporting long-term fat loss.

There has been some concern that protein muscle mass will be so depleted on a fast that there will be dangerous muscle-wasting. While it is true that there is more protein metabolism and lean muscle breakdown in the first few days of fasting—about two to three ounces of protein loss per day—after approximately two to three days, protein loss slows down to about one-half to one ounce per day to provide for a still small ongoing need for glucose as the body shifts to fat metabolism and ketone production for its primary energy needs. Between days three and ten, the use of ketones steadily increases so that by day ten of fasting, the energy needs of the body are derived almost exclusively from fat. Furthermore, the loss of protein and the depletion of blood sugar throughout a fast are more comfortably regulated by ensuring that the fasting person maintains maximum rest. If the person attempts too much activity on a fast, there will be more rapid, consistent, and potentially dangerous muscle loss and blood sugar decline.

As I have mentioned, when fat is broken down to produce energy, a class of compounds called ketones are produced. This produces a state in the body called ketosis. Ketosis is an acidic state that is generated whenever there is a significant breakdown of fat for energy in lieu of carbohydrates and protein. One of the common ketones that is produced is acetone, the main component of nail polish remover, so it is quite common that when you smell the breath of someone on a fast, it can smell like nail polish remover. These ketones also can be seen in a routine urinalysis.

The metabolism of fat during the fasting state has generated another cloud of controversy that must be addressed. There are unwarranted medical concerns about fasting that ketosis could damage the kidney and brain, possibly leading to loss of consciousness and even more dire consequences. However, both scientific studies and the extensive clinical experience of hygienic physicians like myself who have supervised thousands of fasts have shown these concerns to be unfounded. In fact, when fasting is done in a supportive environment with proper hydration under total resting conditions, just the opposite is observed. Kidney and heart function often dramatically improve as weight and blood pressure drop. In an extensive study of hypertension, medically supervised water-only fasts averaging 10–11 days significantly lowered both systolic and diastolic blood pressure (the top and bottom numbers of a routine blood pressure measurement), enabling people to eliminate the need for blood pressure medication.[9] Rather than a loss of consciousness, there is often a dramatic improvement in the acuity of special senses, vision, hearing, and so on. People wearing glasses will sometimes remark how they experience moments of absolutely perfect eyesight without their glasses.

In addition, in the fasting state the brain makes a unique adjustment that ensures its stability even in the absence of food intake. Brain cells are one of two directly glucose-dependent cell types in the body. The brain is truly the conductor of our remarkable body-mind symphony, and its energy needs are top priority. Because of the brain's critical role and its need for glucose/energy, as the body in its evolutionary wisdom responds to the fasting state in which glucose is not available, brain cells are capable of utilizing ketones directly for energy. It has been suggested that the ketone beta-hydroxybutyrate is the most abundant ketone used by the brain during fasting, accounting for roughly two-thirds of the brain's fuel supply, and the ability of the brain to utilize this ketone body has permitted humans to survive prolonged periods of starvation.[7] This ability is unique to healthy brain cells, and it explains how the brain and body can thrive during extensive periods of fasting. I have supervised fasts as long as two to six weeks for certain pathological conditions, and it is notable that while there is fatigue and an increased need for rest, a person is still remarkably stable in body and mind. An interesting observation is that when brain cells become cancerous, they lose the ability to utilize ketones for energy. As a result, if people with brain cancer are maintained on sugar-free diets—or even more powerfully, water-only fasting—cancer cells and tumors in the brain may be starved, shrunk, and even destroyed to some degree.

Promoting Detoxification and Elimination

To understand the role of fasting in detoxification and elimination, it is necessary to take a closer look at the fat reserves of the body. Not only is fat an available energy reserve, but it also serves as a vehicle for the storage of waste and toxic fat-soluble chemicals to which we are routinely exposed. Let's examine this a little bit closer.

Every second of every day, the cells of the body are taking in nutrients and eliminating the waste and by-products of routine metabolism. In addition to this internal toxemia, a variety of chemical poisons come into the body from the outside (e.g., pesticides, pollution, additives in foods, toxic foods, prescription drugs, and so forth) that also need to be eliminated from the body. The body uses energy to direct and control this eliminative process within some well-defined range of normal. So toxic metabolic end-products are typically maintained in the body within different acceptable ranges of normal. That's why, when you do a blood test, certain metabolites like uric acid and urea are reported in relation to a normal reference range. Typically, the toxicity that develops routinely is not eliminated immediately or completely. So, in an attempt to protect itself, the body will take whatever toxic load it can't immediately eliminate and attempt to store it out of the way of blood circulation to protect vital organs and tissues. Here's where we see another role of fat. Many environmental toxins and even internal waste products are fat-soluble (able to be dissolved in fat). So not only do fat cells of the body provide a primary source of energy, but they also work like a garbage dump, hiding and storing our toxic load.

When fat is being utilized in fasting, it is typically the volume of fat cells rather than the number of cells that is changing. As the volume of fat shrinks, fat as well as the toxic debris stored in fat tissue will also be mobilized from these cells back into general circulation, building the body's toxic load and increasing the need to remove it. Here's where fasting exerts a profound power and benefit. Fasting is an energy-conservation process. Since energy is not being used in the procurement, digestion, and utilization of food, the energy that is harbored in the fasting process can be diverted to enhance the mobilization and elimination of waste. This mobilization of waste from storage areas and the circulation and removal of this waste through organs and tissues of elimination, is what is accurately referred to as detoxification and elimination.

The body usually adjusts its blood supply to meet the conditions at hand. I remember big holiday meals with my Italian family. After consuming massive quantities of food, the blood would pool in the digestive tract to promote the digestion of all that food, pulling blood away from the brain, leading to me and others dozing off at the dinner table.

You may have had the experience of trying to exercise too soon after eating. Again, since blood is diverted to the gut and away from the muscles during digestion, this can cause cramping due to the reduced oxygen supply to the muscles. In fasting, since blood is not needed for the work of digestion, there is a significant increase in blood supply directed to organs of elimination, for example, the kidneys. As a result, urinary output is considerably increased during fasting, making it especially important to monitor water intake and hydration. (This is also why the filtration rate of the kidneys and other measures of kidney function need to be evaluated via urine and blood tests prior to fasting to determine if someone is a good candidate for fasting care.) Typically, a minimum of one and one-half to two liters of water (50–70 ounces) should be consumed daily during a fast.

The respiratory surface of the lungs and the skin are the largest organs of the body, so it is very common to see discharge, drainage, and symptoms of elimination via these organs, including mucous discharge, cysts, rashes, and boils. On the other hand, with very few exceptions, since there is no consumption of food or fiber on a fast, fecal elimination is virtually nonexistent. The following story will illustrate the eliminative action that the body is capable of performing in the fasting state.

Fasting Story #1

Some years back, Buddy was a high-powered, stressed-out attorney from New York. He ate a conventional diet loaded with excesses of animal protein, fat, and refined sugar, consumed a fair amount of alcohol, and drank loads of coffee. He started to develop some joint pain in his hands. He was not aware that his lifestyle and food choices were contributing to his discomfort, so he did what most people would do—he started taking some over-the-counter, non-steroidal drugs like aspirin and Tylenol.

While these drugs gave him some temporary relief, they were not addressing the cause of his problems. The joint pain got worse and started affecting other joints in his body. He became progressively more dysfunctional. Taking his doctor's advice, he began rounds of the anti-inflammatory steroid medication prednisone. Again, since causes were being overlooked and only symptoms were being treated, temporary relief gave way to more systemic joint damage and pain.

The systemic destruction and pain increased to such a degree that Buddy ended up immobile in a wheelchair and was subjected to what was supposedly the gold standard of arthritic therapy at the time, the injection of gold salts. At this point, he became aware of fasting and embarked on what became a 52-day fast. Now, understand that it is rare for a person to come in to a fasting center and know for how long they will fast. More typically, this is a day-to-day decision of the monitoring doctor in conjunction with the client, based on the extent of the underlying pathology, age of the person, past clinical history, and the daily reactions of the client.

Typically, as the weeks of fasting progress, the body gets somewhat weaker as energy, in a sense, is pulled from the outer muscular layers of the body into the internal core of the body to promote the even deeper internal work of healing and repair. As we discussed, the body will do all it can to promote increased elimination, and in this case, Buddy had a panorama of skin lesions and discharges as part of his healing crisis. At one point, you could wipe gold salts from the medication he was given off the surface of the skin.

Following the fast and an extensive period of refeeding and recovery, Buddy adopted a predominantly plant-based lifestyle. He never experienced significant joint pain again, even into his seventies. Yet there were times when the pressures of his life would drive him off track, and he would go back to less-supportive eating and lifestyle habits that would provoke joint pain again. At those times when he began to feel any joint soreness, however, he would fast several days, get his eating and stress under control, and nip the inflammation and pain in the bud.

Interestingly, the body will use any natural opening it has to promote elimination, e.g., the vagina in women, the respiratory system through the lungs and mouth, or some new opening it creates if it needs to. The following story illustrates this point.

Fasting Story #2

A young teacher from Canada came to me some years ago diagnosed with neurofibromatosis. In this disease there are multiple small fibrous tumors (fibromas) along the nerve fibers throughout the body and brain. One of her larger tumors was located at the base of the brain, blocking its main blood supply, so she had a shunt surgically implanted to allow blood leaving her heart to bypass this blockage and feed the brain directly.

Because of these small tumors, she had constant small epileptic-like seizures that made her life unbearable. She was on high dosages of Dilantin and phenobarbital to control the seizures. These drugs are hard on the liver and produce a toxic state in the body. Although the intensity of the seizures was lessened by the drugs, the phenobarbital kept her in a semi-comatose state with no energy, so that when she came to me, she had been bedridden for some time. She was carried into my center very weak and fragile and put in bed as if poured off a spoon. It broke my heart to see this young professional woman in her early 20s just a fading shadow of what she could be, what she should be. She had no affect, no smile, just a blank shell in a dormant state of nonbeing.

After a period of vegan, whole-food, plant-exclusive nutrition and vegetable juices to help her withdraw from the medication, she was put on a fast that lasted 30 days. Again, the length of this fast was determined on a day-to-day basis taking into account the reactions, physiological responses, and vital signs that were monitored daily. Many people come in with a finite period of time to both fast and break the fast, but fortunately, this young woman's mother and family were committed to the vegan lifestyle and clinical fasting, so she had the time to fast as long as clinically necessary. During the fast, she became more and more coherent and energetic, even as the days of abstinence continued. Around the 25th day of the fast, her neurological system expressed a flurry of short, frequent seizures related, in my opinion, to the previous patterning and increased activity of her nervous system and potentially tied into a healing crisis. In the midst of this crisis, consistent with an attempt to eliminate the toxic load on her body after years of toxic medication and the assault on her liver, her belly button opened up and drained black bile from the abdominal wall. After an extensive period of refeeding, I carried her around the property of the retreat until she got the energy to walk on her own. Her seizure activity was virtually nonexistent, and she was drug-free. It was an incredible feeling to see her living and loving life. Her smile and the joy she radiated was an absolute joy to behold as we wove our way through the perfume of gardenia bushes and orange blossoms that decorated the property of the fasting center, sharing the sweet taste of Honeybell tangelos.

Unfortunately, when she went home, she and her family were browbeaten, pressured by her previous medical doctors, and relentlessly chastised for even doing a fast. She was put back on a variety of medications, subjected to a botched surgical procedure to remove a small tumor in her ear that resulted in deafness, and after a series of medical crises, interventions, and mismanagement, she was dead in two years. Although time has a way of dissolving the hard edges of past emotion, I can still feel the pain and anger that I first felt at her untimely death. It still brings tears to my eyes.

The body clearly recognizes what belongs in it and what doesn't, and it will do everything in its power to eliminate any and all threats to its integrity. This work requires energy. When energy is available, the body executes the action(s) necessary under the direction of its own innate wisdom to carry out the inborn genetic directive of health and healing. In fasting, not only are the processes of detoxification and elimination enhanced, but the body also demonstrates an intelligent and very selective control over these processes.

During a fast, the body will utilize what it needs least to provide support for what it needs most. It needs heart, lungs, kidneys, bowels, and so forth, but it doesn't need cysts, tumors, stones, and growths. So, through the aforementioned process of autophagy, it will break down a tumor or a cyst, take from it what it can use to support the vital organs of the body, and eliminate the rest. That's why we often see cysts, tumors, and stones break down and dissolve during fasting. As fasting is prolonged, this autophagic process is an additional attempt to produce a small amount of glucose from these extraneous tissues so as to conserve and spare protein and muscle mass in the process. I have monitored women with uterine fibroids or ovarian cysts that significantly shrink and dissolve after several weeks of fasting. Some of these changes can sometimes occur in relatively short periods of fasting. One woman came to me with fibrocystic breasts that looked like they were full of shrapnel on a mammogram. After just seven days of fasting, the breasts were virtually clear. Swollen prostates, kidney stones, and inflamed joints all respond remarkably well to the autolysis of fasting.

My Personal Fasting Story

My own personal life provides a profound example of healing and recovery promoted by water-only fasting. In the early 1970s, prior to going to chiropractic college and embarking on the intense time commitment and educational experience I knew was before me, I decided to take a trip to the old country—Italy—to visit long-lost relatives and connect with my roots. I had just come through a period of major physical and emotional upheaval in my life: years of trying out a new vegetarian way of life, some short periods of water fasting, and experimentation with all the various drugs and pharmaceuticals that were on the streets of New York City in the late 1960s and early 1970s. I knew that when I returned from Italy I would be leaving the only universe I had ever known—my family, my friends, and a close, heart-tugging emotional relationship—when I relocated to what in my New York state of mind was the wasteland of the Midwest, in this case, Davenport, Iowa, to begin my professional training.

I headed out to my ancient homeland in southern Italy to a small town called Gravina de Puglia, which loosely translates as the Garden of Chickens. This was a charming, quaint town where the ancient cobblestone streets were so narrow that a passing car could almost be trapped, stuck in the embrace of the houses and walls that bordered its thoroughfares. Both my maternal grandmother and grandfather were from this town, which in Italian culture meant that I was somehow related to most of the people living there. For a brief period of time, I, the long-lost returning son, was the King of Gravina, the King of Chickens.

Understand that as I made the rounds through my growing population of new relatives, in Italy, it also meant that I had to eat everywhere I visited, and these weren't just meals, they were banquets. In fact, I cut my visit short because I just couldn't eat anymore. I was trying to hide food under the tables, in my luggage, anywhere I could. All these endless hours of visiting and partying lead to an extreme level of exhaustion and overeating. The aforementioned background of drug use and emotional and physical upheaval, coupled with the extraordinary amount of overeating and mounting exhaustion, set the stage for what happened next.

I remember it vividly. Shortly after returning to New York, I was in a movie theater on the Upper East Side of Manhattan. I started to experience intestinal rumbling and stabbing abdominal pain that compelled me to flee from my seat and rush to the bathroom. For the first time, I noticed food matter explosively leaving my body in an undigested form exactly as it went in. It was only downhill from there. For the next week, everything I ate came out of my body undigested, and I lost about 30–40 pounds. My height and weight back then were 6' 1" and 175 pounds, and I think you can appreciate that going down to about 135–140 pounds was a frightening transformation in such a short period of time. I was literally dehydrating to death. If it wasn't for the full beard I had at the time, I would have looked like my face had fallen off. I wasn't a doctor then, and I really don't know how much of a difference that would have made, but I was full of fear.

Think about it. If you had a serious health crisis or an unexplainable set of painful symptoms that lasted for a week, you would probably be afraid. I was watching my body fade away, and I was stuck with the dilemma of what to do. I could have sought medical emergency care, gone to a hospital to get some IV fluid replacement, and probably be put on rounds of antibiotics. But based on the reading I had done, I took a leap of faith and decided to put myself in the back bedroom of my parents' apartment in the Bronx, and I stopped eating. I decided to fast on water only, whether I lived or died. Remarkably, I actually gained a few pounds during the first few days of fasting as my body stopped dehydrating to death.

Based on what I know now, you can go for a substantial period of time without food, but you can't go more than a few days without water, so I had to ensure adequate water intake. In my parents' apartment, the bedroom where I was camping out was separated from the kitchen by a living room. So to get the water I needed, I had to navigate from the bedroom through the living room into the kitchen. Because of my family's concerns for my health (and probably my sanity, too), a number of the members of my Italian family—parents, grandparents, aunts, and uncles—congregated on the couches and chairs in the living room, waiting to see what was going to happen next. So as I, this wraith-like human being, made my staggering journey across the living room into the kitchen, I could feel this gauntlet of concerned family members making the sign of the cross. (I'm sure you've heard of religious fasts. Well, this was a religious fast for the entire family.) Interestingly, on the 12th day of this fast—yes, that's 12 days without any food whatsoever—I had a strong desire to eat bananas. I ate some. They stayed down and were digested perfectly. From that time forward, everything I ate was digested well. That led to normal, healthy bowel function and steady weight gain. The fast had completely resolved the affliction that had plagued me. I continued to eat a simple, plant-exclusive diet of fruits and steamed and cooked vegetables, and I returned to healthy body weight over the next six months.

What makes fasting so beneficial is that while many pathological conditions are improved, including autoimmune diseases (e.g., lupus, rosacea, rheumatoid arthritis), asthma, high blood pressure, ulcers, irritable bowels, colitis, allergies, and depression, it also leads to significant fat and weight loss. In the early days of fasting, weight loss can be as much as two pounds per day; it will taper off to some degree in the latter stages of more extensive fasts. In one human study, weight loss caused by fasting was initially rapid, as much as one and one-half to two pounds per day during the first week of fasting, followed by one-half to one pound per day by the third week of fasting. As much as a 20% loss of body weight occurred by 30–35 days of fasting.[10] It is not always true, but usually the more obese the individual is at the start, the more dramatic the initial weight loss is. I have seen people lose 20 pounds in two weeks of fasting, and as much as 30 pounds or more in a month. Perhaps most importantly, fasting significantly eliminates the risky abdominal (belly) fat and visceral fat around body organs, which is associated with the greatest risk of heart disease, diabetes, and cancer. Contrary to most fad diets that cause reactive fat gain after the dieting period, the visceral fat that is dissolved in fasting does not return, especially if you follow the fast with a whole-food, plant-exclusive diet without added salt, oil, and sugar.

If there are two mistakes that are commonly made after fasting, they are eating too much too soon and moving too much too soon. The refeeding period after fasting is crucial for the success of the overall fasting experience; food needs to be gradually reintroduced. In fasting centers, a common recommendation by supervising physicians is that the person take half the time of the fast to ease back into eating. So, if you fast seven days, you should take another three to four days to break the fast. If you fast two weeks, you should take another week to break the fast. Fasts are most successfully broken over a period of days with a succession of diluted and full-strength fruit and vegetable juices, vegetable broth, fresh fruit, fresh vegetables and salads, and raw and cooked vegan meals.

If healthy, low-calorie-dense, low-sodium, plant-based eating and lifestyle habits are not maintained after fasting, there can be significant reactive weight gain because of the fast's elimination of all calories and the aforementioned starvation response. Briefly, there is a kind of ledger sheet, an internal recognition system that the body uses to match its caloric intake to its caloric output. If you're restricting your intake of calories but burning a lot of them in physical movement, the body will slow down your resting metabolism rate to hold on to future calories more forcefully, and you can begin to gain weight on less and less food intake. Therefore, resting as much as possible is recommended during the fast. Increasing physical activity during a fast is not only potentially dangerous, but it can also promote excessive reactive weight gain after the fast.

Physical activity also should be gradually reintroduced after a fast. Doing too much too soon can cause undue physiological stress to the body and even potentially provoke unforeseen damage or disability. Depending on the length of the fast, I typically recommend short periods of walking, swimming, biking on a stationary bike, or exercising on a rebounder for about four to five minutes at a time a few times per day for the first few days after fasting. After this period, activity can be extended several minutes per day over time until you've built up to about 30–45 minutes per day.

Fasting is not a mystical process. Yes, it has been used by a variety of spiritual traditions as a tool for introspective evaluation and spiritual growth. But fasting is truly just a profoundly simple process of deep physiological rest. That's the main reason fasting is only recommended in a resting state. Typically, other than going to the bathroom and simple activities of daily living, no other physical activity is allowed. The goal is to harbor as much energy as possible for the healing work at hand. That means rest on every level, including all the senses, so while watching TV, listening to music, and playing on the Internet are okay during a fast, the more time spent being quiet, serene, and introspective, the better. Making part of your fasting experience a digital fast away from the constant involvement with electronic equipment and data processing is also a good idea. It is so beneficial to give your eyes, your ears, and your brain a total break in the action—and this not an easy thing in our culture.

We are so inundated with information and stimulation that we are constantly being pulled outside of ourselves. The thought of spending time with, and within, ourselves can sound like a daunting, almost frightening task. However, it is in this introspective time that information about what motivates our cravings and desires can be revealed. Sometimes, only by slowing everything down and stepping back from the chaos and distractions around us can we question and change the patterns and choices of our lives. We need to afford new choices an opportunity to breathe and take root in our brains and neurological systems, making it easier for us to establish constructive, healthier choices over time. For this reason, fasting also is a profound tool for creating a more mindful, self-aware life and for dealing with addictive behavior. Many people have confronted and resolved the compulsive abuse of drugs and food by fasting, which promotes a stability in brain chemistry that even helps with the pain of withdrawal from addictive substances. It's never easy, but I have utilized the fasting process to help people resolve the typically debilitating pain and craving of opiate withdrawal from heroin, Dilaudid, and other drugs, including cocaine, with significantly less pain and discomfort than is usual.

Short periods of fasting, from two to five days, are also extremely useful for changing food habits and addictions to salt, sugar (refined processed candy, ice cream, cookies, and pastry products), other refined carbohydrates (refined breads and pasta), gluten, meat, and dairy products. If you recall, there are about 24 hours of sugar reserves before the body delves into its fat and protein reserves while fasting. So, in reality, you have not even begun a fast until about the second day of abstinence from food.

Unfortunately, there are too many people, including some physicians and scientists, who have created confusion by blurring the distinction between fasting and starvation. It is important to know that they are not the same thing. As we have discussed, in fasting the body is, in a sense, eating and living off protein and fat reserves. Because the body has adequate reserves, vital signs (body temperature, pulse, and blood pressure) are stable and well maintained; they will tend to drop, but will stabilize at a lower point. Fasting is the epitome of order and stability. In contrast, when the body goes beyond its reserve capacity, it enters the world of starvation. In starvation, chaos is the rule. Vital signs plummet and become completely unstable, without regulation or control. Understand that when you fast in resting conditions, with adequate hydration and proper supervision, fasting is a relatively safe and healthy process promoting recovery and weight loss.

There are, however, people who are not good candidates for fasting. People with contraindications include those who have an extreme fear of fasting, people who are anorexic or bulemic, people with metastatic cancer or wasting disease, pregnant diabetic women, nursing mothers, people taking medications other than thyroid and reproductive hormone replacement, and people with specific metabolic genetic defects like porphyria, in which there is difficulty processing porphyrins (chemicals affecting red blood cell production and energy production/utilization in mitochondria, the energy factories of cells).

As we have discussed, during fasting the body can express eliminative activity and healing crises through a variety of acute symptoms involving the skin, kidneys, intestines, liver, lungs, and other body organs and systems. While these actions are in the best interest of the body, most of us have been brought up to be afraid of these vital actions or to not recognize them as such. We have been conditioned to fear acute symptoms of disease, such as fever and discharge, even when these symptoms are typically the most direct expression of the body's inborn ability to protect and heal itself. If this fear surfaces during the fast, it can create stress that is debilitating and counterproductive to the fasting process. This is one of the reasons fasting is usually recommended to be done under the supervision of physicians who have been trained in fasting care. When we supervise fasts, there is typically a lot of hand-holding, counseling, and monitoring of the fasting process. This helps the faster have a better understanding of their symptom picture and what is going on clinically so that much of their fear can be put to rest.

When there is a condition of advanced cancer or metastatic cancer that has spread from some other primary site, fasting may not be in your best interest. Under these conditions, the body may already be wasting away, and fasting may actually hasten the death process. I have witnessed fasting dramatically reduce the pain and suffering of some people with advanced forms of metastatic cancer, improving quality of life, but it did not support or improve their chances for recovery, and in some cases, it may have even hastened impending death. However, some cancers, e.g., lymphoma, have responded quite well to fasting.

With the exceptions of thyroid medications and reproductive hormone replacement therapies, it is not in your best interest to fast with medication. If you think about it, medications are toxic to the body, and the last thing you want to do is take in potentially toxic or irritating substances when no food is coming in. This could impose major physiological stress on the body and potentially lead to severe disability and breakdown.

Many people often equate juice programs and other forms of restrictive caloric approaches with fasting and detoxification and opt for those. But while these approaches may lighten the digestive load on the body, making more energy available for some detoxification, elimination, and healing, they are not fasting programs. A juice diet is a diet, not a fasting process. Since carbohydrates are still coming in on a juice program, the diet does not inspire the intensity of autophagy, detoxification, elimination, and healing that occur in water-only fasting. Remember, however, that fasting requires complete rest. If you have to work or do any other consistent physical activity, you should not water fast. Under those demands for activity and energy, a short-term program of vegetable juice and/or green smoothies or a regular pattern of intermittent fasting may be a better choice and have some major benefit for optimizing fat and weight loss.

Intermittent Fasting

In intermittent fasting, the pattern and timing of your food use is modified to promote the reduction of weight and body fat while limiting the conversion of excessive calories and glucose into fat storage. While this is not a true fast, it provides controlled periods of eating and food restriction within a 24-hour day or for several days per week. For optimal fat and weight loss, it is best to consume calories during the day while eating very little at night, so in typical intermittent fasting protocols, food is consumed during an 8–12 hour period and restricted for a 12–16 hour period. Commonly, people will fast from 7:00–8:00 p.m. until anywhere between 8:00 a.m. and 12:00 p.m. the next day, creating cycles of 12 hours fasting/12 hours eating up to 16 hours fasting/8 hours eating. An alternative approach to this 24-hour variation is to eat normally for five days and reduce calories to 25% of your normal daily calorie intake (approximately 600 calories for men and 500 calories for women) on the remaining two days per week.[11]

The incredible benefits of fasting make it a remarkable tool and an indispensable component of any long-term weight-loss program. Fasting promotes fat breakdown, detoxification, and repair like nothing else. Just understand that fasting is not a weight-loss program per se. At best, you will fast a very small part of your life, while you'll eat throughout the bulk of your life, so what you choose to eat and do in your life on a regular basis is more significant for your long-term weight regulation than brief, isolated periods of fasting. However, even short periods of fasting, in the range of three to seven days, can promote some initial weight loss and help you jump-start a long-term, successful weight-loss program. Since fasting also enhances the balance and function of the hormonal (endocrine) system, regenerates the immune system, and significantly improves metabolism and the metabolic efficiency and function of organs that play a major role in weight control including the liver and digestive system, it can promote improved calorie use and fat loss over time and dramatically improve your opportunity for successful long-term weight control.

Also keep in mind that chronic, excessive inflammation provokes and reinforces disease and weight gain, and fasting, even for short periods, can be one of the most powerful approaches for resolving inflammation and the complications of autoimmune disease. For example, in the United Kingdom, fasting with a follow-up plant-based diet significantly resolved the complications and biological laboratory markers for rheumatoid arthritis. After four weeks, a test group that had completed a seven- to ten-day water-only fast followed by a gluten-free vegan diet had a significant decrease in the number of swollen joints, a decrease in the duration of morning stiffness, an increase in grip strength, and a remarkable decrease in the biomarkers for inflammation and rheumatoid arthritis, including erythrocyte sedimentation rate, C-reactive protein, and white blood count.[12]

For all these reasons, some short period of fasting is recommended in the one-week, two-week, and three-week weight-loss programs discussed in Chapter 15. Remember: the body-mind changes evoked by the fasting process make it one of the most efficient and powerful tools to jump-start any new health program in general, and a significant and successful, long-term weight- and fat-loss program in particular.

CHAPTER 11

COMPASSIONATE EATING FOR ENVIRONMENTAL BALANCE, ANIMAL RIGHTS, AND WEIGHT LOSS

By embracing certain lifestyle choices more consistently, you can establish new ways of thinking that foster significant, beneficial changes in your health and awareness. This is especially so when you adopt a vegan, plant-exclusive nutritional approach that eliminates the use of all animal-derived foods and products. It is important to understand, however, that the vegan approach is more than just an eating plan. It is a lifestyle commitment and philosophy that promotes compassion as well as the sanctity and the supreme value of conscious life.

This mentality and model of compassion is so needed now at a time when we seem to be inundated and infected by a pandemic of greed, strife, violence, and war. When we are stimulated, seduced, and pulled outside ourselves by an endless sea of information, media noise, and mindless distractions, it is extremely easy to lose ourselves and sink into a quicksand of emotional and spiritual bankruptcy. It is necessary, therefore, to find a way to ground and stabilize our technological advances, financial and economic resources, and energy demands for a greater awareness and expression of peace, empathy, forgiveness, and love. We must adopt lifestyle choices that promote a compassionate way of thinking and acting that does not become lost in the agendas, greed, and disconnecting separatism of partisan governments, religions, and special-interest groups—groups that all too often spout anthems of fear masquerading as religious dogma and factions seething with violence and aggression, nursed on centuries of hate and primarily concerned with the propagation of their own power and control.

It is vital to promote the expression of compassion, love, and forgiveness that sees others as ourselves and embraces the sanctity of life over the ideologies and beliefs of political systems and religions. Only through a greater understanding and expression of our ingrained capacity for empathy and compassion can a "life above all else" philosophy be set in motion. Only then can we truly realize that no one has the right to assault or abuse other defenseless species or segments of our human population, and only then can we stop the ignorance and fear that fosters persecution and killing, whether of other creatures for our food, sport and accoutrements, or other people simply because they have different skin colors, different views of God, or different sexual orientations and desires.

Some scientists, philosophers, and even metaphysical traditions suggest that all reality is a sea of connected energy, endless fields of electromagnetic energy merging, interacting, and colliding with the consciousness of all the living creatures perceiving and interpreting their content. Quantum physics tells us that any notion of separation of people or other species is an illusion, one that is an ill-conceived map based on a short-sighted, fragmented view of the world, incapable of matching the territory of wholeness that is fundamental to all life on our planet. If you continue to follow a map of disconnection and discord, you will never be able to navigate the territory of integration and well-being that is truly within your reach.

The truth is that we are all one. We are each other. Trying to separate any of the interconnected, interdependent energies of anything on planet Earth is like reaching into the ocean with your bare hands and trying to separate the individual waves as they flow one to the other. A vegan, plant-exclusive lifestyle is the first, best, and most profound path to living this truth of connection and to applying this truth to the problems of fat and weight gain.

Massive Destruction of Animal Life

We eat way too much meat and dairy in America. We've become like the cartoon family popular in my early years, the Flintstones. When Fred, the patriarch of the Flintstone family, pulled up in his footmobile at the drive-through for his big Bronto Burger, the massive size and weight of the meat would tip his whole car over. According to *Time* magazine, Americans consume more than 600 million Big Mac hamburgers each year and an equal number of Burger King Whoppers. That's 1.2 billion burgers at just those two franchises! Americans also consume 27 billion hot dogs each year and 20–30 chickens each second.

It's a killing field out there, folks. There is a massive destruction of animal life. Trillions of animals (including fish) are tortured, genetically modified, and slaughtered annually to satisfy a vulgar, disgusting appetite for their fluids, organs, and flesh. Too many of us have lost the compassion for creatures around us. Instead of being enlightened caretakers of our planet and the creatures, humans, and animals that are more defenseless than ourselves, we are all too often instruments of killing and destruction. As a result, in my opinion, this directly promotes the spiritual bankruptcy that undermines the moral and ethical advancement of our culture.

Don't misunderstand me. I'm not spouting some dogmatic religious viewpoint. True spirituality is not about religiosity. I am not a religious person, and I am not interested in addressing anyone's religious beliefs. That's your personal business, and you have a right to participate in any religious practice you so choose. Spirituality is about how you see your-self in relation to the people and life around you. It is about transcending your own self-centered interests and agendas while demonstrating compassion, empathy, and harmlessness for your planet and neighbors of all species.

We are all connected, humans and animals. Unfortunately, past history and the modern global perspective fosters the absurd and scientifically untenable view of nonhuman animals as "things" without complex minds to support their agency to make choices and display self-recognition and without the ability to maintain deep social, intellectual, and emotional lives. This continues to deprive these beautiful creatures of any sense of inherent value and independence and reinforces the idea that they are here solely for our corrupted needs for food and entertainment, making them defenseless targets of captivity, torture, and wanton killing. Fortunately, there are organizations like the Nonhuman Research Project and enlightened attorneys like Steven Wise and others who are petitioning for animal rights in the legal system to highlight the autonomy of individual animals and challenge the grounds of their confinement. These organizations, along with other writers and activists, continue to creatively reinforce how important it is for all people to recognize animals as individuals with identities, families, histories, and a sense of self.[1,2] For the sake of humanity, it is essential that we recognize the intrinsic value of all land and sea animals, upholding their right to dignity as well as our own.

If we maintain lifestyle and eating habits that foster violence and killing, a not-so-subtle license for violence and killing becomes etched into the consciousness of our culture. The more we accept and support industries that promote violence and death, the more we feed and condone a pervasive cultural mentality of abuse and violence.

The repercussions of this mentality are all around us, and if it weren't so twisted and disturbing, it would almost be laughable. For example, in movies it always amazes me how so much concern and censorship, especially in the United States, is focused on visual displays of nudity and/or intense lovemaking, even if it is portrayed in a truly tasteful manner between people who really care about each other. However, constantly exposing people of all ages to omnipresent displays of rampant graphic violence, bloodshed, and killing online and in video games, TV shows, and movies is no problem. I personally would prefer having anyone, especially our young people, see true positive emotion and love rather than relentless displays of abuse and harm. The slang words that describe our genitals and common curse words like the F-word are not the most obscene words in the English language. The most obscene word in the English language is "kill." When killing and violence against any defenseless creatures are condoned, all expressions of violence, including spousal and child abuse, are not far behind, making it more difficult to foster the peace, serenity, inner balance, and harmony that are essential to any experience of well-being, including healthy weight regulation.

There is no person reading this book or walking this planet who needs to have their protein needs or weight-loss requirements satisfied by this cycle of harm and killing, by this vibration of violence. Life feeds life. I truly feel that you cannot continue to eat death and hope that abundant health and life will follow.

We have clearly discussed how dietary excesses of animal foods foster obesity and the major epidemics of our culture. In a matter of speaking, the animals that we eat and kill are exacting some measure of revenge. The more we choose to kill and eat them, the more they are killing us. Our food choices do not exist in a vacuum, however. Yes, they are a concern for personal health and weight loss, but more and more data strongly suggest that the preoccupation and obsession with animal consumption also has serious adverse implications for energy use and global environmental destruction. I hope, therefore, that it is increasingly more obvious that the program that is the most successful for weight-loss should also foster the highest level of personal health, the greatest support for the well-being of the animals around us, and the greatest respect, health, and balance for the planet itself.

Deforestation, Greenhouse Gases, and Global Warming

Because of the way the environment, economy, and health of our people are going, the consequences of what you and I choose to put on our plates is no longer confined to the borders of our kitchens or the boundaries of our own individual skins. The consequences of these choices have far-reaching effects on the world and people around us.

For decades, farmers in Central and South America, the site of 60% of the rainforests on planet Earth,[3] have been paid to engage in an agricultural method called "slash and burn," which involves burning the rainforest down to the ground to plant a single crop, often grass to graze cattle for import into Western nations like the U.S. Approximately 70% of the Amazonian rainforest is devoted to cattle production so that millions of pounds of beef can be imported yearly into the U.S. in order that we can have that infamous 99-cent hamburger, meanwhile losing millions of acres of glorious rainforest trees each year. The Consultative Group on International Agricultural Research, funded by the U.N., has indicated that the slash-and-burn agricultural practice contributes to the loss of almost 20–30 million acres of rainforest each year.[4] The continual loss of these trees is even more problematic when you consider that 50% of the world's rainforests had already been destroyed by 1990. This devastating practice is a mindless assault that will almost ensure that the rainforests will be gone within the lifetimes of our children and grandchildren.

Rainforest trees contribute to the normal temperature regulation of our planet by beneficially absorbing carbon dioxide (CO_2) and emitting recycled oxygen (O_2) from their photosynthetic production. These trees have a huge surface area compared with trees in other parts of the world, so they absorb CO_2 and produce O_2 in a big way. Over time, forests build up a huge supply of carbon in their trunks, roots, stems, and leaves. However, when the land is cleared in deforestation, a large amount of that stored carbon is released back into the atmosphere by the burning and decomposition of the trees, negatively affecting the temperature control of our planet. Tell me how good your hamburger tastes when you're suffocating to death as you eat it with your children and grandchildren.

There has been a lot of discussion and controversy about the process of climate change, but understand that a certain amount of global warming is a positive, essential biological process. There is a canopy of natural gases in the atmosphere, including carbon dioxide, methane, and nitrous oxide, that work like the ceiling of a greenhouse to trap the heat produced by the sun and warm the surface of the earth. The effect produced by these so-called greenhouse gases is necessary for maintaining the temperature of the earth within optimal limits that support all life on the planet.

However, destruction of the rainforests and oceans associated with certain realities of modern life contributes to an amplification of the canopy of gases, leading to consequences—abnormal global warming and catastrophic climate change—that negatively affect all life. Industrialization, population growth, and mounting demand for animal food production in modern society have markedly increased the need for energy and the increased burning of fossil fuels (i.e., oil, coal, and gas). In addition, the insatiable demand for animal food and the consequences of animal agriculture have significantly boosted the atmospheric concentration of methane, which exerts the greatest radiating force and is the most significant contribution to increased global warming. The annual methane emissions from animal agriculture alone cause more global warming than all CO_2 emissions from all fossil-fuel sources combined, a fact rarely mentioned in discussion of climate change.[5]

The amount of CO_2 in our atmosphere is currently about 415 parts per million—the highest it has ever been in the past three million years of human history—having increased 50% in just the past 200 years since the beginning of the industrial age. Currently, the temperature of the Earth is one degree Celsius higher than preindustrial times, and if it rises even another half a degree, it will cause catastrophic climate changes. Therefore, anything that increases greenhouse gases poses a threat to the welfare of all humanity and our planet. Any solution must include efforts to phase out the burning of fossil fuels, but more importantly to rapidly curtail the animal-food production practices that promote the liberation of carbon dioxide from the deforestation and burning of trees while creating massive grazing areas that are less able to sequester and remove carbon from the atmosphere. Currently, animal agriculture (the harmful incarceration, torture, and killing of animals on factory farms for meat and dairy food production) uses 37% of the ice-free land area of our planet for grazing animals, land that becomes depleted by grazing and thereafter is only able to sequester 2% of land carbon.

In an effort to reduce the risks associated with the escalating use of fossil fuels, there has been much discussion and action by world leaders to develop alternative energy sources, including wind and sun. There also have been recommendations to drive less and create more energy-efficient hybrid cars, including the further development of electric cars. Yet, while this discussion of alternative energy sources is crucial to our future survival, the conversation has been dangerously short-sighted.

Over the past decade, the Intergovernmental Panel on Climate Change (IPCC) of the U.N. and its research arm, the Food and Agriculture Organization (FAO), have suggested that the only way to prevent catastrophic climate change is to abruptly stop the burning of fossil fuels, without any meaningful mention of the impact of animal agriculture and land-use change (deforestation and using land for grazing). They continue to fail to address that when fossil fuels (coal and oil) are burned, not only do they produce climate-warming CO_2 emissions, they also produce the emission of sulphate aerosols that reflect the sun and have a cooling effect on global temperature. As a result, if you abruptly stop the burning of fossil fuels, you will lose the cooling effect of sulphate aerosols, and the current trend of abnormal global warming will be magnified, producing catastrophic effects more quickly. The cessation of fossil-fuel burning needs to be phased out gradually while we abruptly stop the dominant contribution of animal agriculture and animal food consumption to abnormal global warming.

Unfortunately, due to faulty analyses by the FAO and its questionable partnership with the International Meat Secretariat and the International Dairy Federation that foster the promotion of livestock farming, the contribution of fossil-fuel burning to abnormal climate change has been woefully exaggerated by the IPCC while the contribution from animal agriculture has been dangerously underestimated. This conflict of interest compromises the accurate collection and interpretation of data and has shifted the focus of world leaders and countries across the world away from animal-food consumption as the most significant cause of catastrophic climate change.[6]

Approximately one-third of all fossil fuels burned on our planet are burned in the production of food obtained from the bodies and fluids of farm animals. According to the FAO, the significant contribution of fossil fuels in farm-animal food production includes using them to produce mineral fertilizers for feed products; to run equipment, technologies, and all phases of animal production in massive animal factories; and in the production and transport of processed and refrigerated animal products.[6] Incredibly, according to a rigorous global sensitivity analysis, the current level of animal-food production accounts for 87% of all greenhouse gas emissions, which is significantly more than all of the world's cars, trucks, trains, and planes combined.[5]

Research from the University of California at Irvine indicated that the meats in our diets (beef, chicken, and pork) cause more of the three main greenhouse gases (CO_2, methane, and nitrous oxide) to spew into the atmosphere than does either transportation or industry.[7] And according to the FAO, the waste and the intestinal fermentation and resulting belching of livestock—especially cattle and sheep—play a leading role in emissions of methane, which, in fact, makes a significantly greater contribution to global warming than CO_2.

Furthermore, livestock contributes more than two-thirds of all nitrous oxide emissions. Farm animals can generate 130 times the amount of feces produced by the entire human population. This waste is typically untreated and can generate huge amounts of nitrous oxide, which is 300 times more potent than carbon dioxide for promoting an exaggerated greenhouse effect.[8] In short, while all foods, including fruits and vegetables, have some environmental costs, nothing comes close to the devastation of beef production. Producing a pound of beef generates more than 36 times the greenhouse gases generated in producing a pound of asparagus, 49 times that of a pound of apples, and 57 times that of a pound of potatoes.[9]

As much as they are popular today, organic meats and meat from free-range animals also contribute to the problem. While organic meats may come from animals that are better fed and housed and are not treated with the drugs typically used in more conventional animal factories, they obviously still involve violence and killing, and they still feed the problem of greenhouse gas production from their land and fuel demands as well as their waste production. Free-range animals require even more grazing land than housed animals and render even less available land for the sequestration of atmospheric carbon.

Abuse of Land and Water Resources

I previously stated that a significant portion of the escalating animal-agriculture-generated greenhouse effect comes from the loss of carbon-dioxide-absorbing trees and other plant cover on land where feed crops are grown and harvested. The magnitude of this problem can be more clearly understood when you consider that nearly one-third of the entire landmass of the Earth is used for grazing livestock. However, the drain on our natural resources goes even further: more than half of all our water resources are devoted to raising animals for food.

The impact of this drain on our water supply becomes clear when you understand our natural water-cycling system. Trees, via their massive root systems, both draw water into the soil and pull it up from the soil to release it into the atmosphere as water vapor. The water vapor released into the air condenses in the form of clouds to fall again as rain. When trees are cut down for livestock food production, the stripped land can no longer produce rain. Crops fail, topsoil dries out and is blown away, and deserts begin to form. Through this process, thousands of acres of land worldwide become deserts every hour. This can lead to food scarcity, abnormal climate changes, and a potential loss over time of a number of plant and animal species.

In addition, between 1970 and 2014, there has been 60% decrease in the number of wild animals on planet Earth, and 80% of this mass extinction is due to habitat destruction primarily caused by humans clearing land for the demands of animal agriculture. This loss of biodiversity is the lasting, painful cost of habitat destruction that upsets the beauty and balance of nature.

The manipulation of the animal food industry has gone even further to increase health risks, promote obesity, and stimulate environmental catastrophe. Prior to slaughter, cattle are often put on a special feed that's loaded with corn to cause the meat to become marbled with fat. This marbling makes the meat more tender so that it's more appealing (and more marketable) to the meat-loving, fat-loving public. It has some of the highest saturated fat and cholesterol content of all food sources, making it the riskiest for promoting heart disease, inflammation, and reactive weight gain. In order to provide the enormous demand for corn, megafarms devoted solely to its production have been established in the Midwest. Such monocrop farms deplete the soil's nutrients, weakening it to such an extent that the health of the plants themselves is compromised, becoming more prone to damage by organisms in the environment. To address this problem, these plants are treated with huge amounts of pesticides and herbicides that increase the toxic load of the plants, the toxicity of the land that absorbs these pesticides, and eventually the cattle that magnify and store this toxicity in their fat tissue. When you also consider that feed corn is one of the most genetically modified crops on the planet, these animals are adding significant amounts of pesticides and genetically modified corn into our food chain. Both of these factors can increase potential weight gain.

Furthermore, the pesticides used in these Midwest corn farms run off into the Mississippi River and eventually into the Gulf of Mexico, where they create a dead zone that spreads for thousands of miles. This expanded pool of death is full of poison and devoid of oxygen, so all sea life is suffocated and destroyed. As it turns out, there are thousands of these dead zones across the planet where pesticide abuses in connection with the production of animal foods have occurred.

Food Subsidies

Unfortunately, the destructive use of land, water, and fuel reserves needed for animal food production also has a negative effect on the availability and distribution of healthy food for the population at large. A large portion of the crops currently grown is used to feed farm animals and is unavailable for the needs of the human population, and it takes significantly more land and water to produce adequate amounts of foods for animal feed compared with that needed to nourish people on a 100% plant-exclusive diet. In fact, it takes approximately 100 times more land to produce a gram of protein from beef compared to that needed to grow wheat and rice. Livestock consume 80% of the plant food grown while providing just 15% of the food (including seafood) that humans consume, in addition to occupying 37% of the ice-free landmass of planet Earth for grazing land. This massive depletion of available plant food, energy, and land resources limits the opportunity to feed our ever-growing global population the high-energy plant food that is in its best interest.

Meanwhile, more than 14 million children go to bed hungry every night, and that's not in a third world country, but in the U.S.

Throughout the world, 9,000 children die of food scarcity/starvation every single day.[10] Just think about that for a moment. Every day when you get up, another 9,000 children are so malnourished that they are doomed to die. Sadly, these are children who never even get close to the bare minimal amount of food that could sustain them, food that could easily be made more available with less dependency on animal foods. These children never get a chance to be children. They suffer and die to the dirge of their wailing parents' anguish, parents who watch the life drain from their offspring, helpless to stop this rolling tide of death. Make no mistake, it is all connected. Animal rights are intricately tied to human rights.

Yet Western governments like the U.S. continue to recommend high-fat, high-protein diets that are loaded with meat and dairy products—diets that have been shown worldwide to increase disease and obesity. Why would these custodians of the people and public health make such risky recommendations? Partly because of the unholy marriage that continues to thrive between the government and the meat and dairy industries. But why would the government want to be in bed with these industries? Because the meat and dairy industries are intrinsic parts of the economic landscape and have been feeding the political structure of the government for quite some time with financial contributions. These industries are not known for their charity work; they want something in return, something that men and women have wanted since the beginning of time: money and/or power.

Because of the huge expenditure of land, water, and fossil fuel resources necessary to produce animal and dairy products, government subsidies are necessary to control the flow of these products into the marketplace and to lower the cost of these products so the public can afford them. Without subsidies, the cost of a pound of beef in the marketplace would be more than $30 per pound. Who's going to buy beef at $30 per pound? No one—so government subsidies keep these industries alive.

Since the time of the New Deal programs in the 1930s, subsidies have been in place to protect farmers by setting prices and economic controls around the contingencies of supply and demand. Farmers have been subsidized to produce surplus crops for reserve and/or to keep their land idle, being paid for not growing anything at all. This provides a way to keep too much food from reaching the marketplace so that their livelihoods would not be compromised by low market prices. In the case of animal food production, livestock and dairy foods are destroyed if supply exceeds demand, so that huge volumes of surplus cheese, other dairy products, corn, and livestock raised on subsidized grain that farmers are paid to overproduce are routinely destroyed.[11]

Unfortunately, the largest subsidies go to foods that are most significantly linked with obesity: corn (for high-fructose corn syrup production and animal feed) and other feed grains (oats and barley) for meat and high-fat dairy-food production. Nearly two-thirds of government farming support goes to animal foods that government health agencies suggest we limit, while less than 2% goes to the fruit and vegetable production that most significantly supports human health and optimal weight/body fat.[12] Since 2014, subsidies from the USDA have totaled more than $80 million, with $20 million in 2020 alone. Furthermore, the wealthiest 1% of farm operations receive nearly 25% of the total subsidies from the USDA, and the wealthiest 10% of farm operations receive two-thirds of all subsidies.[11] The result is that the richest farmers and corporate agribusinesses producing feed grains for sugar and animal food production benefit the most from subsidies. Farms that grow fruits and vegetables, which rely most heavily on the greatest number of farm workers, receive virtually no federal support at all.[11]

The total cost that the animal-agriculture system imposes on taxpayers, animals, and the environment is about $414 billion annually, with retail sales of these food products tallying about $250 billion.

That means that for every dollar of product sold, meat and dairy products impose almost two extra taxpayer dollars in hidden costs for all of us.[12] Furthermore, U.S. subsidies can have devastating effects on international trade. Small farmers in poor countries can't compete with subsidized, lower international prices when they sell their unsubsidized products. As a result, millions of people are forced to stay impoverished. For example, the U.S. corn subsidies from 1994–2003 flattened Mexican corn prices by 70%, leading to a 50% increase in Mexican unemployment and a 20% drop in the Mexican minimum wage.[12]

Since our government provides such massive financial subsidies and incentives to the animal product industry to artificially lower the sticker prices for meat, dairy, and eggs, it continues to allow this industry to survive and maintain its stranglehold on the minds and eating habits of the public. And since farmers growing plant-based food for people receive virtually no government assistance or financial support, it is much harder for produce farmers to compete with the prices of animal products and refined foods. Consequently, it is often more expensive for the consumer on a limited budget to make healthier, more environmentally friendly vegan choices in the marketplace. You can still get a 99-cent hamburger, but it costs $6 for a pint of raspberries. It is obvious that if we really want to solve the epidemics of disease and obesity, more attention and money must be given to subsidize fruit and vegetable production and significantly less to an animal product industry that supports death and environmental destruction.[xiii]

[xiii] Put your mind at ease. Large supermarket chains, health-food stores, and farmers markets in your communities are making more and more high-quality produce and packaged food options more affordable and available. Low-cost options for all produce, whole grains, legumes, and even plant-based meat- and dairy-substitution products are more available now than ever. In the pages that follow, I will share some of these foods and products with you. With some modest attention and effort on your part, you can shop more comfortably on any budget and embrace the food options that will promote optimal health and weight loss.

Interconnectedness and Personal Choices

Unfortunately, we have all been sold the erroneous notion that we need to eat large amounts of animal protein to maintain health and healthy weight. We have been enslaved by this worship of protein while, in fact, eating large amounts is the best approach for promoting chronic disease and reactive weight gain. There is no reason for the well-being of our health and of the Earth to consume anything but a plant-exclusive diet. We have a kinship with our planet and everything and everyone living on it. While a shimmering, pulsing, genetic architecture defines the uniqueness of individuals and species, it also is expressed in similarities and connections between the family of man and the diversity of other animals and life forms. The recognition of this connection to life outside ourselves is the essence of being vegan and the essence of spirituality. As was expressed in the remarkable show *Cosmos,* accepting our kinship with all life on the planet is a soaring spiritual experience.

Keep in mind that all life is not just connected, it is interdependent. Every cell of the body is a microcosm of the whole body. Every individual is a microcosm for the entire body of the human population that peoples the earth. Every species is a microcosm of all species that inhabit the earth. The entire history of human creativity and survival, as well as the selective survival experiences of all other species, are etched into the genetic environment of each and every one of us. Some also suggest that humanistic qualities of compassion, empathy, kindness, forgiveness, and love have evolved as selective survival tools, fostering the survival of a more supportive, productive society as surely as does the evolution of superior senses, enzyme systems, and other adaptive outcomes of natural selection.

So please understand, by making positive nutritional and humanistic choices fundamental to the vegan, whole-food, plant-exclusive lifestyle, you are responsibly promoting your own personal success as well as the life and well-being of everything around you. I implore you to embrace the following idea deep within your consciousness and heart: neither the Earth nor any living creature on it has to be brutally treated or killed for you to achieve your optimal health and weight-loss goals. The vegan approach promotes a remarkable ethical and moral win-win situation that is the most conscious spiritual path you can take to further the evolution of all conscious life for generations to come. Do not underestimate the magnificent power of these choices and the impact that you can make personally. Echoing our interconnected reality and the importance of compassionate personal choices, we can reinforce the idea that each individual's moral progress is a social progress, an ethical advancement detectable in the history of civilization.

Because of the fundamental connectivity of all life, it is my firm belief that our individual choices must respect and promote this connection. As a result, I truly believe that our individual health relies on an ongoing commitment to three basic love affairs that create the best versions of ourselves:

- self-love, exemplified by personal lifestyle choices that work to eliminate and prevent disability and disease and promote the highest level of performance and function;
- the love of all conscious life around us; and
- the love and support of the planet itself on which we live.

There is only one eating plan that supports these three love affairs, and that is the compassionate, vegan, plant-exclusive nutritional approach. The vegan lifestyle is also the most humane and successful approach to long-term weight loss while promoting the sanctity of life and eliminating the environmental burdens and changes that challenge the very existence and survival of our planet. The current personal and environmental threats make the beautiful words of Simon and Garfunkle mere reverie; "the writing of the prophets" is way more than on the subway walls. It is written on the burning ocean floor, suffocating algae, disappearing forests going up in smoke, depleted soils, vanishing species, tortured creatures, starving children, and poisoned air. Our house is on fire and more than 85% of this unconscionable blaze is due to animal food production and consumption. The only solution is to shut down the killing machine and eat plant-exclusive. That's where hope lies in wait and echoes the sound of silent resurrection.

I end this chapter with a poem I wrote a few years back that addresses the mindless reality of separation and suffering that I have discussed and the need to embrace the consciousness of interdependence. This poem was inspired by a restaurant I discovered in Florida called The Butcher Shop, whose obvious agenda truly touched a sore nerve and brought these thoughts and images alive for me.

The Butcher Shop

Sometimes

Life seems

like such a butcher shop,

carving the flesh

of defenseless children and animals

to drench trees and fields and oceans

with the blood of innocence,

tortured souls

find comfort

hugging their own severed limbs

as they bathe in the sweet heat

of their own spilt blood,

the mystery of outside world

just the space

between stars

twinkling notes of doubt

in the black amnesia of heaven.

Yet, all suffering is separation
painted from the palette of ego
hiding out in bodies and perceptions
it holds hostage
that took shape
in the flirtation of separation
from god within,

Love and forgiveness
the only true religion
the only answer
from our one holy Spirit,
and since all others are ourselves
we are compelled
to forgive others and ourselves
for what we really did not do
what has truly never been done
except in the electric circus
in our own minds,
but fight to believe
still exists
in the birth of all universes
that explode
in all our big bangs,
till we journey back
to the place we never left,
the formless ecstatic embrace
of divine light....

PART
3

PLANT-EXCLUSIVE
APPLICATIONS
AND OPTIONS

CHAPTER 12

PRACTICAL NUTRITIONAL
STRATEGIES

A ll too often, when someone decides to shift to a plant-exclusive diet and eliminate processed foods, it can feel like an annoying, difficult, restricted journey of deprivation. It can seem as though at every turn someone is telling you what you can't eat or what you can't do. Let me ask you a question: Do you like feeling deprived? Of course not. In all my years of counseling people, I have yet to find anyone who truly loves deprivation. And very often, if someone repeatedly tells you not to do something, there's a part of your brain that just can't wait to do it, and can't wait to do it in their face. An intriguing, and sometimes extreme, fascination for things or behaviors can arise when you feel forced or pressured to deny yourself those things.

Unfortunately, the deprivation mentality may foster ongoing behavior that can put you at risk by preventing you from making choices that are in your best interest. It is imperative to replace any sense of deprivation with choices and creative substitutions that eliminate any sense of restriction and help you experience and maintain enjoyment and satisfaction as you transition into a healthier way of eating. Whether you are eating meat, dairy products, refined breads, cookies, cake, or whatever, you will see that a diverse, plant-exclusive eating plan provides a remarkable opportunity for delectable tastes, meals, snacks, creative substitutions, and even desserts that will excite you, turn you on, dissolve any sense of self-denial, and help you eliminate dangerous addictive eating habits while supporting health and weight loss.

Put a Rainbow on Your Plate

Give yourself the opportunity to experience the bounty of nature, foods of the highest nutritional value blossoming with the greatest variety of colors, tastes, and smells. It has been known for quite some time that certain chemicals give fruits and vegetables their color and their texture. What makes watermelon red or oranges orange? What we have learned is that the same chemicals that give produce its color and texture also give us the best protection against disease and aging. These are not the variety of well-known vitamins and minerals, but rather a panorama of cofactors like phytonutrients and antioxidants that generate their own health benefits while also enhancing the action of classic vitamins and minerals.

For example, the flavonoids that color citrus fruit, the skin of beans, and berries may slow down the aging process and reduce the risk of heart disease. Flavonoids have been shown to significantly reduce several known risk factors for cardiovascular disease, including total cholesterol, LDL cholesterol, and serum triglyceride levels.[1] You may have heard of resveratrol, an antioxidant found in red grapes, which has prompted a variety of professionals to recommend drinking a glass of red wine per day or taking a resveratrol supplement. It is not just the excesses of cholesterol or LDL cholesterol themselves that promote the risk of heart disease. When LDL cholesterol is oxidized, it is converted into a dangerous free-radical scavenger that can damage blood vessels, promote vascular blockage, and increase the risk of heart and brain disease. Resveratrol acts as an antioxidant to reduce the oxidation of LDL cholesterol, decreasing the risk of heart disease and strokes.[2]

However, resveratrol is in the skin of red grapes; it does not have to be consumed with a toxic chemical like alcohol. You would be better off eating red grapes or drinking a glass of red grape juice, though you won't get the same buzz. (We are definitely a primate that likes to get a buzz with our antioxidants!) Other sources of resveratrol include peanut butter, blueberries, raspberries, mulberries, and raw dark chocolate (without refined sugar or dairy).

I do not recommend taking resveratrol supplements. Whole-food sources provide a smaller, more manageable dose of resveratrol that is naturally combined with other synergistic factors that only whole foods can provide, a benefit not available in resveratrol supplements. This is important to consider since the high dosages found in supplementation may promote some deleterious effects. In a study of men in their 60s, resveratrol supplements decreased the beneficial impact of exercise on cardiovascular health, blunting the decrease in LDL cholesterol and serum triglycerides and the increase in oxygen uptake that usually follows exercise training.[3] Remember, simply because something is good, more is not necessarily better. In fact, often when it comes to nutrients, less is more, and more is potentially harmful or even toxic.

The greatest assortment and quantity of antioxidants, the nutrients that quench the action of disease-promoting free radicals, exist in fruits and vegetables. ORAC (oxygen radical absorbance capacity) scores, which measure the capacity of different foods to absorb and neutralize free radicals, are the highest for berries and beans and are high across the board for greens and a variety of other fruits and vegetables. These "superfoods" are not only fundamental in any healthy vegan diet, but because of their micronutrient content and ability to reduce inflammation, they also are incredibly valuable for long-term weight loss.

Because of the relationship between color and nutritional value, you don't need to be a biochemist to build a healthy meal; you just need to put a rainbow on your plate. Fill your plate with a multicolored cornucopia of fruits and vegetables. What's the color of the cuisine in most fast-food joints and hospitals in America? It is basically white, brown, and gray. You know it can't compete with the rainbow. What happens to the color of fruits and vegetables when you overcook them? It gets bleached out as some of the value and quality is lost, so you want to eat your fruits and vegetables in as close to the raw state as you can. If you do cook them, lightly steam or sauté them; do not incinerate or embalm them. Table 4 describes a color-coded rainbow chart of a wide variety of fruits and vegetables.

Nature's Rainbow: Fruits and Vegetables Color Your Plate

- **Red:** Tomatoes, red peppers, watermelon, beets, radishes, apples, cherries, raspberries, strawberries
- **Orange:** Carrots, mangos, peaches, apricots, sweet potato
- **Orange/Yellow:** Citrus fruits, papaya, banana, yellow cherries
- **Yellow/Green:** Yellow peppers, corn, green beans, squash, Yukon gold potato, avocado, cabbage
- **Green:** Spinach, kale, collard greens, lettuce, bok choy, broccoli, Brussels sprouts, Swiss chard
- **White/Green:** Cauliflower, garlic, onions, mushrooms, scallions, asparagus, cucumber
- **Purple/Red:** Purple cabbage, eggplant, grapes, blueberries, plums

---

Table 4. The colors of nutrient-rich fruits and vegetables.
Rainbow colors indicate the diversity of the wide range of vitamins, phytonutrients, and antioxidants in various whole fruits and vegetables.

Another point to keep in mind is that minerals in food are more resistant to the effects of heat and cooking than vitamins in food and supplements. If you make a vegetable soup, for example, the mineral content of the soup will be somewhat maintained and intact. However, vitamins are more fragile and more prone to damage by heat and oxidation, so the vitamin content can be quite compromised in heavily cooked soups and vegetable dishes. Again, I recommend that you eat a large portion of your vitamin-rich fruits and vegetables in the raw or lightly steamed state.

Be Mindful and Give Yourself the Time to Change

As you transition into a more vegan, whole-plant approach and begin to incorporate new plant-exclusive choices and substitutions, be patient, and remember that these changes will not occur overnight. Your tastes and food preferences are conditioned by condiments, additives, and unique chemicals in foods that can program cravings and addictions that make change quite difficult. In addition, the choices that you are making now have grown out of the long history of your diet; their repetition has made them a part of your behavioral repertoire. Therefore, it can take some time for your taste sensitivity and brain to adjust so that you can become accustomed to and appreciate simple, natural, healthy food, which is critical for extinguishing addictions and for new choices to become part of your life. Over time, they will weave their way into the behavioral tapestry of your brain and nervous system.

Cheese, refined sugar, and salt are examples of foods and additives with addictive properties, as I well know from personal experience. Having been raised in an Italian household, refined sugar, salt, and cheese were significant parts of my diet, and eliminating cheese was a daunting task. I grew up eating cheese on top of cheese on top of cheese, fresh Italian cheeses (ricotta and mozzarella) made daily by shop owners who used milk from their own dairy farms in New York and New Jersey. This stuff came out soft and dripping warm milk, a mind-blowing, seductive cheese that would melt in your mouth. It took a long time to extinguish that craving and build new, healthier choices into my diet, and many of my clients echo that story. In fact, it was the hardest food for me to eliminate, harder to get off of than sugar or meat. In all honesty, to make things easier for me during the transition to a vegan diet, I opted for using processed plant-based cheeses made from soy or fermented nuts, tapioca, concentrated oils, salt, and other additives. While I reasoned that these products would satisfy my taste for cheese, keeping me and others who used them in the fold of vegan consciousness and doing less harm to animals and the environment, the truth is that they contain ingredients that pose major health risks. I do not recommend them now, and they are not on the WFPE, SOS-free eating plan. These products are highly processed and made from ingredients and additives that have no place in a healthy diet promoting optimal weight and body fat. Worse, many of the plant-based cheese substitutes are made with substantial amounts of coconut oil, which is more than 90% saturated fat (significantly more than meat, butter, and lard) and can cause risky elevations of cholesterol and cardiovascular disease.[xiv]

Examining the chemistry of dairy and how it interacts with the body reveals a reason for its addictive nature. The major protein in milk is casein, which in the body is converted into something called beta-casomorphine-7.[4] Casomorphins are protein fragments with opiate-like effects similar to endorphins (the natural opiates in our brains) and pharmaceutical opiates like heroin, Vicodin, and Oxycontin. So, cheese and other dairy products, including milk, ice cream, yogurt, and butter, trigger a slight opiate response, a subtle kind of high, and when you remove them abruptly from the diet, there can be an opiate-like withdrawal that increases craving and makes it that much harder to stop eating them.

Eliminating dairy products is made even more difficult because of another characteristic of casomorphins: they also act as direct histamine promoters in humans, triggering allergic and inflammatory responses.[5]

[xiv] In certain recipes and food preparation presented in Chapter 14, the combination of dulse flakes (seaweed) and nutritional yeast can impart a mild cheese flavor that is more optimal.

This assault on the immune system can interfere with satiety signals, promote overeating and compulsive food use, and compromise your long-term, successful weight loss.

Sugar and salt are also highly addictive foods. We have already discussed how refined sugar elicits a cocaine-like pleasure response that sets up a dangerous "pleasure trap."[6] (See Chapter 5.) Eliminating it abruptly provokes withdrawal symptoms and discomfort that reinforce craving, increased use, and potential addiction over time. Also, as I mentioned previously, the excessive use of salt in our diets is a classic example of how taste sensitivity can be blunted by additives in our food, thereby driving you to add more and more salt and salty condiments to compensate for your diminished sense of taste. Rest assured that as you embrace a predominantly natural, plant-exclusive diet, your taste sensitivity will improve, and you will more than adequately satisfy your daily needs for sodium without adding additional sprinkles.

Most of the sodium consumed in our culture comes from packaged, processed, and restaurant foods.[7] Unfortunately, that's also true for a lot of vegan and vegetarian packaged food, since a large amount of sodium is often added to these items, too. Note that if you are eating canned or packaged products—and let's face it, many of us do to some degree—you must be careful. Many, if not most, canned and packaged foods often have too much added salt. However, for many products there are now low-sodium and sodium-free options readily available. Read the labels and keep your sodium intake from packaged and canned foods below approximately 800 mg per day. Instead, take most of your sodium from your whole, plant-based foods.

As a side note, if you are craving salt, it could relate to a vegetable/mineral deficiency, and the increased consumption of more sodium-rich vegetables, like celery, zucchini, Swiss chard, and organic tomatoes, can help remedy the situation. A low level of sodium in your blood also can relate to exhaustion and a suppression of the adrenal glands, which are the glands of stress and metabolism. These glands release the steroid hormone aldosterone that plays a role in sodium balance in the body. Factors that promote stress and exhaustion can tax and deplete the adrenals, resulting in a dysfunction of sodium regulation, the elimination of excessive sodium from the body, and a craving for salt. When dealing with the removal of added salt in your diet, a helpful strategy is to use an assortment of herbs, vegetables, and spices like many of the healthy plant-based ethnic cultures do. A generous use of garlic, arugula, onions, mushrooms, basil, oregano, turmeric, ginger, sage, rosemary, dill, thyme, etc., can add significant, delicious flavors and nutrition to any dish and will help you make the transition to salt-free cooking and a low-sodium diet much easier.

Transitioning away from dairy products, sugar, and salt means that you have to be a little bit patient and give yourself the time for your taste sensitivity to improve. It will not happen overnight, but good food has good taste. Spend your food dollar on the best-quality plant foods you can find. You deserve it. Spend $3 on an incredible mango if you have to; you won't be eating expensive meats or dairy or processed foods, so spend your food dollar on the best produce you can find. The huge range of vegetables and fruits available these days offers a variety of delightful, delectable flavors. Many people have gotten so used to highly salted and chemically seasoned foods and goaded into overeating because of this stimulation that they have lost the ability to experience the nuances and true tastes of natural food. When you try simple, less-salted, plant-exclusive foods yet find them to lack flavor, you have met the problem—and it is you, or more specifically, your desensitized taste buds. However, as your taste buds' sensitivity improves, the taste of simple, plain, whole, natural foods will blow your mind.

I don't choose to eat this way because I want to deprive myself, but because it turns me on and excites me. I love to eat. Eating should be a personal and social pleasure in addition to satisfying our basic biological needs. When I eat, I want to be so blown away by the taste of natural food that I can't wait to eat it again. I want to look forward to eating and experiencing the diversity of flavors, colors, and textures that nature's bounty provides. I want to feel a level of satisfaction, energy, and vitality that nothing but this food can provide. Even if you're not there yet, just know that as time passes, you will get to a place where you can eat salad with little or no dressing and love it!

Patience, time, and commitment to healthy food choices is the required mantra. Just know, deep within your being, that the feelings and experiences of satisfaction, energy, well-being, and vibrant, healthy body weight are available to you whenever you choose to embrace them. And as you experience this energy and vitality, it will reinforce your drive to continue on this path.

Also, understand that an aware, mindful relationship to food and eating and an increased appreciation of the foods that are in your best interest are critical for successful weight loss. A simple strategy to improve this relationship is to slow things down, literally: eat more slowly. In our hectic culture, the average time of a midday meal in a place like New York City is just a matter of minutes. But remember that digestion does not start in the gut; it starts in the mouth. The more time spent chewing, the more one's digestion is improved. While drinking small amounts of water during a meal can help ensure adequate hydration in your day, drinking liquids is not typically recommended at mealtimes. Liquids can urge you to chew less and swallow food whole, making digestion more difficult. Liquids also can dilute and interfere with the strict chemical environment required by digestive enzymes, compromising the digestive process, and this interference with digestion can negatively affect the availability and utilization of nutrients, thereby compromising any weight-loss program. You rarely see animals in nature eat and drink at the same time. So, if you drink anything at meal time, a small amount of plain water is definitely the only drink of choice. I can't tell you how many people I have helped to eliminate problems of reflux and gastric upsets just by getting them to eat more slowly and to stop drinking at mealtimes.

Furthermore, eating should be a time of reverence. It is a time when all that we are is nurtured, not something to do mindlessly while watching TV or reading the pages of the sports section. By slowing things down, we can become more aware of what we are using food for, what the Buddhists call mindful consumption. As we become more attentive to and thoughtful about our food use, we can more effectively understand the role that food plays in our lives and dramatically improve our experiences with food consumption. This is essential to long-term, successful weight loss.

A Simple Exercise

Try the following exercise in mindfulness centered around food use. It will help you slow things down and bring your awareness completely into present time.

- Sit down at the place where you typically eat with an apple in hand. Sweet Pink Lady apples are great for this exercise, but any apple, fruit, or even vegetable will do.

- Close your eyes and feel the shape and texture of the fruit.

- Visualize the sturdy tree that gave birth to this fruit. See the farmer nurturing the soil that fed this tree. Feel the vibrant energy of the farmer and the earth as it brought this piece of nature's bounty to maturity.

- Bring the fruit to your nose and mouth. Smell the apple, and let the aroma of the apple fill your brain and evoke any images or memories you may associate with this experience.

- Take a small bite of the apple, and feel the sweet juice gently explode in your mouth.

- Allow the piece of the apple to rest on your tongue as you experience its texture and sweetness completely in your mouth.

- Then, slowly chew the piece until it completely liquefies in your mouth, and its sweet nectar runs down your throat.

- As it enters your body, visualize the juice and life of the fruit circulating and nurturing your body.

- Repeat these steps with several bites of the apple, and allow this patient, mindful approach, even if for just a few moments, to become a part of the various meals of your life any time you can.

CHAPTER 13

SIMPLE MEAL PLANS

N ow that I've provided the essential background and foundation for this exciting journey into the world of whole plant food and its impact on weight and body fat, let's see how easy it can be to implement a WFPE, SOS-free diet plan into your lifestyle. Although this is not a cookbook, I am committed to sharing some recipes and meal plans with you that I have found to be the tastiest, quickest, and easiest to prepare at home for you and your family.

Breakfast

Breakfast is a perfect time to incorporate fresh fruit in the diet. This can be done simply by having a bowl of organic, seasonal fresh fruit all by itself. I recommend the combination of at least two to three kinds of fruit.

Fruit should be eaten when it is in season. In fall and winter, there are many varieties of apples, grapes (green, black, and red), bananas, several varieties of pears, citrus (oranges, grapefruits, tangelos, tangerines, kiwi), some berries, persimmons, and pomegranates available. However, when it comes to many luscious fruits, spring and summer are truly the seasons that abound with a cornucopia of peaches, plums, apricots, cherries, melons, mangos, and berries. Invest in organic fruits whenever possible to get the cleanest options with no pesticides and to support the growers who provide them.[xv]

If you have been eating a more conventional diet and are dealing with insulin resistance or adrenal dysfunction, fruit alone may not be substantial enough initially to maintain stable blood sugar and satisfy your appetite in the hours between breakfast and lunch. In that case, I recommend some celery, cucumber slices, crisp romaine lettuce leaves with fruit, and/or a small palmful of almonds or walnuts (one to two ounces). This will boost your satiety and keep you stable until lunchtime while providing some additional high-quality protein and omega-3 oils. Almonds from California and Italy are nonirradiated; choose those for the highest-quality raw almonds or raw almond butter. Cooked cereals (e.g., oatmeal, buckwheat, quinoa, or brown rice) in addition to fresh fruit also can be a stabilizing influence at breakfast.

Green vegetable smoothies containing some fruit continue to be a popular option for people on the go and can be an effective way to start your day. Deep greens such as kale, collard greens, mustard greens, bok choy, dandelion greens, and spinach have tremendous value in our diets. Remember all those greens your grandma tried to give you? Grandmas knew where it was at! Unfortunately, as much as I may recommend greens to you, and as much as you may agree that they are very important, as a rule you're probably just not eating enough of them. Let's be realistic: how many people really dive into these greens on a daily basis? The fact is that greens are the smallest part of the typical diet of all people in the U.S. and other Western nations. So, in addition to including them in cooked (steamed or sautéed) and raw forms, green smoothies are an effective way to get more deep greens in your diet. This is especially true for children and adolescents; smoothies can be an easy way to enhance the variety and quantity of greens in their diets.

Here are some some of my favorite breakfast options.

[xv] See Chapter 20 for a discussion of toxins in food.

Green Smoothies

All you need to make green smoothies is a high-speed blender. Although expensive blenders like a Vitamix or Blendtec are commonly used, a less expensive Nutribullet or The Beast work just fine for home use.

My Favorite Green Smoothie

This smoothie in the morning will keep your blood sugar, hunger, and energy stable until lunchtime without cravings.

Ingredients:

$\frac{1}{2}$ cup organic pineapple (frozen or raw mangos or apples can also be used)

$\frac{1}{2}$ cup fresh or frozen berries (raspberries, blueberries, strawberries)

$\frac{1}{2}$ cup kale, swiss chard, and/or bok choy

$\frac{1}{2}$ cup spinach and/or parsley or arugala

2 tablespoon of chia, hemp, or ground flaxseed (see Notes)

3–4 small slices of fresh organic ginger

1–2 pitted Medjool dates for sweetener (optional)

1 teaspoon of maca powder (optional)

Small amount of liquid to blend (see Notes)

Add all ingredients to the blender and blend until smooth.

Notes:

- Chia, hemp, and ground, powdered flax seeds provide your daily omega-3 oil needs. Whole flax seeds tend not to digest as well as the other seeds and need to be ground up first.

- For liquid, there are three options to add to the container for smooth blending. You can use distilled or any form of fresh distilled or spring water, unsweetened organic almond or soy milk without carrageenan or added oil, or raw, organic coconut water.

- Maca powder provides additional high-quality antioxidants and hormone-stabilizing effects that keep appetite suppressed and energy and blood sugar balanced and stable.

Hot and Cold Cereals

Gluten-free oatmeal made from slow-cooked steel-cut oats (or even just rolled oats) can be served with or without unsweetened, oil-free almond, soy, hemp, or rice milks and topped with berries to make a great breakfast. Berries are one of the highest antioxidant foods, and they will satisfy your need to put something sweet on the oatmeal without lathering it with higher-glycemic, calorie-dense options like sugar or maple syrup. A wonderful, tasty option is to add frozen berries and mangos as well as cut-up apples to your oatmeal as it is cooking. This invests the oatmeal with the delicious, warm sweetness of these fruits. When the oatmeal is done, you can add a tablespoon of chia, hemp, or ground flax seeds, and add some ground cinnamon or pumpkin pie spice. Other gluten-free hot or cold cereals can be made from buckwheat, rice, millet, or quinoa.

Unfortunately, many almond, soy, hemp, and rice milks have carrageenan as an ingredient. Because carrageenan can disrupt the healthy bacterial environment of your gut (the microbiota), causing dysbiosis and provoking inflammation, potential weight gain, and stress to the immune system, it is not recommended. If you decide to use plant milks, make sure they do not have carrageenan, added sugar, oils, or other ingredients other than just the main ingredient and water. Always read ingredient lists and nutrition labels to ensure you're choosing the purest plant milk available. Several unsweetened milks (soy, almond, and rice) do not use these ingredients and are recommended, and plant milks can also be made easily at home, utilizing recipes available online and in many vegetarian and vegan cookbooks.

Gluten-Free and Whole-Grain Products

If or when your bread monster rears its hungry head, sprouted-grain and or gluten-free English muffins or breads can be used. Enjoy them plain or with raw almond butter or avocado as a spread. Just keep in mind that the calorie density of any bread product is higher than ideal, so they should be used sparingly in an ongoing weight-loss program.

Lunch

For many people, because of hectic schedules and time constraints, salads are an easy, convenient, and delicious lunchtime option. I recommend a large salad meal for any meal—and notice I didn't say a side salad!

Salad Is the Meal

I recommend putting as many green leafy and vegetable items in your salads as possible. Use at least three different leafy greens from the variety of lettuces (including romaine, Boston, bibb, and red leaf) plus spinach, arugula, broccoli, cauliflower, a variety of sprouts (especially sunflower greens, snow pea greens, buckwheat, and mung bean), onions, mushrooms, multicolored peppers, grated carrots, beets, cabbage, savory herbs, beans (red or black), and one to two ounces of a food with some protein or fat, such as nuts, avocado, sodium-free olives, or tofu. For an additional treat, I recommend cutting a baked white or sweet potato into your salad. This can really make your salad pop and is a singularly great taste sensation.

Salad dressings can be purchased commercially, but almost all of them have too much added oil, salt, and sugar, and those that don't are just chemical concoctions. Dressings are easy to make at home, or you can just use some of the fantastic flavored balsamic vinegars that are available commercially. Here are three salad dressing recipes that will delight your senses and make salad-eating something to really look forward to. Each makes enough for four large salads.

Dr. Frank's Sunshine-Ginger Dressing

Ingredients:

> 2–4 ounces freshly squeezed lemon juice or apple cider vinegar
>
> 4 ounces raw cashews
>
> 1 cucumber
>
> 2–3 celery stalks
>
> 3–4 thin slices raw ginger
>
> 2–3 slices fresh turmeric
>
> 6 ounces freshly squeezed carrot or orange juice
>
> ½ red bell pepper

For all dressings containing nuts, it is best to put the recommended quantity of nuts in the blender, add an amount of water to completely cover the nuts, and blend the nuts to a smooth consistency in a high-speed blender first before adding any other ingredients. Then add all other ingredients and blend again until smooth.

Green Goddess Dressing

Ingredients:

> 4 ounces lemon juice, apple cider vinegar, or balsamic vinegar
>
> 2 ounces raw cashews
>
> 2 ounces raw walnuts
>
> 1 whole cucumber
>
> 3–4 celery stalks
>
> 1–2 small cloves fresh garlic
>
> Small handful curly Italian parsley
>
> 1–2 ounces fresh basil

2 ounces fresh spinach

4 ounces freshly squeezed organic orange juice

3–4 slices fresh ginger

Blend until smooth.

Date Mustard Dressing (the biggest crowd-pleaser)
Ingredients:

2 ounces raw cashews

2 ounces walnuts

2 cups water

1–2 tablespoon unsalted stone-ground or creamy yellow mustard

¼ cup apple cider vinegar

3 pitted Medjool dates (or 6 Deglet Noor)

Blend the cashews, walnuts, and water until smooth, then add remaining ingredients and blend again until smooth. This dressing is also fantastic as a sauce for steamed vegetables and baked potatoes.

Between-Meal Snacks

If you have the problem of insulin resistance, which is common among people with weight issues, sugar cannot effectively enter your cells. As a result, your cells will be starved for sugar, and you will experience craving between meals. Until insulin function is stabilized, you will crave sugar and fat. So, what do most people do? They usually opt for the endless variety of sweets, refined/processed foods, diet bars (typically loaded with an array of sweeteners and additives), sodas, coffee, chocolate, and other stimulants, which only reinforce insulin dysfunction, adrenal exhaustion, and more craving.

The following snack combination has helped many people reduce craving and compulsive food abuse in between meals:

3–4 raw walnuts

3–4 celery or carrot sticks or cucumber slices

apple slices of your choice (preferably a green apple)

1 small salt-free, gluten-free cracker (optional)

Make sure that you eat all of these together. Even if you don't eat all of it, have a little taste of each of these items together. This combination of items is good for several reasons. They stabilize blood sugar very well, they're tasty, and they are all crunchy. (You know how much we all like that oral crunchy thing!)

If nuts present a problem for you, replace them with a few salt-free olives or avocado. A few ounces of plain tofu or plain unsweetened coconut-, soy-, or almond-milk yogurt will also work in lieu of nuts. A few ounces of hummus or dips like guacamole or bean dips can also be viable between-meal options.

This snack strategy works better and is healthier than the typical quick-fix choices people usually make. It will especially satisfy the mid-afternoon energy slump that many people experience that can be associated with a drop in adrenal function consistent with the natural shift in the circadian rhythm of the endocrine system. This prevents craving for refined sugar-laden cookies, cakes, and candy and for caffeine-rich products like coffee, chocolate, and sodas, which only reinforce more adrenal exhaustion, and sugar-craving.

Dinner

Conventionally, most people eat the biggest meal of the day at night for dinner, and it is quite common for people to go out to dinner and to socialize around food in the evening hours. However, it can be argued that we have an inborn directive linked to the body's natural circadian rhythm to consume the larger-calorie meal closer to midday, while evening hours are actually better-suited for smaller meals as we wind down and prepare for sleep at the end of the day. Other health systems, such as Oriental medicine and Ayurveda, propose that the strongest digestive fire, our peak digestive efficiency, actually occurs midday and not in the evening hours, supporting the idea that our biggest meal should be closer to lunchtime, not dinnertime.

In my experience, weight loss is typically more dramatic and consistent when you eat according to this pattern. So, as you begin a new lifestyle approach and weight-loss program, whenever possible, try front-loading your daily calories more in your midday meal and taper off with fewer calories over the rest of the day.

With that in mind, if you ever have a craving in the evening after dinner—and many of us do like having something sweet as a dessert after dinner or as an evening snack—it is in your best interest to consume only satisfying, low-calorie snacks as a protection against reactive weight gain. Fruit is ideal for this purpose. My best simple recommendation is to eat a small amount of fresh fruit, e.g., grapes, berries, apple slices, or grapefruit segments.

In addition, as a regular change in the timing pattern of your food intake, intermittent fasting can spark healthy metabolic changes that promote easier weight loss and weight management.[xvi] Try finishing your evening meal between 5:00–7:00 and then have your breakfast between 8:00–10:00. By doing this, you will be eating in a window of about 10 hours and fasting for about 14 hours, which will promote lowered blood sugar, reduced insulin release, and a more normal, healthy release of growth hormone. As a result, your body will better move from sugar and energy storage to fat metabolism and weight loss.

[xvi] See Chapter 10 for more on intermittent fasting.

The general structure of your dinner menus should be based around the following:

- Begin with a salad smaller or equal to the large salad eaten at lunch.

- After that, include at least two to three dark greens and veggies, steamed or sautéed in vegetable broth or balsamic vinegar—never oil. There are many to choose from: kale, collard greens, mustard greens, Swiss chard, spinach, broccoli rabe, broccoli, bok choy, cauliflower, zucchini, other squashes, asparagus, cabbages, or Brussels sprouts. Other veggies are also recommended, but focus on the dark ones first.

- For your main dish, a wide variety of additional tasty options are available, including various vegetable stews or casseroles loaded with grains, legumes, and potatoes; whole-grain pasta dishes; and organic, gluten-free burgers. Recipes for some of these options, including gourmet raw-food options, are presented in the following chapter.

As we have discussed, it is most important to be concerned with foods that provide low calorie density and high nutrient density. By eating a whole-food, plant-exclusive diet free of salt, oil, and sugar, it is not necessary to waste your time and energy worrying about portion control. If you follow my recommendations, you can just eat until you are full.

Special Considerations for General Meal Planning
A Word About Nuts

Notice that I only recommend one or two ounces of nuts in any single day. Remember how I said that the healthiest diets average about 600 calories per pound? Nuts range from about 2,400–3,200 calories per pound because as much as 70% of their calories is derived from fat. As a result, it's very easy to raise the fat content and calorie density of the diet if you overeat nuts.

Nevertheless, nuts provide significant health benefits for heart and brain health and are an important fat and protein option for any healthy vegan diet. My four favorite nuts are walnuts, almonds, Brazil nuts, and filberts (hazelnuts). These nuts provide an array of antioxidants like vitamin E, flavonoids (found in the skins of almonds and walnuts), complete proteins, selenium, and folic acid. The king of nuts is the walnut. Walnuts have the lowest saturated-fat content, the highest vitamin content, and a more concentrated form of omega-3 fatty acids than some of the other nuts. Just keep in mind the one- to two-ounce limit per day. Avoid eating them out-of-hand; instead, chop them up and use them as an addition to your salads or breakfast bowls. Another strategy that works very well is to buy one-to two-ounce paper cups and divide whatever quantity of nuts you buy among the cups, stored in your refrigerator. Whenever you want nuts, you can just take out one of thes cups and confidently maintain portion control.

The Use of Soy Products

There has been some controversy about the use of food products made from soybeans in vegan diets because of the potential impact of genistein and daidzein, soy phytoestrogens which resemble body estrogens, on cancers of the breast, endometrium, ovaries, and prostate. Elevations in the production, drug intake, and circulation of natural human estrogens have been linked with an increased risk of cancer in the breast, ovaries, and endometrium in women, leading to some concern that an increase of phytoestrogens may similarly contribute to cancer risk. However, a vast body of evidence strongly indicates that this concern is unwarranted and that soy products have significant positive effects of on health.[1]

In the human body there are two different estrogen receptors, alpha and beta, to which estrogen can attach, exerting a variety of effects. Estrogens produced in the ovaries and fat cells or taken as hormone replacement drug therapy preferentially bind with the estrogen alpha receptor, sending signals to hormone-positive cancer cells to grow. Phytoestrogens in soy products, however, bind with a 1,600% greater affinity to the estrogen beta receptor, which exerts an anti-estrogen, anti-cancer effect. Soy phytoestrogens can also bind to the alpha receptors, blocking body estrogen from attaching to them while producing only 1/10–1/100 the cancer-signaling capacity of body estrogen. thereby significantly reducing cancer risk.[1] Soy products also decrease the level of circulating estrogens by blocking the conversion of other steroids into estrogen,[2] and genistein has been shown to block the binding of the body estrogen estradiol to breast cancer cells, thereby inhibiting cancer cell growth.[3] Furthermore, soy phytoestrogens not only reduce cancer risk by blocking cancer-promoting receptors in the breast; they also stop the excessive production of body estrogen by blocking the estrogen-promoting enzyme aromatase in breast cancer cells.[4] Cancers of the uterus and ovaries are also mediated only by the alpha receptors, so soy products don't have negative effects on them. In fact, phytoestrogens are linked to protective effects, and studies have shown that women who ate the most soy products had 30% less endometrial cancer and almost 50% less ovarian cancer.[5]

In some of the largest soy studies to date, extending over many years, even small amounts of soy products (one-half to one serving a week) were associated with significant decreases in mortality from and recurrence of breast cancer.[6,7] And an extensive review of five cohort studies including over 11,000 subjects concluded that soy definitively does not increase breast cancer but in fact decreases the occurrence, recurrence, and death rate—in every single study.[8] The benefit and effectiveness of soy products is further vindicated by epidemiological studies and observations of Chinese and Japanese women in Asia, who consume diets rich in soy foods yet have remarkably low breast cancer rates.[9-11]

There has also been some controversy and confusion about the potential negative goitrogenic impact of soy products on the production of thyroid hormones and thyroid function. To briefly reiterate what I discussed previously, thyroid hormones are essential to fat, sugar, and energy metabolism, and when these hormones are reduced, there can be reactive weight gain even with lowered calorie intake. In addition, when thyroid hormones are low, the brain attempts to stimulate thyroid function by increasing the release of thyroid-stimulating hormone (TSH) that can promote an enlargement of the thyroid known as a goiter. There is some evidence that soy in the diet can modestly raise the levels of TSH (a marker for lower thyroid function), but there was no evidence of any negative effects on the production of thyroid hormones or thyroid function.[12]

In an extensive review of both healthy adults and patients with low thyroid function, there was no significant evidence that soy foods had any negative effect on people with normal thyroid function and adequate iodine intake. However, in patients with already existing low thyroid function and in whom iodine intake is deficient, there is some evidence that soy foods may promote some decrease in thyroid function, requiring an increase of the dose of thyroid hormone.[13] Consistent with these data, iodine deficiency greatly increased antithyroid effects of soy products, and iodine supplementation is protective of any negative impact of soy on thyroid function.[14] The consensus of the evidence base is that people with low thyroid function can consume modest amounts of soy food products and experience the benefits in their diet as long as they maintain adequate iodine in their diets. As we mentioned previously, the daily need for iodine is 150 micrograms daily for adults, which can be obtained by including the seaweeds dulse and nori in your diet or by taking iodine in supplemental form.

Edamame (immature soybeans) and soy milk made from just organic soybeans and water are considered whole soy foods that can be eaten several times a week. Enjoy soy milk on your morning cereal and in recipes calling for plant milk, and choose edamame as a side dish or snack.

Other common soy foods are processed. Tofu is made of soybeans that are boiled and crushed, treated to separate the curds and whey, and pressed into blocks; tempeh, miso, and natto are fermented. Fermentation of soy products has been shown to provide additional health benefits to your diet because it significantly reduces phytates and converts the phytonutrient isoflavones in soy into their most active form.[1] The natural process of fermentation also provides a diversity of probiotic organisms to your gut microbiota that can decrease gut inflammation, gas, and bloating.

In light of the benefits of soy products, foods made from processed soybeans can be included in the WFPE, SOS-free eating plan. However, my weight-loss program eliminates as much processed food as possible, so I recommend tofu, tempeh, miso, and natto be eaten in moderation, only about four to six ounces of organic, non-GMO soy products per week, if you choose to use them at all. Try dishes such as scrambled organic tofu for breakfast or tofu/tempeh stir-fry with vegetables (without oil) for lunch or dinner.

Other soy-based items (some soy milks, soy cheeses, soy-based meat substitutes, etc.) are made with hyper-processed soy protein derivatives and soy protein isolates; these are to be avoided entirely. Also, always keep in mind that soybeans are one of the most disturbingly genetically-modified (GMO) crops on the planet, heavily sprayed with the toxic herbicide glyphosate, so it's critical to make sure that any soy products you buy are 100% organic and GMO-free.[xvii]

[xvii] It's interesting to me how the subversive forces of our food industry and government have filled people with fear and continue to tell them to avoid soy products at all costs, while milk, dairy, animal products, processed foods, and refined sugar, which are much more notorious for heart disease and cancer risk, fly under the radar. I hope that this starts to bother you as much as it bothers me. Let's be realistic. The epidemics of heart disease, cancer, and obesity in the U.S. are not due to the overconsumption of soybeans!

The Use of Organic Greens and Vegetables

In my discussion of deep greens, I have consistently recommended organic greens. This is an extremely important consideration for long-term weight loss. Leafy greens, cruciferous vegetables like broccoli and cauliflower, and plants like celery, cucumber, carrots, and squash all grow close to the ground with relatively short root systems. When they are sprayed with pesticides, toxic chemicals get on the surface of these plants, but also are taken up by their root systems into the bodies of the plants. This toxicity can, with repeated use over time, contribute to a wide range of hormonal imbalances in all mammals, including humans, and may provoke the overproduction of fat, feeding the epidemic of obesity. [xviii]

Furthermore, it is important to consider that cruciferous vegetables, including cabbages, Brussels sprouts, cauliflower, kale, mustard greens, and collard greens, contain chemicals called isothiocyanates, which can be goitrogenic (capable of interfering with thyroid-hormone production).[9] Yet the nutritional value of these foods is very high and remarkably beneficial for any health and weight-loss programs, so you don't want to avoid these foods completely. As discussed previously, the good news is that when these plants are steamed or cooked, the isothiocyanates are altered, and any potential negative effects on thyroid function are significantly reduced or completely eliminated. Therefore, if there is any suggestion of a sluggish thyroid or a history of thyroid problems, I would recommend eating these vegetables in the cooked state and less in raw green smoothies or raw-food preparations.

The Use of Animal Products

I recommend never eating or using any animal products at all. In fact, their use is directly opposed to my compassionate weight-loss program and vegan lifestyle. I have emphatically reinforced the need and power of the WFPE, SOS-free approach for optimal health, weight and body

---

[xviii] This is discussed extensively in Chapter 20.

fat. But people have been sold the unthinkable idea that eating lean meat is in their best interest for health and weight loss, which has provided an extreme false sense of security to dieters opting for fish and lean meat. This is a dangerous illusion. As I have mentioned previously, cholesterol is a major part of the cell membrane of all animal cells and is therefore a significant component of the muscle meat of all animals—and it's primarily in the lean meat, not in the fat. Commercially sold salmon and other fish also contain considerable mercury and PCB contamination, and there is potential arsenic contamination in chicken.

Focusing your diet on plant-exclusive protein sources such as deep greens, nuts, legumes, whole grains, and minimal amounts of soy products is truly the way to go for overall health and successful weight loss. But if you currently feel compelled to make a more gradual transition and include some animal products in your diet, it is critical that they be an extremely limited part of your diet, meaning no more than a few ounces per week. Here's a strategy that will help you control the quantity of animal protein as you hopefully transition fully into a completely WFPE, SOS-free approach. Open your hand with your thumb extended and then fold the remaining fingers down tightly until your fingertips touch your upper palm. The part of your palm that you can still see should be the maximum size of the portion of animal protein that is ever on your plate in any week. On the other hand, the amount of salad and veggies on your plate should be the size of a good-sized, open-armed hug. What happens in countries like the U.S.? Salad is about the size of our palms, and the animal protein is exploding off the plate. A local restaurant in my community advertised a remarkable deal on a 48-ounce steak. Does anyone ever really have to put three pounds of meat on their plate? You may as well bring the cow to the table, take the head off, and eat your way through the carcass. It is inconceivable.

If you work with the idea that meat or any other concentrated foods are the small part of the meal, and the salad and veggies the biggest part, you will feel satisfied at a much lower calorie density. I discussed this earlier, but it is worth mentioning again. If you take a dish of pasta, for example, and replace half the pasta with a nonstarchy vegetable like broccoli or spinach, you will significantly reduce the calorie content of the meal while significantly increasing the nutrient value of the meal, and you'll still feel satisfied. However, I do want to emphasize again that this program is not about focusing on calorie reduction. *It is about eating well, not eating less.* Plant-based foods loaded with nutrients are so low in calorie density that they build in calorie protection naturally, and are better than any other eating plan on planet Earth for providing satisfaction, enjoyment, and long-term weight loss. Just have fun with it!

CHAPTER 14

RECIPES FOR SUCCESS

The recipes that follow are some of my personal favorites, ones that can be part of your lunch or dinner repertoire. Some are my own creations, but many were developed by Collin Cook, the head chef of retreat centers that I have directed over a number of years in South Florida, and by other talented vegan friends and family members. These recipes will bring excitement and diversity to your meal planning while significantly promoting long-term weight loss.

The Black Beans (Frijoles Negros) and Channa Masala recipes come courtesy of my dearest friend and partner, Jayney Goddard. Jayney is one of the coolest vegans I know, and her bean recipes are—in the words of my old neighborhood—simply to die for. Jayney is a longtime vegan and a highly trained homeopath from England. She also is the founder and President of the CMA, The Complementary Medical Association, an organization in the United Kingdom that has been at the vanguard of promoting evidence-based, complementary, holistic health care, animal rights, and whole-food, plant-exclusive (WFPE) nutrition. She publishes a remarkable newsletter, leads vegan health retreats, and provides online training courses in business practices, vegan lifestyle, and stress-response management/resilience for lay and professional audiences. She also is the author of a remarkable recent best-selling book on plant-based age reversal, *Rewind Your Body Clock*. (www.jayneygoddard.org)

Soup

Dr. Frank's Tuscan Veggie Soup
Rich, hearty, and delicious, this soup is even more incredible the next day or two.
Serves 4–6.

Ingredients:

3 quarts water, low-sodium veggie broth, or your own homemade salt-free broth

6 medium carrots, cut small

6 stalks celery, cut small

1 bunch scallions and/or leeks

1 16-ounce can white cannellini beans, drained

4 small gold potatoes or turnips, peeled and cubed

8 ounces mushrooms (white, baby bella, shitake, and/or portobello)

12–16 ounces kale or mustard greens, chopped

6 cloves of garlic, minced

2 ounces raw ginger, minced or grated

2 ounces dill, chopped

1. Add all ingredients to a large pot and bring it to a boil. Simmer about 45 minutes or until the hardest ingredients (the carrots and potatoes) are done.

Entrées

Mushroom Chili with Cashew Sour Cream
This hearty chili will satisfy, nourish, and warm you and your guests!
Serves 4.

Chili Ingredients:

4 cups diced onions

2 cups seeded and diced red bell pepper

3 cups seeded and diced green bell pepper

1½ pounds baby portobello (crimini) mushrooms, minced

2 15-ounce cans no-salt-added, organic kidney beans (or 4 cups home-cooked beans), drained and rinsed

2 15-ounce cans no-salt-added, organic pinto beans (or 4 cups home-cooked beans), drained and rinsed

1 15-ounce can no-salt-added, organic black beans (or 2 cups home-cooked beans), drained and rinsed

2 14.5-ounce cans no-salt-added diced tomatoes

1 15-ounce can no-salt-added crushed tomatoes

1 13.6-ounce can unsweetened lite coconut milk (or cashew cream)

½ cup minced garlic

2 tablespoon smoked paprika

3 tablespoon chili powder

2 teaspoon garlic powder

2 teaspoon ground cumin

1 teaspoon ground black pepper

pinch cayenne pepper (optional)

1 bunch Italian parsley, chopped

Cashew Sour Cream Ingredients:

1 cup raw, unsalted cashew pieces

½ cup water

¼ cup lemon juice

1 tablespoon onion powder

1. First, make the cashew sour cream: add all ingredients to a high-speed blender and blend until smooth. Refrigerate until ready to add to the chili.

2. For the chili, sauté the onions, bell peppers, and mushrooms in a medium sauce pan until tender. Drain off any remaining liquid and set aside.

3. In a large pot, slowly simmer the beans, diced tomatoes, crushed tomatoes, lite coconut milk, and garlic for 45-60 minutes or until the beans are fully cooked. Season with the paprika, chili powder, garlic powder, cumin, black pepper, and cayenne pepper.

4. Add the sautéed mixture to the bean-tomato mix and simmer for 10–15 minutes to blend flavors. Stir in the chopped Italian parsley.

5. Serve topped with sour cream to taste.

A Note About Beans[xix]

All too often, when I talk about the virtues of adding beans and other legumes to the diet, people smile and shake their heads affirmatively, as if they are in agreement with everything I'm saying, all the while saying to themselves, "Yes, beans, but what do I do with them?" For many people, beans are like little rocks in a bag, and they don't have the foggiest notion about how to prepare or use them in their diet. Learning how to cook beans and legumes will diversify your vegan diet while expanding your opportunities

---

[xix] For beans and for all of your canned foods, make sure the cans say three things: organic, no salt added, and BPA-free. BPA is found in the metal casings of cans and is an obesogen and estrogen mimic that promotes cancer risk and reactive fat and weight gain. (See Chapter 20.)

Recipes for Success 207

to incorporate these remarkable high-fiber, high-protein, low-fat, high-antioxidant foods into your life. They can also be sprouted and added to salads and cooked dishes.

As we have previously discussed, legumes (including beans, lentils, and peas) make a significant protein contribution in a vegan, WFPE diet. However, many people often complain that they have difficulty digesting these valuable foods. This is because raw legumes contain small carbohydrate molecules called oligosaccharides that are indigestible and are fermented by your extensive gut microbiota to produce gas, bloating, and digestive distress. Beans also have a trypsin inhibitor, an antinutrient that blocks the digestive enzyme trypsin from adequately digesting the protein in beans, promoting more distress and potential inflammation. However, by soaking raw beans at least 12 hours before cooking, the indigestible oligosaccharides will be drawn out and discarded in the soaking water. Then, by simmering them in lots of fresh water (about 6 cups to one pound of beans) until they are mushy to the modest pressure of a fork, any remaining oligosaccharides and the trypsin inhibitors will be removed or deactivated, making the legumes easily digested. If you are not used to eating beans, it is best to start with small quantities, perhaps focusing on smaller, more easily digestible legumes like lentils, and adding more and different beans and sprouted legumes over time to ease these foods into your routine.

Penne à la Vodka, Vegan Style
This is a favorite recipe created by my son, Dante.
Serves 4.

Ingredients:
2 medium white onions, chopped

32 ounces of organic frozen peas

2 16-ounce jars salt-free, low-oil organic marinara sauce or your own homemade version

1 13.6-ounce can unsweetened lite coconut milk (or cashew cream)

8 ounces fresh basil leaves, chopped

16 ounces gluten-free rice, quinoa, or legume penne pasta

1. Sauté chopped onions until soft, adding the peas for the last minute or two. Set aside.

2. Cook the pasta according to the package instructions. Drain and set aside.

3. Add the lite coconut milk to the marinara and simmer over medium heat for 5 minutes.

4. Add the pasta and basil to the sauce, stir to combine, and cook for an additional 2 minutes. Remove from heat and add the peas and onions.

5. Stir to blend and serve.

Black Beans (Frijoles Negros)
Feeds 2–4 hungry people.

<u>Ingredients:</u>
1 small red onion, finely diced

1 stalk celery, finely diced

2 large cloves garlic, crushed and left to stand for 10 minutes

1 15-ounce can no-salt-added, organic black beans (or 2 cups home-cooked beans), drained and rinsed

1 very small dash apple cider vinegar

16 ounces organic, no-salt-added vegetable stock

1 tablespoon cumin

pinch chili flakes

3 bay leaves

1. Sauté the onion and celery until soft in just a small amount of the stock.

2. Add garlic and continue to sauté for 1–2 minutes, then add all other ingredients. Bring to a simmer—do not boil. You may need to add more stock as the beans cook to keep them covered. The idea is to cook the beans very slowly so that the flavors really integrate. So, just simmer gently for 45–60 minutes until the beans are fully cooked and top up with stock as necessary.

3. Serve with organic brown rice and a green salad and or some steamed green vegetables, and warn your guests about the possibility of stray bay leaves. Top with raw cashew or nondairy sour cream. (See chili recipe above.)

Chef's Note: The reason the garlic is left to stand for 10 minutes after crushing is because the allicin in the garlic reacts with the oxygen in the atmosphere and creates a whole host of beneficial organic compounds which are much more potent than garlic that has not been left to oxidize.

Channa Masala
Serves 4.

Ingredients:

1 15-ounce can no-salt, organic chickpeas (or 2 cups home-cooked chickpeas), drained and rinsed

1 small red onion, finely diced

16-ounce can chopped organic tomatoes

2 large cloves garlic, crushed and left to stand for 10 minutes

16 ounces organic, no-salt-added vegetable stock

2 heaping teaspoons medium-strength curry powder

1. Sauté the onion until soft in just a few tablespoons of the stock, then add garlic to soften.

2. When they are soft and most of the stock is evaporated, add the curry powder to the onion/garlic mixture and sauté for a minute or two to release the full flavor. (Traditionally, Indian spices are sautéed with the onion and garlic.)

3. Add the tomatoes and remaining stock, and simmer until the liquid is reduced by half.

4. Add the drained chickpeas and continue to simmer for about another hour, adding more stock if needed so that it doesn't become too dry.

5. Channa masala is ready when all flavors have really opened up. Adjust seasonings and serve with organic brown basmati rice and salad or steamed greens.

Scrumptious Sweet Potato Latkes
Makes 12–15.

Ingredients:

8 ounces organic baby spinach

2 organic sweet potatoes, grated

½ cup of ground flaxseed

¼ cup diced cilantro

½ teaspoon smoked paprika (mild)

½ teaspoon onion powder

½ teaspoon curry powder

zest and juice of 1 lime

1. Preheat oven to 400°F (200° C) and line two baking sheets with parchment paper.

2. Place the spinach in a large nonstick pan on medium heat and sauté in a small amount of sodium-free veggie broth for a few minutes until wilted. Do not add water and keep the pan uncovered.

3. Add the grated sweet potato to a large bowl and massage to soften.

4. Add the wilted spinach to the sweet potato along with the ground flaxseed, cilantro, spices, lime zest, and lime juice. Mix together by hand.

5. Shape about ¼ cup of the mixture into a tight ball and place on the baking pan. Repeat with the rest of the mixture. Flatten the latkes a bit so they are 2"–3" wide and ½"–1" thick.

6. Bake for 20 minutes, flip, and bake for an additional 10 minutes. Serve immediately.

Chef's Note: These are fantastic for breakfast, lunch, or dinner. Serve plain or top with hummus, guacamole, or other plant condiments, or serve them with steamed greens sprinkled with lemon juice to give them a nice kick. The latkes can be frozen either before or after baking; store in an airtight container or bag.

Brilliant Burgers

These are simply the best WFPE, SOS-free burgers! Courtesy of Candy Myles.

Makes 8–10 burgers.

Ingredients:

1 cup of diced onions

4 cloves garlic

8 ounces crimini mushrooms, diced

1 cup spinach or kale, chopped fine

1 cooked Hannah sweet potato (cream-colored ones with cream-white flesh)

1 cup uncooked rolled oats

2 16-ounce cans black beans (or 4 cups home-cooked beans), drained and rinsed

½ cup chopped cilantro or chopped Italian parsley

2 tablespoons of mild sodium-free or low-sodium taco sauce

1 tablespoon cumin

1 tablespoon smoked paprika

1 tablespoon oregano

1. Cook onions and garlic until lightly browned, then add mushrooms and kale or spinach and continue cooking until mushrooms are cooked.

2. While the above is cooking, mash the sweet potato, beans, oats, seasonings, and herbs together in a large mixing bowl.

3. Add the sautéed veggies to the bowl and mix by hand.

4. Scoop out and form patties and cook over medium-low heat for 10 minutes per side.

5. Alternatively, you can place them on a baking sheet lined with parchment paper and bake at 400°F for 20 minutes. Flip and cook 10 minutes more on the other side.

Chef's Note: If you wish to freeze these, do so before baking.

Weight Control in the Raw

I have emphasized the value of eating a panorama of raw fruits and vegetables, and now it's my intention to turn you on to some novel, interesting, and easy ways to expand your raw-food options. These easy-to-make recipes are a brief introduction to raw-food preparation at home. If you are going to do raw-food preparation on a regular basis, consider getting a dehydrator, a great addition to your kitchen appliance collection. And remember: when making raw foods, be sure to dehydrate them at 115°F or less to retain all their vital enzymes and other nutrients. Try these out, have some fun, and enjoy!

Raw Salads and Entrées

Kale Caesar Salad

Serves 2–4.

Ingredients:

½ bunch curly green or lacinato kale

¼ head Napa cabbage, thinly sliced to resemble Parmesan shreds

½ cup Caesar dressing (recipe below)

handful of onion flax croutons (recipe below)

fresh lemon wedges

1. Rinse and chop greens and place in a large mixing bowl.
2. Top with Caesar dressing and onion flax croutons. Garnish with lemon wedges and serve immediately.

Caesar Dressing

Creates 2 cups.

Ingredients:

½ cup cashews

¼ cup lemon juice

2 cloves fresh garlic, peeled

2 pitted Medjool dates (or 4 Deglet Noor)

¹/₂ teaspoon black pepper

1 tablespoon dulse flakes

1 teaspoon salt-free, stone-ground mustard

> 1. Combine ingredients in a high-speed blender and process until smooth.

Onion Flax Croutons

Like many raw recipes, these delicious croutons require a dehydrator. Look for other salt-free, raw recipes to try like crackers, fruit rollups, etc.

Ingredients:

¹/₄ cup water

¹/₈ teaspoon black pepper

1 tablespoon Italian seasoning

¹/₄ yellow onion

1 garlic clove

¹/₂ cup golden flaxseeds, ground

> 1. Combine all ingredients except flaxseed in a blender. Blend until smooth and pour into a small mixing bowl.
> 2. Add the ground flaxseed and mix well until a thick, batter-like consistency is achieved.
> 3. Spread thinly on a silicone or Teflex liner placed on a dehydrator tray. Gently score into 1" squares using a tool that won't cut the tray.
> 4. Dehydrate for 12 hours at 115°F.
> 5. Flip over and dehydrate for 2–3 more hours or until crispy.

Chef's note: Times for dehydration vary quite a bit depending on the moisture in the foods and the temperature and humidity where you live, so dehydration times in these recipes are variable. Check the foods as they dry and adjust times as needed to get the perfect, even results you want.

Spiralized Pesto Primavera

If you don't have a spiralizer, you can still enjoy this recipe. Many supermarkets now sell veggies already spiralized, or you can use a peeler to make very thin ribbons. Another option is to grate the vegetables using the largest side of a common box grater.

Serves 2.

Ingredients:

½ medium zucchini

½ medium yellow squash

1 large carrot

1 handful chopped spinach

1½ to 2 cups diced cherry tomatoes

1 cup Pesto Sauce (recipe below)

1. Spiralize or grate the zucchini, squash, and carrot and place in a large mixing bowl.
2. Add spinach, cherry tomatoes, and Pesto Sauce. Toss and serve.

Pesto Sauce

Yields one cup.

Ingredients:

2 cups chopped baby spinach

2–4 ounces fresh basil

¼ cup walnuts

2 tablespoons lemon juice

¼ teaspoon nutritional yeast

1. Combine all ingredients in a high-speed blender. Blend ingredients for a moment, then stop and use a spatula to scrape down the sides.

2. Continue blending and scraping the sides down as needed until the sauce is smooth. Store in the refrigerator.

Living Loaf with Ketchup Glaze
Serves 2.

<u>Ingredients:</u>
½ cup ground sunflower seeds

½ cup ground brown flaxseeds

¼ cup minced almonds

¼ red onion, chopped

2 stalks celery, chopped

1 cup crimini mushrooms

1 garlic clove, peeled

1 tablespoon fresh parsley, chopped

Raw Ketchup (recipe below)

1. Use a high-speed blender to grind the sunflower and flax seeds; place in a large mixing bowl. Do the same for the almonds, pulsing gently until they are in tiny pieces, and place into the bowl.

2. Place the rest of the ingredients in the empty blender and blend into a purée.

3. Add the purée to the bowl with the seeds and almonds. Mix together until well blended.

4. Spread on a nonstick surface such as a silicone mat or Teflex sheet on the dehydrator tray so the loaf is 1" high and 6" x

6" square. Dehydrate for 12 hours at 115°F, and then flip over. Dehydrate for 2 more hours.

5. Spread the Raw Ketchup on the top and dehydrate for another hour. Serve immediately or refrigerate until ready to be eaten.

Raw Ketchup
Yields 2 cups.

Ingredients:

½ cup sun-dried tomatoes (soaked overnight, drained, and rinsed)

6 pitted Medjool dates (or 12 Deglet Noor), chopped

¼ cup water

¼ vine-ripe tomato, chopped

2 tablespoons raw apple cider vinegar

2 tablespoons raw agave nectar (optional)

1. Combine ingredients in a high-speed blender and process until smooth.

Chef's note: You may want to soften the dates by soaking them for several hours, then draining. If you do, reduce the water in the recipe slightly to adjust for the added moisture in the soaked dates.

Mashed Cauliflower with Mushroom Gravy
Serves 2–4.

Ingredients:

½ head cauliflower, roughly chopped

½ cup water

½ teaspoon black pepper

3 ounces psyllium husk flakes

Mushroom Gravy (see below)

1. Blend cauliflower in a food processor while slowly adding the water until smooth.

2. Add the remaining ingredients and process until thick and fluffy. Be sure to stop occasionally and wipe the sides with a spatula to prevent lumps.

3. Scoop onto a plate and create a well in the middle. Pour in as much gravy as your heart desires, and enjoy.

Mushroom Gravy
Yields 2 cups.

Ingredients:

1 cup crimini mushrooms

¼ cup cashews, soaked overnight, drained, and rinsed

½ cup water

1 teaspoon salt-free seasoning

1 tablespoon psyllium husk flakes

1. Combine all ingredients in a high-speed blender until smooth.

Tikka-Alive Masala
Serves 2.

Ingredients:

¼ head cauliflower, chopped

¼ red bell pepper, diced

½ medium zucchini, chopped

½ medium yellow squash, chopped

Raw Masala Sauce (see below)

1. Combine ingredients in a large mixing bowl and toss with Raw Masala Sauce.
2. Serve.

Raw Masala Sauce
Yields 1–1½ cups.

Ingredients:

¾ vine-ripe tomato, chopped

1 garlic clove, peeled

1 teaspoon paprika

½ teaspoon garam masala

½ teaspoon curry powder

½ teaspoon ground cumin

½ teaspoon ground coriander

¼ teaspoon black pepper

¾ yellow onion, chopped

1. Combine all ingredients except the yellow onion in a high-speed blender and process until smooth.
2. Add the yellow onion and slowly pulse until well-minced into the sauce.

Taco Salad with Ranchero Dressing
Serves 4.

Ingredients:

¼ cup walnuts

¼ cup almonds

¼ cup sunflower seeds

¼ cup red bell pepper

⅛ yellow onion, chopped

2 teaspoons paprika

4 tablespoons of no- or low-sodium vegetable broth

Mixed greens, tomatoes, and/or avocado

Ranchero Dressing (recipe below)

1. Combine first seven ingredients in a food processor and pulse until the consistency of ground beef is achieved.
2. Serve on top of a bed of mixed greens with fresh avocado, tomatoes, and a side of Ranchero Dressing.

Ranchero Dressing
Yields 2 cups.

Ingredients:

¼ cup cashews

3 ounces sunflower seeds

¾ cup water

2 tablespoons lemon juice

1 teaspoon dill

2 tablespoon apple cider vinegar

2 teaspoon onion powder

1. Combine all ingredients in a high-speed blender and process until smooth and creamy.

Desserts

Lemon Basil Avocado Pudding

Serves 4.

Ingredients:

2 Hass avocados, pitted and skin removed

3–5 pitted Medjool dates (or 6–10 Deglet Noor)

3 tablespoon lemon juice

fruit of 1 lemon, peeled and deseeded

2–3 fresh basil leaves, thinly sliced

1. Combine avocados, dates, lemon, and lemon juice in a high-speed blender and process until smooth, stopping and wiping the sides down with a spatula to ensure that all the date pieces are well-blended.
2. Serve chilled and garnished with fresh basil.

Jill's Black Bean Brownies

What? Making brownies from black beans? While it may sound bizarre, these super-healthy brownies, loaded with antioxidants and anthocyanins, will blow your mind! This recipe is courtesy of Jayney Goddard's mom, Jill Lucas—just goes to show that moms always know best!

Yields 8–9 brownies.

Ingredients:

1 tablespoon of ground flax seed

3 tablespoons water

1 16-ounce can organic black beans (or 2 cups home-cooked beans), drained and rinsed

10 pitted Medjool dates (or 20 Deglet Noor)

½ cup raw cacao powder

1 teaspoon organic vanilla extract

¼ cup water

1½ teaspoons organic baking powder

1. First make the flax egg: Mix 1 tablespoon ground flax seed with 3 tablespoons water. Let it sit for 10–15 minutes until it thickens and gets slightly viscous, like an egg white.

2. Preheat oven to 350°F and line an 8" x 8" baking pan with parchment paper.

3. Combine black beans, dates, cacao powder, and vanilla extract with 1–2 tablespoons or more of water in a food processor. Blend until smooth.

4. Add the flax egg and baking powder and blend again.

5. Spread batter evenly in the prepared pan and bake for 20 minutes. Check to see if the top is brown and slightly firm. If still soft, continue baking 5 more minutes or until done.

6. Take brownies out of oven and let cool for 20 minutes to set.

7. Cut, serve, and enjoy!

CHAPTER 15

JUMP-START WEIGHT/
FAT LOSS PROGRAMS

I have emphatically and unequivocally promoted the plant-powered approach for consistent long-term weight loss success over the inevitable failures of quick-fix fad diets that engender short-term weight loss while mortgaging your health future in the process. Everyone starting a new weight-control program wants the gratification and positive reinforcement of some immediate success. So, it is important to emphasize that the low-fat, WFPE, SOS-free diet and supportive, lifestyle choices that I am recommending will promote significant, healthy weight loss within days of starting this program.

However, to enhance and jump-start the initial results of this program and begin to build a foundation for long-term success, this chapter presents 7-, 14-, 21-, and 30-day programs that have been time-tested on thousands of people I have worked with in health centers over decades of clinical practice. These programs incorporate a combination of detoxification and nutrition that can help resolve food cravings and addictions while improving metabolic efficiency and hormonal balance. They can also help your transition and commitment to the plant-exclusive diet and lifestyle plan that is essential for your success. Just keep in mind that these programs are not mandatory. They are not a necessity. They are just presented as viable options or opportunities to more intensely address the toxic consequences of poor diet and lifestyle choices that may have been a big part of your personal history.

By incorporating fasting, juicing, and raw food components, these jump-starts can more quickly reduce food addictions and compulsive-eating that create roadblocks to diet change and fat/weight loss. The short periods of water fasting can be done at home *as long as you can commit to rest during the fasting period, are not on any over the counter or prescription medication other than hormone replacement therapies, do not have a complicating disease condition, and have the support or endorsement of your primary health care provider.* If you do not satisfy these conditions, or if you are not comfortable with the idea of fasting and food restriction, or are maintaining a busy work and family schedule, I recommend that you just do the regular program or the one- and two-week programs using more raw food, smoothies, and juices without water fasting.

These programs also include intermittent fasting that varies your daily pattern of food consumption and food restriction. Typically, I recommend that dinner be eaten around 5:00–7:00 p.m. with breakfast between 7:00–9:00 a.m. or later. This will provide a pattern of eating that includes eating in a window of 10–12 hours and fasting 12–14 hours each day, which eliminates late-night eating to further improve metabolism and weight/fat loss.

7-Day Jump-Start Program

My 7-Day Jump-Start Program consists of 24–48 hours of water fasting followed by two days of fresh, organic green juices and smoothies and three to four days of raw fruits and vegetables. *If you are on any medication other than hormone replacement with thyroid medication or female hormone replacement therapy, you should not fast.* Instead, just work with the food, juice, and smoothie components of these programs. Fasting should be done in as much of a resting state as possible with no exercise/physical activity other than 15–30 minutes of gentle stretching and gentle walking daily and minimal activities of daily living. This also means you should give your senses as much rest as possible with minimal use of computers, TVs, phones, etc. In fact, a digital fast is a wonderful, supportive accompaniment, reducing the chatter of your life and allowing you time for introspection and self-discovery. Water intake is essential; approximately 50–70 ounces of distilled water is recommended daily.

Days 1 and 2

Water fast, sipping on approximately 50–70 ounces of filtered or distilled water. Rest physically and give yourself a sensory rest by minimizing phone, TV, and computer use.

Days 3 and 4

Breakfast
Green smoothie (See Chapter 13.)

Midmorning
Fresh juice made from romaine lettuce (2–4 leaves), carrots (4), cucumber (1–2), celery (3–4 stalks), and snow pea and/or sunflower sprouts if available. I recommend the Breville Elite Juicer, which is an inexpensive cold-press juicer that works well.

Lunch
Smoothie similar to breakfast. You can replace pineapple with mango or apple or other seasonal fruit. Use the same greens.

Midafternoon
Same juice as midmorning

Dinner
Smoothie similar to breakfast and lunch

Days 5–7 (Raw Food)

Breakfast
Fresh mixed melons (watermelon, honeydew, cantaloupe), berries, and other seasonal fresh fruit

Lunch
Large mixed salad, completely raw and unprocessed. Add unlimited amounts of sunflower sprouts, bean sprouts, and 2–5 ounces (¼ to ½) of a Hass avocado or 2 ounces of nuts (almonds, walnuts, etc.).

Dinner
Large mixed salad as above, alternating the avocado and nuts between lunch and dinner.

14-Day Jump-Start Program

My 14-Day Jump-Start Program consists of three days of water fasting (depending on your comfort level) followed by three days of fresh organic juices and smoothies, four days of raw food, and four days of raw and cooked foods.

Days 1–3

Water fast, sipping on approximately 50–70 ounces of filtered or distilled water. Rest physically and give yourself a sensory rest by minimizing phone, TV, and computer use.

Days 4–6

Day 4: *Breakfast, Midmorning, Lunch, Midafternoon, and Dinner*
Vegetable juice made from romaine lettuce (2–4 leaves), cucumber (1–2), celery (3–4 stalks), and sunflower sprouts, if available. (60 ounces of juice per day)

Day 5: *Breakfast, Midmorning, Lunch, Midafternoon, and Dinner*
Vegetable juices made from romaine lettuce (2–4 leaves), carrots (6–8), cucumber (1–2), celery (3–4 stalks), and snow pea and/or sunflower sprouts, if available. (60 ounces per day)

Day 6: *Breakfast, Lunch, Midafternoon and Dinner*
Green smoothie (See Chapter 13.) (64 ounces per day)

Days 7–10 (Raw Food)

Breakfast
Fresh mixed melons (watermelon, honeydew, cantaloupe) or fresh, in-season fruit plate

Lunch
Large mixed salad, completely raw and unprocessed. Add ¼–½ small Hass avocado or 2 ounces of nuts (almonds, walnuts, etc.) and unlimited amounts of any available sprouts including sunflower, snow pea, alfalfa, broccoli sprouts, etc.

Dinner
Large mixed salad, alternating avocado or nuts between lunch and dinner

Days 11–14 (Raw and Cooked Food)

Breakfast
Fresh mixed melons (watermelon, honeydew, cantaloupe); fresh, in-season fruit plate; or cooked rolled or steel-cut oats

Lunch and Dinner
A large salad with avocado or nuts (amounts as above), steamed or broth-sautéed veggies, and either a baked white or sweet potato or some brown rice or quinoa with lentils or beans. (Tip: Whenever you want butter on a baked potato, use avocado—nature's butter. Mashing one-quarter (2–3 ounces) of a ripe Hass avocado into a baked potato is a total turn-on!)

Following a Jump-Start, it is important to continue the progress you have begun by incorporating a wide variety of fruit and vegetable options (always without added salt, oil, or sugar) into your daily routine. The tastes and experiences of these foods will inspire you to stay on a better track. The more consistent you are, the more these new, healthy changes will become a part of you and the more successful you will be at continuing to take weight off and keeping it off over time.

21-Day and 30-Day Weight-Loss Programs

If you would like to extend the 7-Day or 14-Day Jump-Start Programs, here is a week of follow-up menus that you can use to create highly successful 14-, 21-, and 30-day weight-loss programs. These menus and recipes can be can be repeated or mixed and matched to create additional weeks, and they will give you a good idea of how to structure your meals after you have completed your Jump-Start Program.

Extension Day 1

Breakfast
Gluten-free oatmeal, fresh fruit (mixed seasonal, fresh fruit including at least three to four different fruits and organic mixed berries)

Lunch
Large salad with baked sweet potato

Dinner
Salad and steamed or broth-sautéed veggies (kale, spinach, asparagus) with quinoa and beans (red, black, garbanzo, or any other variety)

Extension Day 2

Breakfast
Fresh fruit (as described above), cooked oatmeal, millet, or buckwheat

Lunch
Large salad with avocado and beans, like red kidney beans

Dinner
Salad and steamed or sautéed veggies (broccoli, mustard greens, carrots) with brown rice and sautéed organic tofu

Extension Day 3

Breakfast
Fresh fruit, oatmeal with berries

Lunch
Large salad with hummus or black beans

Dinner
Salad and steamed or sautéed veggies (bok choy and broccoli rabe) with Penne à la Vodka Vegan Style (See Chapter 14.)

Extension Day 4

Breakfast
Fresh fruit, oatmeal with berries and 1 tablespoon organic ground flaxseed

Lunch
Large salad with guacamole and baked white or sweet potato

Dinner
Salad and steamed or sautéed veggies (snow peas, cauliflower, spinach) with vegan chili

Extension Day 5

Breakfast
Fresh fruit, gluten-free English muffin with avocado or almond butter

Lunch

Large salad with an SOS-free burger (See Chapter 14.)

Dinner

Salad and steamed or sautéed veggies (such as collard greens, red peppers, zucchini) with brown rice and your favorite beans

Extension Day 6

Breakfast

Green smoothie and fresh fruit

Lunch

Large salad with Dr. Frank's Tuscan Veggie Soup (See Chapter 14.)

Dinner

Salad and steamed or sautéed veggies (kale, Brussels sprouts, spinach) with baked sweet potatoes

Extension Day 7

Breakfast

Fresh fruit, buckwheat grits with berries

Lunch

Large salad with 2 ounces walnuts

Dinner

Salad and steamed or sautéed veggies (broccoli, yellow squash, bok choy) with Channa Masala (See Chapter 14.)

CHAPTER 16

EATING OUT IN THE REAL WORLD

As hectic and busy as our lives have become, eating out and getting takeout (or take-aways for my European readers) have become a way of life for many of us and our families. This is the "real world" that many of us inhabit. I have included this chapter to address this very real concern for people who are transitioning to a vegan, WFPE, SOS-free diet.

There's a lot to take on board when you are making these important healthy changes in your life, so my hope is that this information will help you negotiate situations that are often over-looked by many physicians, health coaches, and counselors. I feel that it is extremely important to give you realistic, helpful, practical guidance as to how to find delicious, healthy food when you are out so that you can continue on your health and weight loss journey without risking self-sabotage—which is all too easy if you don't know what to choose in restaurants. However, please keep in mind that while it is useful for you to learn how to eat out in your local communities and on the road, I recommend doing as much food preparation at home as possible, for the sake of maintaining better control of whole-plant options without added salt, oil and sugar, for optimal quality of nutrition, and for family socialization and bonding.

There are other considerations that make this information even more relevant. All too often when people attempt the WFPE diet, they feel imbued with a sense of deprivation because they have a limited perspective on just what a whole-plant diet is all about. People will often act as if the diet is nothing more than romaine lettuce and a baked potato. Obviously, this would not work for anybody over time. If you didn't die from disease you would die of boredom. However, the truth is that with the amazing cornucopia of phenomenal options in vegan, WFPE, SOS-free nutrition, you are limited only by your lack of imagination. When you open your mind to the creative options and substitutions that are available, the transition to a healthy lifestyle will be easier and much more fun while significantly increasing your chances for successful weight management.

I have previously discussed eating a diverse array of plant-exclusive foods including fresh fruit, greens, rainbow veggies, whole grains, legumes, nuts, and limited amounts of processed soy products along with analog foods like plant milk, nondairy cheese, and very limited amounts of meat substitutes for people wishing to make a more comfortable transition to a low-fat, WFPE, SOS-free diet. The key word is diversity. Interestingly, if you look at many of the lean, healthy, long-lived cultures throughout the world, you will see is that their cuisine centers around this same plant-exclusive list of food options. In many cases their traditions include a long history of eating plant foods low in processed fats and refined carbohydrates. So, why reinvent the wheel? When you decide to eat out, take advantage of what these cultures have been eating for centuries and adopt some of their cuisines for your own culinary fun, enjoyment, and successful weight loss.

In this chapter, I am going to take you on a journey through some menu options available in many easily found ethnic restaurants. My goal is to excite and inspire you with the wealth of creative dishes within your reach that can truly help you realize the unlimited possibilities of a vegan lifestyle, all as you establish healthier weight and body image. I will be listing these meal items exactly as they appear on the menus of many restaurants. Depending on where you live, there may be different menu options than what I share with you. However, the following dishes are a good representation of what is typically available in these restaurants.

All cultures have some "caveat" items in their cooking, whether it's too much oil, salt, sugar, or spices. As a result, when eating out, it's more difficult to stick to the highest ideal of SOS-free food preparation. But infrequently, as you are transitioning or when you choose to accept some small dietary modifications, these ethnic foods can offer better WFPE options than do most mainstream American restaurants. I will address these caveat items directly, focus on dishes that give you the greatest opportunity to reduce unwanted additives, and offer advice for making special requests when you order food. In recent years, restaurants have responded more readily to more widespread consumer demand for heart-healthy menu items, low-sodium items, gluten-free options, and so on. As a result, it is much easier now to successfully request menu modifications than ever before.

Let's start our journey in Asia.

Japanese Food

Japan is composed of a series of four islands in the Pacific. The midsection of these islands is on the same latitude as the Carolinas on the eastern seaboard of the United States, and so, the climate is very temperate and supports plants like rice, various vegetables, and fruits like cherries and persimmons. The Japanese culture has a long tradition of low-oil grain and vegetable cooking that is right on track with the approach I am recommending in a vegan, WFPE, SOS-free lifestyle. In fact, one of the human populations that is famously known for its longevity, having one of the largest percentage of people living past the age of one hundred, is the Okinawans.[xx]

Because Japan has basically an island culture, the Japanese have learned to harvest food from the sea, including fish and a variety of sea greens and sea vegetation. Also, Japanese cuisine is fundamentally a low-oil one, and because each dish is usually freshly prepared, you are given options to customize your meal. For example, many dishes allow you to choose your protein, with tofu among the choices. You can also choose the level of spiciness (heat) and can request that the food be made with no or little oil. Therefore, Japanese cuisine works extremely well for our purposes and provides a high degree of satisfaction and support for healthy weight loss.

Here are notes on some specific menu items.

Japanese Soups

Japanese menus typically feature several kinds of soup, usually a base broth with added noodles, vegetables, and/or fish. The most commonly used broth is dashi, a family of stocks used in Japanese soups. It is the base for miso soup, clear broth soup, and noodle broth soups. Some dashi versions are made with fish, but many versions are made with just vegetables.

Miso is a traditional Japanese seasoning used in many ways, a thick paste made by fermenting soybeans with salt and other ingredients. Miso soup is a culinary staple in Japan made by mixing miso with dashi soup stock. Restaurant versions typically have some seaweed and tofu added to the broth. It can be quite salty, however, too

[xx] A sad commentary is that in recent years the Japanese people have adopted more of the standard American diet loaded with animal, dairy, and refined, processed foods. As a result, they are now experiencing epidemics of obesity, heart disease, and cancer similar to those in the U.S.

much so for a salt-free diet and especially for people with high blood pressure. When ordering soup, check the broth's ingredients with your server.

I prefer the soba soup. Soba soup is made with soba noodles. These noodles are typically made with buckwheat flour, so they are ideal on my recommended eating plan. Soba soup can be ordered as a bowl or as a cauldron for a main dinner item. Just make sure that the soup does not have a fish base. Soba noodles can also be purchased, (sometimes organic versions) in health food and grocery stores for home use and can be served with steamed and/or sautéed vegetables.

Appetizers and Salads

In most Japanese restaurants, the appetizer menus are so extensive that entire meals can be made from them alone. The following appetizers and salads offer great vegan options that you can integrate into your weight-loss program.

• House Salad

The salads in many Japanese restaurants are some of the most unimaginative salads in the history of salad-making, though I will admit that in some Japanese restaurants they have gotten significantly better recently with a wider variety of fresh greens. However, the dressings, often ginger- or peanut-based, can be worth the price of admission. Some restaurants do have mayo-based dressings, though, so again, check with your server.

• Oshitashi

This is a cold spinach salad that is made either with a brown béchamel-type sauce or with tamari (gluten-free soy sauce) and lemon. The brown sauce can be quite salty so I prefer the lemon tamari version.

A Note on Soy Sauce

In Japanese restaurants the soy sauce may come in two different bottles, a red top that is high-octane sodium and a green top that is lower sodium; note that even the green top is intensely salty. Also, restaurant soy sauce is not gluten-free, so if that's important for you, ask for tamari instead, which doesn't include wheat in its ingredients. A better option with significantly lower salt levels is coconut liquid aminos. These are soy sauce-like liquids made from coconuts. They still contain substantial amounts of sodium and can still promote unwanted salt-like effects on fluid retention and high blood pressure, but to a somewhat lesser extent. If you use them at all, do so sparingly. Small spray bottles can be purchased and filled with these aminos and carried in a tote bag or a purse whenever you're eating out. A better choice is to use your favorite SOS-free seasonings.

• Edamame

Edamame is simply immature soybeans in the pod, which are steamed and served salted or unsalted. Always opt for the unsalted variety. This is the most unprocessed form of soy, very high in protein and fiber, and is highly recommended.

Edamame can also be purchased in supermarkets and can be easily steamed to create fantastic Asian-influenced casseroles. Brown rice combined with some grated carrots, mushrooms, seaweed, tofu, and edamame makes a very satisfying and tasty dish. Also, edamame makes a great snack food in the midday or evening. They are crunchy and tasty and satisfy that snacky/crunchy thing that we all like at some time. In fact, I have even gone a step further and brought steamed edamame into the movies in lieu of popcorn!

• **Grilled or Steamed Tofu Steaks**

These are an absolute delight, especially when they come smothered in a wide variety of mushrooms, as they are in some Japanese restaurants.

• **Mushrooms**

Mushrooms can provide remarkable nutritional value and should be a staple in your ongoing eating plan, containing quite a diversity of immune-enhancing and supporting substances. The Japanese have developed the culinary use of mushrooms to a very high art form, utilizing a diverse assortment including shiitake, enoki, maitake, king oyster, and others.

• **Vegetable Roots**

Depending on the authenticity of the restaurant, they may have several different steamed or lightly sautéed root vegetables like burdock and lotus root, which are a remarkable addition and taste treat for any meal.

• **Seaweed Salads**

Japanese seaweed salads are typically made with a combination of the following: wakame, arame, hijiki (which looks like black tubular spaghetti), and some combination of kelp and dulse. Focus on wakame or arame options; it is best to avoid both hijiki because of its high arsenic content and kelp because of its high iodine content, which can promote problems of iodine excess. Also, some seaweed salads have fish products among their ingredients, so check with your server.

A Note About Seaweed

Seaweed can be a valuable addition to a vegan diet, and the Japanese have developed seaweed use to a very high art form. You may be familiar with nori, the seaweed typically used to make sushi; it's ideal for its more moderate iodine content. Seaweeds have a high mineral content, including iodine and calcium, and as a result, they can be supportive of bone and endocrine health, including the stability of the thyroid gland, which plays a major role in the weight-loss story. In addition, seaweeds, especially algae, are the best natural sources of the omega-3 fatty acid DHA, which can sometimes be deficient in people for either dietary or genetic reasons.

Seaweeds can be purchased in an organic form in your health-food stores. If you use them, I do not recommend cooking them directly. Before you use them, soak them in cold water for about 20-30 minutes to get all the surface brine off the seaweed while keeping the leaves intact. Then, let's suppose you're going to put the seaweed into a rice dish. When the rice is almost done, break up the seaweed and toss it into the cooked rice so the heat of the rice gently steams the seaweed. If you cook seaweed directly, it can get too wilted and lose some value.

Entrées

• Vegetable Sushi

All Japanese restaurants have one or more versions of vegetable sushi. A black square of nori seaweed is laid out on a bamboo rolling mat. A layer of rice is placed on the nori and vegetables such as carrots, cucumber, sprouts, avocado, and asparagus are added to the rice. The seaweed is rolled and then cut in pieces and served on a plate or cutting board along with some pickled ginger and a dollop of wasabi.

Any all-vegetable sushi is an ideal choice when dining out, as it has no added salt and is a very clean vegan option; in some Japanese restaurants, you can even ask them to make it with brown rice instead of white rice. (Remember, you always want the lower-glycemic-impact whole grain rather than the stripped or bleached refined version.)

Wasabi is the little clump of green paste served with sushi, a kind of combination of horseradish and hot mustard, and it is smokin' hot. Hot spicy additives and condiments can overstimulate appetite and irritate the digestive tract. If you use the wasabi, you really only need the amount that would fit on the head of a pin. I was out to dinner with someone once who mistook the clump of wasabi for a clump of avocado and popped the whole thing in his mouth. It was so hot that tears streamed down his face, and his life flashed before him as he processed through a lifetime of deep psychological issues! You get the point.

I ate a lot of hot stuff when I was younger and eating more conventionally. However, as I got more and more used to the taste of natural foods, my tastes simplified, and I lost interest in extreme seasonings, additives, and condiments. As you get more and more accustomed to the tastes of simple, natural foods over time, your tastes will change, too, and you will seek out food that is less spicy and salty.

• Itame

This is the word for stir-fried, often meaning stir-fried vegetables, which is an ideal choice when ordered with no or minimal oil. A nice option is that you can get the itame on a bed of brown rice or a bed of soba noodles to make a Japanese version of pasta primavera. Some itame can be made with small amounts of meat that can be substituted with steamed tofu.

• Yakisoba

This is one of my favorite dishes. It includes lightly sautéed soba noodles combined with a variety of sautéed or steamed veggies. You can pick and choose vegetables that you prefer to make this dish exactly to your liking. I love extra broccoli, snow peas, and other greens, so that's what I order. Typically, this dish is made with meat, but you can substitute steamed tofu or just limit it to vegetables, making it a completely vegan delight.

• Steamed Vegetable Gyoza

Gyoza are delightful vegetable-filled dumplings that are often made with some form of refined wheat or rice flour which makes them less than ideal. However, since they are filled with a variety of vegetables, they are an acceptable option on my program.

• Vegetable Fried Rice

Ask to have this prepared without the traditional egg and without oil. The rice and vegetables can be dry sautéed, making it a delicious, viable option when eating out.

Japanese food works very well as an eat-in or take-out option. It's a great choice for business or social lunches, too, because everyone can customize their meals to their liking, whether that means WFPE or with chicken, beef, fish, and eggs. However, my experience is that when you fill up a table with soups, appetizers, seaweed salads, noodle dishes, veggie sushi, and itame, even people who are not vegans or vegetarians are excited to try these plant-based choices.

Japanese food also is a great option for weight regulation. It is relatively light fare with relatively low calorie density. Personally, I don't like that feeling of being overly full, heavy, and weighed down after I eat. When you eat this food, you will not feel overly full or bloated; you will be quite satisfied, stable, and comfortable. This feeling of satiety and stability eliminates any sense of craving and supports a healthier relationship with food and eating out.

Chinese Food

The Chinese culture also has a strong agricultural, plant-based tradition. Unfortunately, China, like Japan, has become increasingly more seduced by the disease-inducing eating habits of countries like the U.S. and the incidence of chronic diseases like heart disease, cancer, and obesity has dramatically increased as a result. This clearly demonstrates how the high-calorie, high-fat, nutritionally bankrupt Western diet correlates with negative health outcomes regardless of unique genetic variations of disparate populations. Long-term research like *The China Study* has shown that the foundation of the healthiest Chinese diet is grounded in an extensive use of plant-based foods.[1] So Chinese food, if approached judiciously, can be a great eating-out option that supports your weight-loss program. The caveat items in Chinese food are oil, salt (sometimes in the form of monosodium glutamate (MSG), and sugar in the Szechuan sauces. With the development of heart-healthy options in many Chinese restaurants and smaller take-out stores today, eliminating these caveat items has become easier.

Soup

When you're in the mood for soup, Chinese vegetable soup is a great option. It is often loaded with vegetables such as broccoli, snow peas, carrots, tofu, etc. It often has a meat base, but if you are willing to wait, many restaurants will make you a veggie-based vegetable soup.

As in Japanese food, a complete meal can be made from the variety of appetizers and greens offered in Chinese cuisine.

Appetizers—Greens

I don't know of any other ethnic food that provides the variety and quality of deep-hued greens found in Chinese restaurants. The major greens offered are:

• Chinese Mustard Greens (Yu-Choy)

This is a Chinese version of broccoli rabe. It is a stringy, deep-hued green that can be ordered steamed. It can be prepared as greens alone or served as a main entrée with big black mushrooms, steamed tofu, and brown rice. Very light, clear garlic sauce is available. My advice is to order the sauce on the side so you can drizzle it on, thereby controlling the amount you want. If the sauce is not served on the side, the dish will often come swimming in sauce, which is not in your best interest.

• Baby Bok Choy

These bok choy are the size of your hand. They can be ordered as a succulent platter of tender deep greens, steamed with brown rice, black mushrooms, and tofu. Tender bok choy is an absolute delight and will melt in your mouth.

• Snow Pea Greens (Snow Pea Tips)

This is a delicacy that is typically known only to the Chinese population. Snow peas grow on a vine that also gives off little tender green shoots. These harvested shoots can be steamed and eaten alone or with other greens, grains, and legumes. Snow pea greens are available at different times of the year, so you will have to check with the restaurants in your community to find out when they are available.

Other Appetizers

• Steamed Vegetable Dumplings

These are made with a refined rice flour. Although it is not ideal, it is still a vegan option that can be used, especially since you will probably not be eating it every day. For very occasional use, some small amount of refined, gluten-free flour should not be a setback.

• Cabbage or Lettuce Rolls

For these, cabbage or lettuce leaves are rolled with a filling of mixed, shredded vegetables and mung bean sprouts. These may be available raw or lightly steamed in Chinese restaurants (and as a raw spring roll in Thai restaurants) and provide a great eating-out option. However, keep in mind that these are different from the deep-fried egg or spring rolls that are also available and should be avoided.

Noodle Dishes

Noodle dishes in Chinese restaurants typically come in two varieties, lo mein or chow fun.

• Lo Mein

These are thin rice noodles that can be ordered with a variety of vegetables as vegetable lo mein. Chinese restaurants are great because you can order the kinds of vegetables you truly enjoy in any rice or noodle dish. I don't need all those little baby corncobs, but I sure want extra snow peas, broccoli, and greens! And I don't know of any restaurant where broccoli comes out as delicious as it does in Chinese restaurants.

• Chow Fun

These wide rice noodles are my favorite—fun with chow fun! Veggie chow fun is a wonderful dish of mixed vegetables and noodles. Noodle dishes can be quite oily, so I recommend asking for low-oil or steamed versions of these dishes. Many Chinese restaurants, including many of the small storefront take-out places, now have heart-healthy, low-salt, low-oil options. Therefore, asking for what you want and need is now easier than ever, and it will allow you to make the appropriate changes in the best interest of your weight-loss program.

Other Entrées

• Buddha's Delight

This an assortment of mixed steamed or sautéed veggies. I recommend getting them steamed with just a light, clear garlic sauce on the side. Again, whether you're eating in or taking out, I always recommend getting any sauce on the side to allow you to drizzle the sauce at your own discretion and maintain control of the amount used.

• Home-Style Tofu

When tofu is added to Buddha's delight, the dish is typically referred to as home-style tofu. Be sure to ask for the tofu to be steamed because most restaurants will typically serve it deep-fried in this dish.

Depending on the restaurant, there may be a large number of other options available. Some restaurants will offer a vegan meat substitute, seitan (a wheat-gluten-based product that is high-protein and low-fat), as a protein option in various dishes. Mock duck, for example, is a common seitan option in Asian restaurants. These substitutions may have some value as vegan alternatives in the short run, but since they are made from gluten and can be high in sodium they are not recommended in an ongoing healthy weight-loss program.

Covering a table with the variety of vegan options in a Chinese restaurant will even inspire the interest and desire of non-vegans to try these plant-based foods. It's a great way to turn on friends, family members, and even business associates to a healthier way of living and eating.

To really help yourself, become more aware of what is available to you in your immediate environment. You will be amazed at what you can find in your own backyard, so to speak. In my studies, I have lived and traveled all over the U.S. When I spend any time in a new place, I know that I'm going to be eating out. Within a few days, I routinely find several places where I can get everything I need and want. I have experienced the best Chinese restaurants in Chinatowns in New York City, Boston, and San Francisco. One of the best Chinese restaurants I ever found was in San Antonio, Texas. You will be amazed at what you can find when you look!

Italian Food

This part of our journey will take us to Italy and the Middle East, two of the many different cultures and their cuisines found around the Mediterranean. As with other areas, salt is a caveat of Mediterranean cooking, but the biggest caveat is *oil*. Before we look at restaurant options for these areas, let's talk about that.

As you can see, I wrote the word oil in italicized letters to emphasize that if you don't address the oil issue in Mediterranean food, you can leave the restaurant feeling like you've had an oil change. Now if you're an older used car like me and you need an oil change, this may feel and even taste good, but it's really not a healthy option for optimal weight and fat loss, and absolutely not on the WFPE, SOS-free program. Understand that what's low-oil to a Mediterranean chef is not low-oil to you and me. To the Mediterranean chef, a half a bottle of oil is low-oil. Just keep in mind the problems we have already addressed with oils and potential weight gain and be prepared to ask for menu adjustments.

I'm starting with Italian food. (Not because I'm biased or anything. Don't let the name Sabatino fool you.) I rarely meet anyone who doesn't like Italian food. In 24 years at the last health center I directed, there were only two people who didn't like Italian food, and they were both asked to leave. (Just kidding.)

Now, when I say Italian food, I'm basically referring to Southern Italian cuisine. It's quite different from the cuisine of Northern Italy which uses more milk, cheese, and meat, simply because the cuisine of Northern Italy is similar to the cuisine of Austria, of which it once was a part. Southern Italian cuisine is typically referred to as the Mediterranean diet. This is a way of eating that is plant-based and loaded with vegetables, grains, pasta, olive oil, and a small amount of fish. The adjustments and options I recommend will eliminate the oil and fish and make it a viable option on my program. I start with the following.

Salad

If you can't get an amazing salad in an Italian restaurant, you can't get it anywhere. They have everything you would want to put in a salad (romaine lettuce, other lettuces, spinach, tomatoes, onions, mushrooms, arugula, and olives). In a pinch, order a Caesar salad, hold the Caesar. You know they have romaine lettuce, but you don't need the cheese or anchovies. For a simple dressing, just ask for some lemon or balsamic vinegar. Another option is to make one of the really scrumptious salad dressings presented in Chapter 14 and bring it with you to the restaurant. Make sure you order the salad on the way in the door so it gets to the table before the breadbasket, because once the bread comes and you get started with that hot Italian bread dipped in oil, you are done. You can wind up eating a half a loaf of bread before the salad even comes! Usually the bread is refined wheat bread, which has a high-glycemic impact and provokes overeating, so it should be avoided. If you do eat some bread, though, be sure to skip the oil.

Appetizer Greens

Depending on your mood, these can be side dishes, appetizers, or the main focus of a main meal.

• Broccoli Rabe

This is Italian soul food. It's my all-time favorite. Whenever I was coming home to see my folks, I would find out if there was any broccoli rabe available so my mother could fulfill her motherly duties and prepare it for me. If you are not from an ethnic household, you should know that when a child of an Italian family approaches within a certain geographical distance of the home, there is a gene that is turned on in the Italian mother that drives her into her kitchen for food preparation. (It's well-known in the scientific literature. It's called the ethnic-kitchen-homing gene. Not really, but it might as well be.)

Enjoying broccoli rabe can be an acquired taste because it can be somewhat bitter, but the bitterness can be mitigated by how you prepare it. The old Italian grandmother's technique for preparing broccoli rabe is to cook the greens in a pot of hot water containing garlic and a teaspoon of olive oil until it's soft, followed by sautéing the greens in garlic and oil. At home, you can eliminate the oil completely by dry sautéing or steaming. After it is cooked, it is best served with copious amounts of fresh lemon squeezed all over the greens. This preparation, followed by the showering of lemon, will cut the bitterness, promote better iron absorption, and transport you to the roots of the old country. The greens can be combined with pasta or, as I prefer it, straight up, no chaser.

• **Steamed Broccoli, Steamed Spinach, and Steamed Escarole**
Italian restaurants typically have a variety of fantastic greens on the menu. My advice is that when you order them, remember to ask for low- or no-oil preparation, because if you don't, they will come swimming in oil. I always ask for steamed greens, no oil, and heavy garlic. (Just make sure that whomever you're eating with is eating just like you; some people don't like to be around people oozing with garlic. Being Italian, I just love, love, love the smell and taste of garlic.) Keep in mind that at home you can dry sauté or sauté in no-sodium-added vegetable broth and balsamic vinegar with a variety of herbs and spices including, garlic, ginger, basil, cilantro, etc.

You can eat these greens as side or main dishes, or as I sometimes do, order some whole-grain pasta and pour these greens on top to make a delectable mixed-greens-and-pasta dish with a plain basil-tomato sauce.

Entrées—Spaghetti and Other Pasta Dishes
Most often, the pasta in Italian restaurants is refined and wheat-based, so it is not ideal. Many Italian restaurants now have whole-grain pasta on their menus, but it will still be wheat-based. Some now offer gluten-free pastas or spiralized vegetable options (such as spiralized zucchini), which is helpful if you are limiting wheat or gluten-containing products in your diet, and many offer gnocchi, a pasta that is 85–90%

potato. Gnocchi is often served with a heavy cream sauce, but you can order it plain, with veggies, or with marinara sauce, just as you would with any pasta.

Spaghetti, of course, is a staple Italian dish, and it's a straightforward choice when dining out. Order a simple entrée of pasta and marinara with a big side salad or steamed vegetables, and you're set. Skip the parmesan, though.

I always recommend eating some greens with any pasta dish. It will reduce the calorie density of the meal and help stabilize blood sugar and portion control. You can order a plain tomato sauce, but many restaurants put sugar and/or butter in their sauces, so a better option may be to get a crushed tomato-basil sauce or the Italian style, with just garlic and/or a hint of olive oil, but again, ask for the lowest oil possible and go heavier on the garlic.

Entrées—Pizza

Do you know anybody who likes pizza? Oh, yes, yes, yes! Typically, most Italian restaurants make their crusts with refined flour, but many restaurants now have whole-wheat crusts and some even have gluten-free crusts. When dining out, I usually just get a veggie pizza without cheese. I like having all kinds of greens on my pizza, so I get broccoli, broccoli rabe, spinach, basil, mushrooms, and onions with tomato sauce on a whole-grain crust. It's amazing.

At home, it's even easier, especially if you start with a pre-made crust. There is an endless array of pre-made, whole-grain crusts sold in both regular supermarkets and health-food stores. This also includes a fair number of gluten-free crusts made from cauliflower, rice, corn, etc. (Look for ones with the least oil and salt and with the cleanest ingredient lists.) Take one of these pre-made crusts, cover it with any good organic, low-sodium, low-fat tomato sauce, load it up with your favorite raw or lightly steamed veggies, and pop it in a 400°F oven. In

10–15 minutes, you've got a pizza to die for. Pizzas are perfect for parties and any fun social gathering—or just for an easy, delicious meal anytime.

With their salads, greens, pastas, and pizzas, Italian restaurants provide an interesting opportunity for great-tasting options that will excite your taste while still supporting your health and weight-loss program.

Middle Eastern Food

Middle Eastern cuisine offers a wide variety of earthy, plant-based options. These options tend to be concentrated in the salad and appetizer parts of the menu, while entrées are typically more meat- and dairy-based. You can easily make a dinner plate by combining several vegan appetizers. If you're eating out with someone, you can each order several different appetizers and share them, which can expand your dining experience and allow you to taste a wider variety of options. The caveat items in this food are basically salt and oil. They're somewhat difficult to control, but do not have to be deal-breakers. Its just imperative that you are careful to request no-oil options.

Salads

• Fattoush Salad
A finely diced and chopped salad made from tomatoes, cucumbers, lettuce, onion, and peppers, accompanied by a mint dressing

• Mediterranean Salad
Romaine lettuce, cucumbers, tomatoes, chickpeas, fava beans, and a Mediterranean dressing (mostly garlic, lemon, and olive oil). Have them leave off the dressing and ask for just some lemon and garlic instead, or use one of the dressings recommended previously.

Appetizers and Entrée Items

Middle Eastern food is one of the best cuisines to share with someone else; its finger-food nature lends itself to comfortable, congenial dining. It's deliciously, deeply flavorful, but it's usually made with liberal amounts of salt and oil. It's a plus that the appetizer-style dips below are usually eaten with raw vegetables or pita bread, allowing you to focus on those with small amounts of the dips. Be sure to ask your server about the best low- or no-oil options. That doesn't mean you have to avoid these delightful foods, however, because there are many easy recipes online that can be made oil- and salt-free.

As with other cuisines, these appetizers can also be a satisfying entrée.

• Hummus

A puréed mix of chickpeas, tahini, garlic, and lemon, usually served with raw vegetables and/or pita bread. Hummus is often served with olive oil on top, so instruct them to not add the oil.

• Baba Ghanoush

Roasted eggplant mashed with garlic, lemon, and salt with additional smoky flavor added.

• Tabbouleh

Made with finely chopped cracked wheat, scallions, and mint. If the tabbouleh isn't premade, ask for the chef to use lemon in lieu of olive oil.

• Sautéed Fava Beans

These are traditionally prepared in copious amounts of olive oil, so ask for a dry sauté instead.

The journey continues to one of my favorites.

Indian Food

India has a long history and tradition of vegetarian and vegan food preparation. The spices and tastes of Indian food are so exotic and different that it offers an incredible way to break from your usual routine while staying on a vegan track that will still promote weight-loss success. The caveats of Indian food are salt, spice levels, and oil, and if you don't address the spiciness issue when you order, you may feel like your face has been burned off. Your server will usually ask you whether you want your food mild, medium, or hot. I always say less, less, less than mild, because what's mild to an Indian chef may not be mild to you. They can always bring the heat to the table with side sauces that range from pleasantly spicy to so spicy that one taste can set your mouth on fire!

Some Indian foods use an animal-derived form of clarified butter called ghee, but this can be avoided by your request, by the choices of dishes you order, and by the regional Indian food you are consuming. Most people are aware of Tandoori Indian cuisine, which is more Northern Indian cuisine. Tandoori cooking has more ghee-based dishes and is not as vegan as Southern Indian cuisine. Southern India is a hotter climate, and the food is much spicier and vegan-based.

Many Indian restaurant menus designate which dishes are vegetarian or vegan. I recommend that you find an Indian restaurant that is either vegan-based or at least has a mix of Southern and Northern dishes. The following recommendations are readily available, strictly vegan options that can be ordered without ghee and mostly gluten-free. Restaurant menus often describe their vegetable dishes temptingly in ways that look entirely vegan, but it's a good idea to double-check to make sure your choices don't include yogurt or paneer, a soft white cheese made from buffalo, goat, sheep, or cow's milk.

Appetizer

• Idli
Steamed rice and lentil cake

Entrées

• Sambhar
Veggies and lentils in exotic spices

• Dal Tadka
Yellow lentils cooked with onions, tomatoes, and Indian spices

• Channa Masala
Casserole of chickpeas in tomato sauce and spices—one of my favorite dishes, high-protein and melt-in-your-mouth. (See Chapter 14.)

• Aloo Gobi
Cubes of potatoes, cauliflower, onion, and bell pepper with Indian spices

• Baingan Bharta
Fresh eggplant, baked and mashed, then cooked with onion, tomatoes, and Indian spices

• Kadai Bhindi Masala
Tender okra cooked with spices

• Indian Fried Rice
Ask for no egg and no or minimal oil.

• Uttappam
These are South Indian-style savory pancakes made with a rice or garbanzo beans, filled with a variety of vegetables, including onions, peas,

mixed vegetables and chick peas, and served with several vegan sauces. They are fluffy and light, an incredible, unique, vegan dining experience. Ask for them to be made without ghee.

• Vegetable Pulao
Pulao, often referred to as vegetable pulao, is an Indian dish made in a pot or pressure cooker containing basmati rice, vegetables, spices and herbs. It is light and fragrant and can be served as a side dish or main course.

• Bisi Bele Bath
Rice cooked with lentils and garden-fresh vegetables

Breads—Roti and Dosai
There are as many as 22 unique Indian breads available including naan, paratha, dosai, roti, chapati, and pappadum, but only dosai and roti are vegan (if not brushed with ghee). The others, notably the popular naan, are often made with yogurt, milk, and/or oil. Be aware that after baking, all Indian breads may be brushed with ghee, and all are typically made with wheat flour, so are not gluten-free. In restaurants that prepare more Southern Indian cuisine, which is more typically vegan and spicy hot, you can get vegan naan, dosai, and roti without ghee or animal products but it may still be brushed with vegetable oil. Although I have cautioned about the overconsumption of breads, an occasional taste is a culinary delight well worth the price of admission.

Roti are whole-wheat flatbreads baked in a clay oven, an excellent choice. Chapatis are roti that are oiled on both sides and cooked again on a griddle, so stick with roti.

Dosai are delightful crêpes made from lentils and rice. These versions of Indian veggie wraps are simply amazing. They are served with various vegetable and coconut sauces that will blow your mind.

• Masala Dosai
Thin, crispy, rice crépes filled with potatoes and onions

• Onion Dosai
Thin rice crépes with a topping of onions

• Spinach Dosai
Thin rice crépes rolled with sautéed spinach. Simply my favorite.

You have probably noticed that I have not discussed desserts. That is simply because desserts worldwide are generally full of eggs, butter, and sugar and because too many of us overdo desserts. In the U.S., it's not uncommon for people to eat a huge meal and then follow it up with the mile-high chocolate cake! Eating sweets after big meals often increases fermentation of sugar, resulting in gas, bloating, distention, and heartburn. Berries or fruit will still be your best bet for a dessert that will keep you on track without provoking sugar-craving and reactive weight gain.

It is important to note that while this chapter provides a good snapshot of wonderful, tasty, vegan options in a variety of ethnic restaurants, it is not comprehensive. Depending on your communities, there also are tremendous vegan opportunities that may be available to you in other cuisines, including Thai, Vietnamese, Ethiopian, and even in more enlightened Mexican restaurants. Thai cuisine in particular has wonderful raw plant-exclusive summer rolls, a plethora of remarkable steamed and sautéed vegetable dishes with tofu, as well as some incredible noodle dishes like vegan (on request) pad Thai. I urge you to search online for restaurants with vegan options in your community and in the areas that you may visit for personal or business reasons. You may be pleasantly surprised by the amazing international options you discover.

Also keep in mind that delicious ethnic foods that traditionally use oil or dairy products can often be prepared at home to strictly meet vegan, SOS-free recommendations. Take advantage of the many excellent recipes available online (but ditch the oil!).

Regardless of where you dine, a useful strategy relates to the fact that most restaurants publish their menus online. By taking advantage of this resource, you can be aware of what's available before you even leave home, and there won't be any surprises about what can be ordered. This is especially helpful when dining out socially, whether with family, friends, or work associates. In those situations, offer to be the one to pick the restaurant, freeing yourself to choose one such as those we've discussed where you know you'll have options to create a healthy, WFPE choice for yourself.

Remember, eating the WFPE, SOS-free diet I recommend is definitely not about deprivation. It is about experiencing a broad diversity of whole, plant-exclusive foods to support a healthier lifestyle. By taking advantage of the experience and expertise of a variety of cultures on planet Earth and the multitude of food options that they have created, you can experience a whole new world of creative options and substitutions while eliminating craving and deprivation. You don't need to reinvent the wheel. Make the most of the history and tradition of plant-based eating that occurs around the globe, and have fun while still promoting your personal health and weight loss. Bon appétit!

4

LIFESTYLE SUPPORT FOR PERMANENT WEIGHT/FAT LOSS

CHAPTER 17

THE ROLE OF EXERCISE AND ACTIVITY: MOVE IT AND LOSE IT

L et me be perfectly frank. No long-term health and weight-regulation program will be successful without consistent exercise and activity. Activity/exercise is a basic biological requirement of life and an essential pillar of healthy lifestyle change and the regulation of body fat and weight. While regular exercise significantly improves a wide variety of conditions that demand the most healthcare dollars, including high blood pressure, heart disease, osteoporosis, type 2 diabetes, depression, and cancer, the relationship of calorie expenditure in movement to calorie intake from food is fundamental in energy metabolism and affects the outcomes of weight and body fat. Exercise also significantly reduces chronic inflammation and oxidative stress that can promote insulin resistance, elevated glucose levels, and C-reactive protein levels, which are a strongly associated with obesity. And as you will see, certain exercise approaches can have direct effects on reducing dangerous levels of body fat.

We are built to move until we die, preferably dying in the act of moving. As you look out at the world, it seems that this mentality is making its way more and more into the general population. More people seem to be working out, walking and jogging in their neighborhoods, and going to the gym. Unfortunately, this could not be further from the truth. While some people may be moving more regularly, a national survey by the Kaiser Group indicated that fewer than one-third of Americans are doing some form of physical activity at least three times per week. People in Western nations like the U.S. have become increasingly more sedentary, and this inactivity continues to exact a serious toll by promoting a variety of chronic diseases, especially weight gain and obesity.

The accepted model of fatness that has been around for quite some time is rather short-sighted. This model suggests that the fat cells you have as an adult were laid down in infancy and childhood, leaving people with the limiting idea that if they were overweight as a child, there isn't much they can do about it as an adult. However, we now know that this bleak, deterministic view of obesity is not the whole story. Many people who were lean as children became overweight as adults, but more interestingly, there are people who were overweight as children who became lean as adults. I personally fit into this latter category. I was overweight as a child. I had all that fat on my body and face that ethnic parents and relatives just loved to pinch and was praised for the large amount of food I could make disappear at mealtimes. Yet, I have maintained a lean body with 10-12% body fat throughout most of my adult life. Others fit this description, too, so there appears to be another piece to this story.

What we now know is that fat cells are some of the most dynamic, changeable, plastic cells of the human body. The fat you have as an adult is a combination of the number of cells and the volume of fat contained in these cells.[1] Fat cells expand and shrink depending on the accumulation, mobilization, and utilization of fat by the body. They can change their size and shape markedly, able to grow thousands of times larger or smaller.

However, the number of fat cells that you created early in your life is resistant to reduction. Even in advanced stages of fasting and starvation, the number of fat cells is relatively stable. Unfortunately, there is also a somewhat dark side to this story; while you typically can't eliminate fat cells that were laid down in infancy and childhood, you can add new ones as an adult. When a certain threshold of fat volume is exceeded in available fat cells, it stimulates those cells to divide, creating more fat cells to house the surplus.

Therefore, it is important to realize that both the number and volume of fat cells can be significantly increased by negative lifestyle factors including poor nutrition, lack of activity, excessive stress, and sleep deficiency. So, if you laid down a large number of fat cells early in your life and were overweight as a child, you may be prone to be fatter as an adult. But why get lost in the past with something that you no longer have any control over? It is much more important to understand that the choices I am recommending you continue to make at all stages of your life, from your present time forward, will significantly decrease your volume of body fat while making further production unnecessary. So, regardless of the number of fat cells you created in your childhood, by adopting the positive lifestyle factors of my program, you can be leaner and healthier as an adult than you were at earlier stages of your life.

Surgical procedures to reduce body fat, like liposuction, will never be the answer. Even if you suck out fat cells, if you maintain lifestyle choices that promote the production of fat, you can continue to increase overall body fat that will replace the volume and number of the fat cells that were removed.

In addition, these procedures only contour the body by removing a small amount of fat in specific areas. If you're overweight, it is essential to make choices that can affect a more extensive loss of systemic body fat. Also, these surgical techniques are not benign throwaway procedures. They are blood-and-guts procedures that engender potential risks and complications associated with anesthesia and infection.

Furthermore, even if you surgically remove fat, you still have to come back to the factors that we are sharing to ensure that you will keep it off. So why put yourself at risk when it is most important and essential to focus on the routine choices you can make to successfully and naturally reduce body weight and fat? Enter the world of physical activity and exercise.

A Triangle of Fitness for Successful Weight Loss

I recommend a triangle of fitness for weight loss that involves a combination of endurance/aerobic training, strength/resistance training, and flexibility/lengthening training.

Endurance/Aerobic Activity

When you walk, run, bike, swim, skate, or dance, you're using your skeletal muscles, the large postural muscles that move your skeleton. These muscles are primarily composed of slow-twitch, red-muscle fibers that fire at a low level of stimulation, so they can always be active and ready to help you stand up against the pull of gravity. Two aspects of these muscle fibers are important for our goals. First, they demand oxygen. Second, they burn fat and glycogen reserves as their energy currency.

Large-muscle activity stimulates the energy factories of skeletal muscle cells, the mitochondria, to more effectively translate oxygen into energy. Exercise promotes the health, genetic development, function, and metabolism of these mitochondria and is a powerful tool for enhancing our energy reserves.[2]

How important for weight control is burning fat as the energy currency of skeletal muscle fibers? Again, there are data that suggest that after the age of 25, Americans are gaining as much as one and a half pounds of body fat per year.[1] In addition, around the ages of 30 to 40, the metabolism can begin to slow down due to the increase in body fat and loss of muscle mass. Therefore, as you get older, it gets a lot easier to hold on to fat and harder to take it off. Have you or anybody you know ever experienced that? No doubt. That means as you get older, you've got to move more, not less. As you get older, however, all too often you tend to feel like you've been there, done that, and want to just rest on your laurels. Unfortunately, your laurels just keep getting fatter and wider. So, what's a person to do? You've got to get out there and move your body. You've got to do some form of physical activity that includes aerobic/endurance exercise.

Remember that exercise significantly reduces adiposity.[3] Since postural muscles burn fat and sugar reserves as their energy currency, these are muscles that you need to get friendly with. When you start walking, for example, these muscles get involved. As you increase the intensity of walking, picking up the pace, you recruit more and more muscle fibers. Since physical activity increases the oxygen demand of these muscle fibers, the body's need for oxygen significantly increases. Therefore, as activity increases, the lungs work harder, and you begin to breathe harder and faster. However, this only gets air into your lungs. It's got to get out into the entire body, so the heart also has to beat harder and faster. This type of physical activity that increases the recruitment of red-muscle fibers, increases your muscles' demand for the oxygen that is provided by your heart and lungs, and increases the burning of body fat is called aerobic exercise, also referred to as endurance activity. Aerobic/ endurance activity is the base—the foundation—of my fitness triangle.

If you push your workout to such an extent that your heart and lungs can't keep up with your demand for oxygen, you will create an oxygen debt, and your workout will become more anaerobic. How do you make up an oxygen debt? You hyperventilate and pant. Short bursts of anaerobic training are not a problem. In fact, short intervals of higher-intensity anaerobic training can even promote a beneficial short-term utilization of elevated blood sugar, especially in diabetics, and decrease the burden on insulin. But if you overtrain regularly, pushing yourself into an anaerobic state, it may create some interference with successful weight loss and may even increase risky abdominal fat.

Why is that? When you work out anaerobically, there is a tremendous need for energy, but since fat-burning requires oxygen, the oxygen debt makes it impossible initially for the body to burn fat for energy. If the body can't get energy from fat throughout your workout, it needs to take advantage of the most convenient source of energy it has. Can you guess what that is? It's blood sugar, always available in the bloodstream and always ready for the taking. As a result, regular anaerobic overtraining can promote longer episodes of low blood sugar and create the condition of hypoglycemia. This creates stress in the body that can influence the glands of stress, the adrenal glands, to release the hormone cortisol and increase abdominal belly fat.

How many people want to increase physical activity and get bigger, fatter bellies? No one. So instead of the no pain/no gain, stressed-out-to-the-max, anaerobic overtraining that many people in our culture feel compelled to do, it is best to work out aerobically in a more moderate way that gives you the best opportunity to more slowly burn fat and stored glycogen reserves. This is referred to as the aerobic training rate, the ideal target heart rate to get the most out of your exercise safely. An individual's training rate can be calculated simply using this formula:

Training Rate (TR) = 60–80% of (220 minus your age)

220 minus your age is considered your maximal heart rate or (MHR).

To simplify, I cut this range right down the middle and give you my 70% rule. So, for example, if you are 40 years old, your MHR is 180 (220-40) and your target training rate is 70% of the MHR: .7×180 = 126. To work out in a way that gives you the best opportunity to burn fat, therefore, you want your pulse to be in the range of 120–130. To make it easy, during your workout, take your pulse (at the wrist or neck) for six seconds and just add a zero to whatever number you get—no multiplication, no division, no muss, no fuss. For the best estimate, take your pulse at the beginning of your workout, then again at mid-workout, and one more time at the end of your workout. This will give you a clear idea of whether you have been in your training zone or not. A simpler strategy that doesn't use these calculations and measurements is to work out at an intensity where you are breathing heavier and can barely carry on a conversation.

During extended aerobic training, you may feel a runner's or walker's "high." This feeling of elation is associated with the release of opiates (endorphins and enkephalins) that occurs naturally in the brain; they are released during pleasurable experiences including exercise, meditation, laughter, and sexual activity. These opiates can also suppress appetite. Therefore, when you finish an aerobic workout, there should be a feeling of elation and a natural loss of appetite for some short period of time, perhaps another 30–60 minutes. If you finish a workout and you are immediately fatigued and hungry, you have probably overtrained (trained anaerobically) and created a state of low blood sugar.

It is your training rate that is important, not that of the people you may be training with. You may walk a nine-minute mile while someone else may drag themselves across the floor, and you both may be training. This is why I sometimes have a problem with exercise classes. In a class, there are usually three groups of people: one group for whom the exercise is not strenuous enough, one group that's training aerobically, and one group that's overtraining, huffing and puffing. Like an aerobic Goldilocks and the three bears, you want to find the pace that's just right for you.

If your goal is to decrease weight and body fat, it is recommended that you get into your training rate at least four to five times per week for a minimum of 20 minutes each. To achieve this, I recommend walking 30 minutes five times per week, or 45 minutes four times per week. This timing allows for a warm-up, a cool-down, and at least 20–30 minutes of fat-burning aerobic time.

I like walking because there is a great aerobic return on your time investment, and it's something you can do at almost any age. All you need is a decent pair of shoes and a piece of ground or a treadmill.

With the possible exception of cross-country skiing, nothing will change your body (especially if you are a woman) exactly the way you want it—firmer hips, thighs, waist, and abdomen—as well as walking will, especially racewalking or at least adopting a modified racewalking gait. A good description of this gait, illustrated with effective animation, can be found online at: https://youtu.be/6205BWkdrUY.

Interval walking will burn even more calories. Interval training is when you walk at pace that gets you to your mid-level training rate for 5–10 minutes, then increase the pace to your highest level of aerobic training (or even a little bit above it) for a few minutes, then come back to your mid-level rate, and repeat this alternating pattern throughout your workout.

When your schedule is really busy and your time is limited, there is evidence from studies in a variety of countries including the United Kingdom, Australia, and the United States that episodes of "short-burst activity" (SBA) can promote a significant improvement in fitness and fat-burning. For example, performing your favorite activity at a moderate pace for 45 seconds followed by 15 seconds of maximum effort/intensity and repeating this pattern a minimum of 20 times three to four times per week can significantly lower high blood pressure, high blood sugar, and elevated cholesterol while remarkably increasing fat-burning. Short-burst activity has also been shown to increase the release of growth hormone, which may slow down the aging process, and to suppress the release of the body's natural appetite stimulant, ghrelin, which can reduce hunger and craving. Episodes of SBA also can even be incorporated into routine housekeeping tasks to transform some of your routine activities of daily living into more dramatic fitness and fat-burning activities.

Your commitment to physical activity should be a minimum of four times per week. This is nonnegotiable. That means even on that week when you feel like you have no time left for anything, you still work out four times. But I'll give you one concession. If you get up in the morning, look in your mirror (you have to do this completely naked because this is a moment of truth) and say, "Damn, look at me: I am perfect, I look so good, I couldn't look any better than I look right now," then three times per week is cool for you. For everybody else, it's four times per week. I have a simple rule of thumb. If your fork can make it from your plate to your mouth, get yourself moving. If you ate that day, you move that day. No question about it, the people who have the most successful long-term weight loss have made a commitment to routine movement and consistent exercise.

We are animals built to move, but we have become way too sedentary. We are animals who are built to run and walk and climb and jump, and when we confine ourselves to sedentary behavior, we are going against our very nature and will pay a serious price on physical, emotional, and spiritual levels. In fact, I will elaborate on this later, but I feel that the epidemics of insomnia and depression that are so common in our culture are directly related to the fact that we just don't move enough.

When it comes to movement, I like to replace the concept of exercise with the concept of pleasurable activity. Do something you like. If you don't like walking, do something else, an activity you really enjoy doing. If you like to swim, swim four to five times per week. If you like to dance, dance four to five times per week. I can tell you to go to the gym, and you may go because "the doctor told me to." Then you realize that you hate the gym, and in two days it's over. There is no reason why you can't have fun with it. You *need* to have fun with it. Let's face it: we are fun-seeking, pleasure-seeking creatures, and you will be more successful in your commitment to exercise if you do something you really enjoy. Just remember, you have got to move. There are no exceptions...well, maybe only one: if you fail what I call the George Burns test, you don't need to include movement in your life.

Do you remember the famous comedian? He always had a cigar in his mouth and was still doing stand-up comedy in his 90s. This is one of the most famous orthopedic tests in science and medicine (well, kind of). Stand up and alternately extend your arms overhead and out to the sides. If your hands hit the side of a coffin, you failed the test and don't need to exercise. That's the George Burns test.

Please understand that this is not just about formal exercising. Move more in your normal activities of daily living. Take the stairs, park your car farther away from your destination so you have to walk more, and so on. The average person in the U.S. spends approximately six hours per day sitting in front of one screen or another—TVs, computers, cell phones, etc. It has been estimated that if you can cut screen time down about two hours per day while increasing simple basic movement, it can translate to about 10 pounds of weight loss per year.

Recently, one of the medical directors of the World Health Organization made a statement that addresses the concerns about sedentary behavior. He said that when you look at Americans today compared with 30–40 years ago, they are spending 600 fewer calories per day in normal activities of daily living. It only takes approximately 3,500 extra calories over and above what your body needs to perform its daily activities to add an extra pound of fat on the body. When you consider how much our portion sizes have increased over the years and you add that to the reduction in calories burned due to the rise in sedentary behavior, it's not hard to understand how the pandemic of obesity has occurred to such a grotesque degree. Move.

Strength/Resistance Training

While aerobic/endurance exercise is the foundation of my fitness triangle, one of the other very important legs of the triangle is resistance training performed with free weights, machines, or bands. As people get older, and as early as age 40, there is a natural loss of muscle mass called sarcopenia. Remember, muscles harbor energy as glycogen, a storage form of sugar. When muscle mass is lost, not only is there a relative increase in body fat, but also the body's ability to store energy is reduced, resulting in more fatigue.

In fact, there is a phenomenon that occurs as people get older, typically referred to as senile fatigue: you get older and more tired. So, you go to your doctor and tell the doc that you feel tired a lot of the time. Your doc tells you not to worry, that you just got older and you've got senile fatigue. You reply that you already knew that. Unfortunately, the doc didn't tell you one of the important things you have to do to fix it. The most effective long-term solution is to increase muscle mass through the process of weight training. When you add muscle mass, you create more energy factories (mitochondria in the new muscle cells), which in turn increase your opportunity for energy production and availability. The increase in muscle mass and energy can dramatically improve metabolic efficiency and significantly enhance fat loss and weight regulation.

A Routine Weight-Training Program

As a routine weight-training program, I recommend eight basic movements, five for the upper body and three for the lower body. These are movements that incorporate the eight major muscle groups of the body.

• Chest

Chest muscles, the pectorals, are best worked with push-ups or with a bench press in a sitting position, on an incline, or lying down on your back.

• Shoulders

Sitting with your back relaxed and lengthened, gently braced against the back of a chair (or standing), hold weights at shoulder height and push up overhead in a shoulder press.

• Back

The latissimus dorsi muscles, running from the spine across the back, are best worked with a rowing-motion apparatus in a sitting position or by reaching up and pulling down an overhead bar that is connected to weights.

• Front of upper arms (biceps)

The biceps are best targeted with biceps curls. Standing or sitting, arms hanging down at your sides holding weights, bend your arms at the elbows curling the weights upwards.

• Back of upper arms (triceps)

Work the triceps with triceps extensions. Bending forward at the waist, hold a weight with your elbow at your waist and the arm bent at a 90-degree angle. In a smooth motion, extend the weight backwards, straightening your arm. You also can use a triceps pull-down Y-rope or Y-bar, holding the rope or bar in front of you with arms flexed, and then lowering the bar or rope until your arms are in a straight, extended position in front of you.

• Front thigh (quadriceps)

Sitting in leg-extension/curl machine, extend the lower leg upward against resistance. Alternatively, perform lunges with or without weights in hand or squat with a weighted bar across your shoulders.

• Back thigh (hamstrings)

Hamstrings can be worked by standing or lying on your stomach with your leg in a stirrup strap and curling the lower leg upwards against resistance.

• Hip extension

The hip is the most common area of fracture in post-menopausal women, so movements that help prevent bone loss in the hip are essential as we age. Using a leg extension machine, stand with your foot in a stirrup that is attached to a pulley system that allows you to lift variable weight resistance and extend the leg back behind the body, stretching and opening up the hip joint to increase the angle between your hip and thigh.

For these exercises, I recommend using an amount of weight that allows you to do 10–12 repetitions of each of the movements, working up from one to three sets for all the muscle groups. The workout will take about 30 minutes and should be done two to three times per week.

The combination of aerobic activity and weight training is not only essential for preventing bone loss in men and women as they get older, but also for significantly reversing the problem of insulin resistance so as to stabilize blood sugar and prevent and/or reverse diabetes. The impact of activity on diabetes is an interesting side note of our weight-loss story. While type 2 diabetes is a genetically predisposed metabolic disorder, the epigenetic impact of diet and exercise is profound. Interestingly, even in people who already have developed diabetes, prolonged exercise over time restores metabolic and cardiovascular function.[4]

Type 2 diabetes is truly a disease of obesity and sedentary behavior. It is promoted and sustained to the greatest extent in people who maintain a sedentary lifestyle. Let me rephrase that in anatomical terms the way I learned it in the Bronx: type 2 diabetes in adults or children is a sitting-on-your-butt disease. That's a big reason why there currently is a huge epidemic of type 2 diabetes, which used to normally be seen in people above the ages of 40–50 but is now showing up in teenagers and young adults. In fact, one of the largest growing groups of diabetics in the U.S. is people between the ages of 18 and 30.

Our children have gotten way too sedentary, in part because physical education has all but disappeared from the public school system, but also because of the troubling, extreme increase in sedentary screen time on phones, computers, etc. In addition to refined-food diets, diminished activity is one of the reasons why, in the past 30 years, the most rapidly increasing group of overweight people in the U.S. has been children under the age of 19.

Increases in body fat/weight gain may be the most significant factor for the growing epidemic of diabetes. In addition, obesity and diabetes are two of the most influential factors in increasing the risk of and mortality from cardiovascular disease, the number one killer in our culture.

As I've explained, insulin resistance is fundamental to the development of obesity and diabetes. Weight training and aerobic activity have a unique, positive impact on the function and attachment of insulin and can reduce the problem of insulin resistance.[3,5] Resistance training also stimulates the growth and function of skeletal muscles, those that move our skeletons. When you work out with weights, there is an increase in the number and sensitivity of insulin receptors on the surface of cells in the muscles activated by resistance training. This increase in insulin receptors increases the number of places where insulin can attach, opening more doors in the membranes of muscle cells and activating more sugar transport vehicles to significantly enhance the entry of sugar into these cells. Therefore, sugar levels in the blood will drop more effectively, reducing the chance of developing diabetes, fat production, and weight gain.

Flexibility/Lengthening Training

As we get older, there is a shortening, tightening, and hunching of the body in general, and in several muscle groups in particular. The increase in back and pelvic pain and the resulting disability that is so common in our culture is promoted to a great extent by weak core strength, the painful shortening of the adductor muscles of your inner thigh, and the hamstrings in the back of your thigh. This can interfere with your workout program and make it much harder for you to control your weight.

So, not only do we want to increase endurance and strengthen, but we also need to increase flexibility by lengthening the body's muscles.

Therefore, the third leg of my fitness triangle is flexibility training. This is where the magical movements of yoga, tai chi, or systems like Pilates have tremendous value. These approaches work directly on gentle stretching, opening, and lengthening. If you do not already practice any of these disciplines, consider starting. The internet offers many online videos you can easily do in your own home, and little or no equipment is needed for most of the exercises. Take some time each day to gently stretch and release the muscles of the lower back, pelvis, inner thighs, and hamstrings. Keeping these areas limber will dramatically reduce the hip, back, and pelvic pain that have become increasingly prevalent in our culture for people of all ages, but especially for people who are more elderly.

Age Is No Barrier

When it comes to getting older, do not let any negative, preconceived notions about age interfere with your commitment to an exercise regimen and your potential fitness success. Regardless of your age, it is never too late to start a regular fitness program. Significant, beneficial increases in muscle mass and decreases in body fat can be achieved and maintained even in your elder years when you commit to an ongoing activity program. In a comparison of MRI scans of muscles of the upper thigh (the quadriceps muscles) of a 40-year-old triathlete, a 74-year-old sedentary man, and a 74-year-old triathlete, it is striking to see that the 74-year-old triathlete's MRI is similar to the 40-year-old triathlete's, with significantly enhanced muscle mass and decreased fat content, while the sedentary 74-year-old shows significant muscle loss and accumulation of body fat.[6]

Additional Benefits: Decreased Body Fat, Decreased Setpoint, and Weight Control

The body seeks and maintains equilibrium and stability. With regard to energy use, weight, body temperature, etc., it finds a level, within a healthy normal range, at which those functions tend to stabilize, which

is called the setpoint. In a sense, the setpoint is part of the body's ther-
mostat that establishes a balance point around which the body's calorie
needs can be regulated, basically evaluating the calories that you're taking in versus the calories that you're burning up. As we have discussed,
aerobic activity involves muscle fibers that, in combination with WFPE
nutrition, burn body fat as their energy currency. The drop in body fat
creates a relative increase in lean muscle mass, enhancing the metabolic
machinery of the body and effectively lowering the setpoint for body fat.

In other words, when you lower body fat through exercise and nutrition, there is an improvement in overall metabolism, so that calories are
more effectively burned rather than retained. As a result, you can actually eat more food and regulate weight more effectively when regularly
exercising, especially when you're eating more plant-exclusive foods that
are low in calorie density. This is important because the mindset associated with weight loss has been associated for so long with the idea of
deprivation. All too often, people with weight issues have become con-
vinced that denying oneself the pleasure of eating is the only path to success. The fact of the matter is that such deprivation typically provokes
craving, compulsive food use, and inevitably, reactive weight gain.

**Please understand that this program is not about
eating less. It is about eating well.**

It is so important to embrace this new perspective. I have had the
unique opportunity of directing several plant-exclusive health centers
that were extremely successful in helping thousands of people lose substantial amounts of weight. In the first few days to weeks of adopting the
program I'm sharing with you, clients would often lose about one-half
to one pound per day, especially if they were previously eating a more
typical conventional Western diet loaded with refined and animal-based
foods. Following the conversion to a vegan, WFPE diet, therefore, you
could lose as much as three to seven pounds in the early weeks. All too

often, someone would come into my office who may have just lost five pounds in a week, and they would complain about the large amount of food that was being served. "But you just lost five pounds," I would remind them. In their mind, if it didn't involve deprivation, they would think that something must be wrong. What was wrong was their mindset.

If you try to lose weight with extensive calorie restriction, all you do is slow down your basal metabolic rate (BMR). Remember, the body has a way of looking at and balancing the calories you are taking in compared with the calories you are burning up. When at rest, the body needs to burn a certain number of calories to maintain the basic functions of the body; the BMR is that baseline number. If you dramatically reduce calorie intake while continuing normal activity, the body has no choice but to slow down its resting metabolism to balance the new challenging stress of reduced calorie supply. Under these conditions, eventually the body can continue to gain weight on less and less food; even small amounts of food, and especially the smallest amounts of refined and processed food, can provoke significant weight gain. In fact, you will seemingly gain weight on air alone. People will remark, "Oh, my god! I haven't eaten anything for six months, and I gained 6 pounds." Unfortunately, as I've already discussed, calorie deprivation can eventually trigger a starvation response, which leads to a loss of satiety signals and reactive overeating. What really needs to be done is to eat plentifully of high-fiber, low-fat, low-calorie-dense plant foods while also jacking up metabolism and energy efficiency with physical activity. By moving more, by eating well, and by avoiding extreme calorie restriction and fragmented diets that trigger the starvation response, you can more effectively reduce compulsive overeating and avoid reactive weight gain.

Eliminating Food Cravings

As I have discussed, when a person has insulin resistance, sugar cannot enter their body's cells, and the cells become starved for sugar. This results in a craving for sugar. Since exercise improves insulin attachment and helps heal and reverse the problem of insulin resistance, it helps eliminate sugar craving. This very positive effect on hormonal balance and function is one of several important reasons why exercise is such an invaluable tool for dealing with food addictions and compulsive food use.

Resolving Depression and Insomnia

Exercise also evokes a series of chemical changes in the body and brain that may reduce depression and anxiety. This is an important part of our story because, as you will see when we discuss addiction, the addictive process can be associated with depression. Consistent physical activity can stimulate the release of neurotransmitters in the brain, especially opiates, serotonin and dopamine, which have antidepressive and anti-anxiety effects.[7-9]

I think it's safe to say that depression and anxiety have achieved a devastating epidemic status in our culture. The causes of depression can be genetic and/or lifestyle-related. The excessive use of stimulants (coffee, sugar, etc.) to mindlessly raise the flagging energy of our exhausted, hectic culture has definitely contributed to the epidemic of depression, simply because all stimulants cause rebound depression.

Unfortunately, the excessive use of psychotropic drugs prescribed for anxiety and depression is a glaring example of unwarranted drug abuse in our culture. The prescription of these drugs is based on the faulty premise that depression is primarily caused by a deficiency of serotonin—due to some compromise of serotonin release, action, uptake, or metabolism—in the synapses (spaces) between nerve cells in the brain. The scientific evidence does not fully support this assumption and, on the contrary, suggests that these drugs incite compensatory changes in the brain that can compromise normal brain function, brain chemistry, and neurotransmitter action, potentially reinforcing and promoting long-term depression, anxiety, and other mental illness.[10]

However, there is finally some truth in advertising. In television advertising for antidepressant medications, they quite honestly state that two out of every three people on these medications are still clinically depressed. What does that tell you? You don't need to be a rocket scientist to know the answer: the drugs are not working! Yet even though the efficacy of these drugs is questionable, so much revenue is generated by their use that they continue to sink their tentacles into the psyche of the public, feeding the coffers of the pharmaceutical industry and the physician pushers who prescribe them. So much money is invested in these medications that it's obvious that they're not going away. However, they are so inefficient and ineffective that a whole new—and significantly more dangerous and even life threatening—class of drugs has been created to amplify the ineffectiveness of the original antidepressants.

What makes this even worse is that one of the largest growing groups of users (and abusers) of medication for depression in the U.S. has been children under the age of 10. There are now more than one million children under the age of five on these medications, even though no studies that have ever been done to show the safety or efficacy of these drugs in children. Even worse, it is well-known that children under the age of 18 who take these meds are significantly more prone to suicide and suicidal thinking. This is something to seriously consider when you realize that in recent years, there has been a more than 50% increase in teenage suicide in America.

Antidepressant drugs do not increase the body's ability to produce the transmitters that improve well-being and emotional stability. They just allow these transmitters to linger longer by blocking the body's ability to break them down. Don't get me wrong: if you were drowning, I would throw you a life preserver to help you float. However, to really help you long-term, I need to teach you how to swim. If you were drowning in depression, some short-term use of drugs that help you just float may be a lifesaver. But in the long run, you need cognitive tools, skills, behaviors, and nutritional choices that allow you to more naturally increase the brain chemistry of well-being so that you are more empowered to swim effectively throughout life.

Exercise is one of these powerful tools for improving your mental health. There is clear evidence that strenuous and consistent exercise significantly reduces depression and anxiety.[11-13] Four months of exercise was shown to have a benefit comparable to typical serotonin-enhancing antidepressant medication but without any of the adverse effects and potential harm associated with these drugs.[13] Exercise naturally and powerfully increases the brain chemistry that improves well-being, pleasure, and emotional stability. It helps balance the pleasure-reward process in the brain, and it can also help you improve your relationship with food and eating, reduce the need for compulsive food use, and enhance your opportunity for successful weight loss.

The same brain chemical that affects emotional well-being, serotonin, also affects our craving for fat and sugar, and it is one of the neurotransmitters involved in promoting restful sleep. When serotonin levels are altered, as they are in depression, there can be an increased craving for fat and sugar as well as a potential disturbance of normal, healthy sleep cycles. Since exercise increases serotonin levels, it can help counteract these cravings.

Also, it's no mystery why people who exercise more regularly typically sleep better: aerobic activity significantly increases serotonin production, promoting better sleep and reducing insomnia. It is now known that sleep deficiency can promote weight gain, so the impact of exercise on the sleep cycle is also important for long-term weight loss. For the most part, you don't need sleep meds or sleep products. These drugs may allow you to achieve some additional sleep, but they do not promote the pattern of sleep that is so important for weight control.

Do not underestimate the full impact of an ongoing activity program in your life. Moving regularly and vigorously is an important directive of your innate intelligence and body wisdom. When you live in a way that is more consistent with your true human nature and embrace exercise routinely, you have the greatest opportunity for emotional and physical well-being. This will promote a healthy and more mindful sensitivity to those factors that promote high-level health in general and the most successful weight loss and maintenance in particular.

CHAPTER 18

STRESS AND WEIGHT GAIN: KISSING STRESS GOOD-BYE

One of the most important yet overlooked parts of the weight-loss story is the impact of stress and stress response management on body fat and weight. The discussion of stress brings us directly into the arena of what is referred to as the mind-body connection, how the psychological and emotional fabric of our lives affects what we experience in every aspect of the physical body and vice-versa.

For the longest time, the idea that our thoughts and feelings could affect the symptoms and actions of the body was only in the musings of artists and philosophers. However, over the past half century, this idea has become firmly enmeshed in the world of science. For quite some time now, there have been whole fields of psycho-neuro-endo-immunology, the study of how our psychology and our nervous, endocrine, and immune systems interact to create what we experience physically and emotionally. This work has yielded physicians and scientists who now think that as much as 80% of everything we suffer with as human beings is stress-related, including heart disease, cancer, and weight gain.

A classic example of this interaction is the extensive and well-documented impact of chronic stress on the immune system.[1] It has been known for some time that during chronic stress, the increase in stress hormones decreases the function of the immune system. This classic effect of long-term stress is often seen in caregivers. When caregivers take care of sick and dying relatives and loved ones, they demonstrate immune suppression with slower wound-healing and increased susceptibility to bacterial and viral infection. The suppression of immunity over time can result in a wide variety of pathological conditions, including allergies, autoimmune diseases, and even cancer.

You might be asking yourself the million-dollar question: how can a stressful event affect the intricate workings of the immune system? The answer to this question is a remarkable example of body wisdom and a fundamental example of how the body is a world of intricate connection and relentless, ongoing feedback and communication.

Nerve fibers from the brain and sympathetic nervous system—the part of the nervous system primarily activated by stress—innervate the cells and tissues of the immune system, including bone marrow, thymus gland, spleen, lymph nodes, white blood cells, and lymphocytes, directly affecting the function of the white blood cells and natural killer cells involved in immunity.[2-5] In addition, the hormone cortisol and the neurotransmitter noradrenaline released during stress can attach directly to white blood cells and affect their function and involvement. Also, chronic stress can promote accelerated cellular aging[6] and inflammation that damages the inner walls of blood vessels to the heart. This damage attracts white blood cells (macrophages) that gobble up LDL cholesterol and become foam cells forming the fatty plaque (atherosclerosis) that promotes heart damage/disease.[7]

When we talk about stress, it can be somewhat confusing, because the word stress itself is a high-level abstraction that has different meanings depending on a wide range of circumstances. For example, a certain amount of stress can be good when it positively motivates the performance of athletes or performers. In fact, the biological concept of hormesis refers to beneficial physical and genetic effects that occur when living things respond and adapt to low levels of toxic and stressful conditions. It's like that old line by the famous German philosopher, Friedrich Nietzsche, "That which doesn't kill us makes us stronger." However, stress can also be associated with the conflicts and pressures of any number of situations, both major and minor: life-cycle changes (e.g., childhood to adolescence to adulthood), lifestyle adjustments (e.g., marital state, home locations, work and retirement, parenting), family and work relationships, and overwhelming traumatic and catastrophic events. All of these circumstances come under the umbrella of stress. To simplify and clarify the role of stress in health and weight loss, I will be addressing what I call the changing nature of stress and your stress response management. To fully appreciate these concepts, I need to discuss the way the body typically reacts to stressful circumstances.

Like all mammals, we have the inborn ability to confront, resolve, and survive threatening and traumatic events in our environment. When we encounter these stressful circumstances, there are basically two options: we can fight the situation head-on, or we can turn around and run away from it. Hence, these options are referred to as the fight-or-flight response and are under the direction of the excitatory part of our nervous system called the sympathetic nervous system.

Although it is not discussed much in the literature and research on stress, there is a third option of response to stressful conditions that is important for human behavior. When you encounter an event that is so overwhelming that you really believe there's nothing you can do about it, you can lie down and play dead, also referred to as the possum or Thanatos response. This survival strategy of "freezing still" is linked to the idea that if you lie down and play dead, your aggressor will think you're out of the game and will pass you by. However, understand that the possum response is a response of hopelessness or overwhelming trauma. It is a surrender to events that you truly believe are out of your control, a deep sense that there's nothing you can do to make a difference. Have you ever had the feeling when you were dealing with some stress in your life, maybe in your family or a relationship, that no matter what you did, it was just not good enough, filling you with a sense of despair and hopelessness? I'm sure the answer is a resounding yes. I know I have.

If you think about it, these three responses basically sum up what happens whenever human experiences and interactions become stressful. Usually, some combination of fighting, running away, and/or surrendering is employed. Yet, the major survival responses are to fight or to run away. To understand this fight-or-flight response, I need you to follow me as we take a journey back in time. Imagine that you are living in a very austere, threatening time in the distant past. As you emerge from your condo cave, you encounter a threatening tribe or animal (much like entering the subway system in New York City). Again, you've basically got two choices: you can fight or you can run away. For either one, your body wants to get as much blood and oxygen into the muscles in the shortest period of time, so the actions of arousal are designed to provide this much-needed oxygen and blood supply. Let's take a look at these actions of arousal.

Increased Muscle Tension

Muscles tense up and get poised and ready for action. Keep in mind that no matter what you experience physically, emotionally, or spiritually, the only way you can respond and act on these experiences in your environment is through the nervous and muscular system. So, in a sense, the response and activity of your muscles is intimately affected by much of our routine behavior. It is also why so much of our physical and emotional trauma and pain can manifest in our muscular system.

Increased Blood Pressure and Heart Rate

The body attempts to pump more blood and oxygen into muscles for action by increasing the pressure of blood as well as the number of times the heart pumps that blood per unit of time. These responses are also related to a very important measure of heartbeat and one of the most important measures of fight-or-flight stress called heart rate variability (HRV). Keep in mind that your heart rate is never constant. It must vary throughout your day based on the demands of your body, e.g. if you are physically active, stressed or at rest. Simply, HRV is the variation of time between heartbeats and is controlled by the autonomic, or automatic, part of our nervous system that works behind the scenes regulating a wide variety of basic life functions. Basically, when you are in sympathetic fight-or-flight mode, as the heart beats faster, the variations in the times between heartbeats is less (lower HRV), and when you are in a more relaxed state, the variations in the times between heartbeats is greater (higher HRV). HRV is a valuable tool to evaluate both the negative impact of chronic stress and/or healthy relaxation strategies in your life.

Increased Respiratory Rate

Breathing becomes more rapid and shallow as the body tries to get more oxygen into the muscles in the shortest period of time. While this restricted pattern of breathing is essential for short-term survival, it becomes counterproductive when stress is more chronic, since it promotes oxygen deprivation and more tension over time. Unfortunately, this short, shallow rapid breathing pattern is the pattern of anxiety and has become the typical pattern for many people dealing with the ongoing tension of our hectic culture. [xxi] Breathing is the most important primal function of the body directly affecting physical and mental health, and unhealthy breathing patterns lead to persistent, subtle tension in the body.

[xxi] The way your breath goes, so go your emotions. Toward the end of this chapter, I will elaborate on the impact of breathing on different states of emotion and share a quick and easy breathing technique that can help you establish a healthy breathing pattern and reduce anxiety and stress in the moment.

Decreased Digestive Function

If you're concerned with some life-threatening circumstance, how concerned do you think you're going to be with getting your next gourmet meal? "That tiger looks like it's going to take my head off; boy, am I hungry." No way! In the stress response, the digestive system is basically shut down as the muscular movement of the digestive system is decreased and the hormones and enzymes of digestion are significantly reduced.

Consider what this means. It means that when stressed, we are least able to digest our food. Yet, when do most of us eat the most? Under stress. And when do we eat the most difficult things to digest, namely high fat and high sugar? Again, under stress, simply because we have associated these foods with comfort and distraction. So, many of us are eating the most difficult-to-digest foods at the times when we are least able to digest them. Is it any wonder, then, why gas, bloating, distention, reflux, and heartburn are so prevalent in our culture? You don't need antacids and anti-reflux drugs; you just need to realize that sometimes the best meal you can have is the one you miss. Sometimes not eating is the smartest thing to do. When stressed, most animals basically stop eating. Humans seem to be the only animals that will overeat in fight-or-flight stress.

Decreased Immune System Function

In the typical fight-or-flight response there will be a short-term suppression and reduction in the function of the immune system. This reduction of immunity may not sound very constructive, but in a sense, the body is trading off longer-term protection for short-term survival. For energy to be devoted to dealing with life-threatening circumstances, it is necessary, and even beneficial, for less energy be expended in any immune response.[7] Notice I said short-term survival, because as we discussed, if the stress becomes chronic, there can be a long-term suppression of the immune system that may compromise health and survival over time.

Increased Cholesterol

While short-term cholesterol elevation in a fight-or-flight moment is not that important, the impact of chronic stress can provoke a significant long-term increase in serum cholesterol levels. As a result, a fair number of milligrams/deciliter of cholesterol on your blood tests are likely to be stress-related, though you will rarely find any physician that addresses this significant contribution. This has been known for quite some time, but it is amazing to me how many doctors are either unaware of it or unconcerned about it.

Decreased Libido and Sexual Function

In longer-term stress situations such as the threat and trauma of relentless financial, work, relationship, and family pressures, how interested are you, really, in putting on your sexiest accoutrement and getting excited about love-time with your mate? Probably not very. When you are overwhelmed by stressors of life, how interested are you in being the best, most-sensitive lover you can be? Probably not very much. These examples are the result of the typical loss of libido and sexual function in fight-or-flight stress conditions. As you might surmise, this is a huge problem for men and women in our culture today, and even though there can be other physical and nutritional reasons for this dysfunction, chronic stress is a major contributing factor to decreased libido.

The human body's responses to fight-or-flight stressors have evolved over eons for our benefit and survival. If you look carefully, you will notice that these physical responses of healthy survival are at the root of the very things that drive most people to the doctor's office on a daily basis: high blood pressure, cardiac concerns, respiratory problems, and a litany of digestive difficulties, plus immune system disorders, musculoskeletal pain syndromes, cholesterol excesses, and an epidemic of libido loss and sexual dysfunction.

On a regular basis, people are trying to medicate out of existence the consequences of the very actions that the human body has created for their benefit, but the truth is that you can't get rid of these responses short of removing your entire brain and nervous system. Since you're probably not going to choose the neurosurgery route, the better question is not why are these problems happening to you, but why has your body found it necessary to chronically create and relentlessly maintain these stress responses?

The Changing Nature of Stress Response

To understand this better, I introduce you to a concept called the changing nature of stress response. Imagine again the trip to the distant past. When you were confronted by a threatening tribe or animal, you would feel the tension, express the actions of fighting or running away in the moment, deal with the challenge, discharge the tension, and move on to your next survival challenge.

Unfortunately, in modern times we are not dealing with clear-cut threats from other tribes and animals. Today's stressors have become more of the gnawing, nagging stressors of interpersonal relationships and the abstractions of human communication. Such stressors tend to linger within us, remaining for long periods of time and maintaining an ongoing presence in your consciousness that interferes with your ability to fully experience the present moments of your life. Instead of discharging the tension in present time, you can get lost in the sorrows and traumas of the past or become worried and apprehensive about your insecure future. As a result, you lose contact with the only moment you have, which is the precious present that you are in, here and now.

Remember, the past was your present at one time, but in the present, the past is only an illusion, a memory shadow of what once was. Thoughts and memories of the past are mere descriptions of experiences that took place in a present that you once inhabited but no longer exists. They no more accurately create the full-bodied experiences and feelings of current life than words or maps are the real objects and territories they attempt to describe. Unfortunately, we often populate the present with the lifeless corpses of past memories. The future will be your present at some point, but nothing about the future is promised in your present because the future is also an illusion that may or may not occur.

The only place you can truly access your life is right now, in this instant. The exciting, constantly changing, unknown magic and mystery of life unfolds moment to moment, providing a remarkable opportunity to fully feel and be the moment and transcend the illusion of separation created by your ego that fears change and mystery, allowing you to realize the true reality of connection to all that is. When you lose contact with your present, you become less and less effective in discharging, changing, and resolving the stressful situations of your life.

For example, have you ever argued with a loved one? Who hasn't? When you argue, your blood pressure goes up. As we've seen, the arousal response has been physiologically programmed to go up, but also to come back down in a short period of time. If you internalize the argument's hostility and incorporate this tension but do not discharge and release it, it will remain in your life from one argument and upset to the next.

When you hold on to the stress of your life, the fight-or-flight response stays turned on. So, the high blood pressure that was initially created for your survival and benefit will then be carried into your future where it can become a condition of chronic disease. The high blood pressure is not the root problem; your inability to effectively discharge the stress in present time is. If blood pressure stays elevated high enough for long enough, it can damage your brain, your heart, and your kidneys, and every step along the way you'll find an army of happy physicians that will gladly treat every one of these problems with pills and procedures. Please remember the following words of research scientist Robert Sapolsky: "Stress-related disease occurs because we often activate a physiological system that has evolved for responding to acute physical emergencies, but we turn it on for months on end worrying about mortgages, relationships, and promotions."[8]

Bottom line: when we talk about stress management, it must begin with bringing our attention into present-time awareness.

Adaptation to Stress and Weight Control

To understand how stress relates to weight loss, it is necessary to examine the body's hormonal and chemical responses to stress. The stressors of life are more than the psychological and emotional factors that are typically associated with stress. I describe stress factors under the umbrella of the three Ts: *trauma, toxins,* and *thought.*

This includes all injury and physical *trauma,* including the inflammation, cell damage, and oxidative stress (free radical damage) caused by eating animal and processed foods. It includes all *toxic* substances you are exposed to, including environmental toxins in our food supply (pesticides, herbicides, and food additives), personal care products, and all the toxic by-products ingested in animal and processed food consumption, including saturated and trans fats; high sugar and the resulting excessive insulin output from insulin resistance; oxidized cholesterol and oxysterols from dairy and eggs in processed foods; heme iron; trimethylamine N-oxide (TMAO); heterocyclic amines; and advanced glycation endproducts (AGEs). And lastly *thought,* which includes all the emotional and psychological factors and worries of our lives.

The General Adaptation Response

To take it a step further, when you encounter any of these stressful circumstances, the body's arousal response is part of a larger, extensive process called the General Adaptation Response (GAR).[9, xxii] Figure 3 presents a general overview of the GAR. In the small boxes depicting the GAR sequence, notice the line of energy availability/use traversing

---

[xxii] Dr. Hans Selye's name for his discovery was the General Adaptation Syndrome. I have chosen to use the word "Response" here instead of "Syndrome" because the process is more clearly understood as a natural body response.

from good health to exhaustion. Energy use peaks during the resistance phase and then crashes to its lowest point in the exhaustion phase.

General Adaptation Response

1. Alarm
Adrenal hormone release:
cortisol, adrenaline,
norepinephrine

2. Resistance
Chronic stress, cortisol
excess, adrenal depletion,
thyroid recruitment

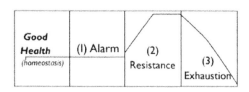

3. Exhaustion
Burnout and reactive
weight gain

Figure 3. The three phases of the General Adaptation Response. The bracketed line in the diagram shows the availability and utilization of energy as the body transitions from the basic state of health/ homeostasis to exhaustion. (Image source: Public Domain)

Let's take a closer look at the phases as the body moves from a stable state of health and homeostasis.

Alarm Phase

This is not a bell but a chemical alarm. In the alarm phase, the stress hormone cortisol and the neurotransmitters norepinephrine and adrenaline are released from the adrenal glands, the glands of stress. The cortisol and neurotransmitters generate all of the fight-or-flight responses mentioned previously. Without these biochemicals, there is no increase in heart rate, blood pressure, breathing rate, etc., and therefore no arousal response or survival mechanism. If you can handle the situation behind the alarm in present time and halt the stress response, thereby minimizing hormone/neurotransmitter production, the situation will be over and no additional reaction will be necessary.

But unfortunately, all too often our modern stressors are the gnawing, nagging variety mentioned earlier that linger on and become chronic, leading to a steady, ongoing adrenal response and release of stress chemicals to continuously resist the ongoing conditions of stress. As a result, you move into the second phase of the GAR, resistance.

Resistance

Dealing with stress is an energy-demanding process, and the sugar in your blood is a readily available source of immediate energy. Recall that the body controls overall blood sugar by storing some of it as glycogen in a savings account in liver and muscle cells and converts the excess into fatty acids in fat cells. The body can lean on this reserve during the stress response. So in the short run, if we deal with stress in the present time of the alarm phase, that's just fine and dandy, and quite efficient.

However, when stress is constant, and we are driven into the resistance phase, there is a chronic stimulation of the adrenal glands and a resulting chronic elevation of cortisol. Under the demands of ongoing resistance, cortisol can excessively draw on your sugar savings account to replenish the bloodstream by pulling glycogen from the liver and muscle and fatty acids from fat cells to provide a consistent level of energy to fuel the chronic stress response.[10] Over time this increased energy demand can deplete blood sugar reserves and may even lead to craving and stressful eating of processed junk food.

To expand on what I discussed briefly in the chapters on exercise and hormone regulation, cortisol has a natural affinity—a love affair—with fat cells in the abdominal region. The chronic elevation of cortisol can stimulate both the genetic expression and activity of the fat-making enzyme lipoprotein lipase in fat cells around your belly.[11] When these fat cells are exposed to the high levels of cortisol and the heightened levels of sugar and fatty acids released in the chronic stress response, they can convert the sugar and fatty acids into fat and dramatically increase the deposition of visceral belly fat. That's why increasing belly fat is typically due to a cortisol-induced stress pattern of weight gain.

Let me emphasize again that abdominal weight gain is the riskiest weight gain of all. When belly fat increases, the risks of stroke, heart disease, diabetes, and cancer also increase, dramatically. Historically, the expansion of belly fat was the typical male pattern of weight gain. This was associated with an increased incidence in heart disease and more heart attacks in men. Women, on the other hand, tended to get more of the saddle-bag, hip-and-thigh pattern of weight gain. Well, guess what? Women may not have caught up to men with equal pay and rights in society, but they sure have caught up with equal stress. More and more women are dealing with increased abdominal fat and so with an increase in the incidence of heart disease. It's a telling fact that heart disease has become the number-one killer of women as well as men in America.

Keep in mind that the body is very wise and capable of doing whatever it needs to do to promote well-being and survival. As stress becomes more chronic, the adrenals become more run-down, burnt-out. The body then will recruit any help it can get to provide backup support for the adrenal glands. It sends out an SOS signal to the hormonal system, aka the endocrine system, to recruit this support. This system answers the cry for help by recruiting the thyroid gland. Therefore, as the stress continues, both the adrenal and thyroid glands are involved. If the stress continues long enough, these glands will become overworked and run-down, the energy reserves of the body will be severely depleted, and there will be no choice but to move into the third phase of the GAR, which is out-and-out exhaustion.

Exhaustion

Understand that when we say the body gets exhausted, it's not just normal fatigue you feel, it's systemic; all of the body's systems are exhausted, including, of course, the thyroid and adrenal glands. Please note that these crucial dancers in the hormonal ballet of the body are not only involved in the stress response, they also are directly involved in metabolism and energy production.

Therefore, when these glands get burnt out, you are less and less capable of losing weight and keeping it off. Interestingly, in addition to stress factors, the exhaustion of these glands is intimately connected to the consumption of refined, high-glycemic-impact foods. If you recall, when you eat refined sugar, there are spikes of blood sugar that can cause exaggerated insulin release and a reactive crash of blood sugar. It is the job of the adrenal glands to counter the crash and move sugar back into the blood to keep blood sugar stable.

Episodes of low blood sugar are in themselves a major stress to the body that stimulate the adrenal glands to release cortisol, mobilizing sugar and fatty acids from liver and fat cells to replenish blood sugar levels. If these extreme blood sugar changes become a routine part of your life, they will lead to an increased burden on the adrenal glands that may result in a rebound suppression of these glands. As a result, the excessive routine consumption of refined, processed sugar products not only exhausts the pancreas and insulin system, but it can also exhaust the adrenal and cortisol system.

In addition, eating is associated in the brain with pleasure. Typically, when you have had enough to eat, a part of the brain called the lateral habenula is activated to reduce food-reward signals and induce the feeling of fullness. Chronic stress can override this natural brain response so that the brain is continuously rewarded and will cause you to continue to eat beyond the point of normal, healthy satiety. In addition, research at the Garvan Institute of Medical Research suggests that eating high-calorie-dense "comfort" foods—those high in fat and sugar—when stressed leads to brain changes and nonstop signals that further promote the craving and compulsive eating of hyperpalatable foods loaded with refined sugar that can provoke weight gain.[12]

If you have reached the all-out exhaustion point, you must be patient. It takes a lot to burn these organs out, and once you do, it takes months of conservative, supportive care to achieve full recovery. Bottom line: all the factors and choices in our lives that increase and reinforce exhaustion interfere with our ability to regulate weight effectively. This speaks to the very heart of our exhausted culture.

Avoid the Roller Coaster of Stimulant Abuse

With the relentless demands and pressures of family, work, financial concerns, and social responsibilities, most of us are not burning the candle at both ends. We're cutting the candle in three or four places and burning it at six, eight, and ten ends. We are a nation teetering on the edge—the precipice of exhaustion. You find yourself constantly saying, "I've got a deadline, the kids, the whatever, so I have no time to address my exhaustion now." Instead, you look for the props. What are the props? All the chemicals and behaviors of stimulation: sugar, nicotine, caffeine in all its forms, and my favorite misnomer of all time, "energy" drinks.

In the big picture, these drinks are not about increasing energy; they are actually products that reinforce exhaustion and depression. Here's why. Whenever you furnish the body with any form of chemical stimulation, that stimulation is only the initial effect. As your body processes and handles these substances, you have no choice but to crash to the same extent that you were stimulated.

One of the most famous hygienic health pioneers of all time, Dr. Herbert Shelton, called this the Law of Dual Effect. Whatever goes up has to come down with equal and opposite force. We've known this about objects since the time of Sir Isaac Newton. But nobody told you that with respect to energy, you're out there writing checks with no money in the bank. Why do you think Dr. Starbucks has such a busy practice in your community? A population of flagging consumers is constantly thirsting for some high-octane fix just to get their motors running. How else can you get four to six dollars for a cup of coffee? Are you kidding me? You have got to be a serious energy junkie to pay these prices for coffee.

Now I know you're probably asking yourself, "What the heck is he talking about? How can he challenge the joy of java?" when stimulant abuse—especially caffeine—is so well accepted throughout the world? Caffeine is the most socially acceptable psychoactive drug on the planet, and while energy drinks, chocolate, and tea have substantial caffeine content, coffee is the primary delivery system via the over two billion cups of coffee consumed daily worldwide. In extreme moderation, are these things a major problem? Not really. But as we say in the old neighborhood, this is not a culture that knows from moderation.

While there are data suggesting that moderate amounts of caffeine consumption may have some positive value, even reducing morbidity and mortality from certain chronic diseases, you must understand that caffeine stimulates the brain-reward system and the release of the neurotransmitter dopamine to provoke craving, addiction, excessive sugar consumption, inflammation, and reactive exhaustion and depression that can't be overlooked. Caffeine can suppress levels of the neurotransmitters adenosine and serotonin in the brain, reinforcing insomnia, chronic fatigue, depression, and sugar craving. Consistent caffeine use will overstimulate the adrenal and thyroid glands and the chronic release of cortisol, adrenaline, and thyroid hormones, triggering a potential increase in abdominal belly fat and, eventually, the potential rebound exhaustion of the glands associated with chronic fatigue, brain fog, and disturbing fat and weight gain. My clinical experience is that when people come off of caffeine, it is one of the worst withdrawals there is, often eliciting headache, pain, nausea, and vomiting. This is a serious drug, folks.

As a result of stimulant abuses, we are a nation of chemically fatigued and depressed people. Yet, if you look at medical advertising, you get the impression that the entire nation woke up depressed one day. Someone forgot to put Prozac in the water supply. What a load of crap. It's an insult to our intelligence. I'm here to tell you that we do have an epidemic of depression, and that it is primarily due to our overwhelming pace, demands, inactivity, stimulant and other lifestyle abuses, and, in a limited number of cases, genetic predisposition.

When people have come to the health centers and retreats that I have directed, they have often come following habitual abuses of various stimulants like chocolate, sugar, coffee, and energy drinks, cruising in on their flying carpets of stimulation. To promote detoxification and healing, one of the first things I would do was pull the carpet out from under them—*whoosh!*—taking all those stimulants away. What do you think would happen next?

Crash!

These people would come down *hard* and spend the next few days stalking the grounds like the night of the living dead. They would grope their way into my office with a pained, strained expression on their face and would confront me with what I call "the dialogue." It would go like this, "What did you do to me? This place is killing me." or "This can't be happening to me, I'm on vacation," as if their body cares that they made a deal with their travel agent. And my favorite line, "I don't think I'm getting enough protein."

The body has an ancient, genetic directive, etched over millions of years of evolution and change, to heal itself if given even a glimmer of an opportunity. The pain, the discomfort, and the symptoms of detoxification are all working to promote healing and recovery. Under these circumstances of exhaustion and withdrawal from stimulants, what you're confronting is who you really are. Which is…what? An exhausted and toxic human being. It's not a sin. It's not a crime. It is what it is. Sooner or later, you and I have to confront the reality of what is, and that's the reality that in your busy life there is too much chatter and too many things demanding your attention, disengaging you from the inner voice we all have that seeks to satisfy our physical, emotional, and spiritual needs. As a result, you often find yourself prone to making a number of choices that are not in your best interest.

Making a healthy choice is up to you. It is within your reach. If you are exhausted, overweight, and abusing stimulants, that choice needs to be to start with getting out of this self-defeating cycle of stimulation and depression. You need to abandon this grand illusion of artificial energy. It's like "The Emperor's New Clothes." You're riding a roller coaster of energy stimulation/dissipation and disability in the amusement park of your life, believing that you are decked out in your funkiest, sexiest clothes with just the right accoutrements, proudly parading an illusion of well-being. I love your heart and soul because you and I are connected. We are truly one. But like the clear-eyed little boy in the story, I can't help but point out that you are completely naked, in pain, living on borrowed time, sick and fatter than you need to be. You need to get off the ride and break the debilitating pattern of energy dissipation and hormonal imbalance that compromises the function of the adrenal and thyroid glands and ensures reactive weight gain and failure. Anything that helps you eliminate factors of exhaustion and manage stress more successfully will increase the opportunity for hormonal balance and successful weight loss.

The Connection of Stress, Immunity, the Intestine, and Weight Gain

The impact of stress on the immune and digestive systems is an interesting and important part of the weight-loss story. For starters, understand that approximately 70% of the immune system is in the intestinal tract. The first line of immune defense is a specific protein immunoglobulin called secretory IgA (sIgA) that is found in the mucous lining of the intestinal tract. All offending agents, including viruses, bacteria, and threatening food antigens, have to get through (sIgA) in order to enter the body.

In addition, the integrity of digestive and intestinal health is maintained by the population of healthy bacteria and yeast that naturally inhabit the intestine, called the microbiota. Chronic stress and excessive cortisol can disturb the balance of intestinal flora and create a state of dysfunctional microbial ecology called dysbiosis. In dysbiosis, healthy bacteria are damaged, resulting in an abnormal overgrowth of unhealthy bacteria and yeast, potentially inducing a state of disease by inflaming and damaging the lining of the intestine and altering your digestive efficiency and immune response. Eventually this damage can result in a "leaky gut," whereby larger, incompletely digested components of food can pass through the damaged intestinal lining, which can trigger exaggerated immune and autoimmune responses, potentially provoking still more stress, inflammation, dysfunction, and disease.

Since chronic stress promotes dysbiosis, irritation, and inflammation of the intestine, it can compromise digestive function. Furthermore, the combination of dysbiosis and damage to the intestinal lining also promotes a decrease in sIgA; this is the most common immune deficiency, and it can result in yeast infection (candidiasis), malabsorption, and food allergies.[13] Furthermore, these problems with absorption and potential food sensitivities and allergies can contribute to autoimmune disease and compromise the availability of essential nutrients, possibly leading to craving, compulsive food use, metabolic disturbances, and reactive weight gain.

A classic example of this is seen in the relationship between gluten consumption and the autoimmune form of hypothyroidism called Hashimoto's thyroiditis. Gliadin is a major protein component of wheat gluten. In certain cases of dysbiosis and allergic sensitivity, the body creates antibodies against this protein. Unfortunately, antibodies made against gliadin/gluten also can cross-react with transglutaminase, an important, naturally occurring enzyme which is involved in energy metabolism and is present in all body cells, with especially high concentrations in the thyroid gland. As a result of this cross-reaction, the cells of the thyroid can be attacked by autoantibodies against transglutaminase, compromising the function of the thyroid.[xxiii]

[xxiii] As a significant side note, Hashimoto's thyroiditis is also promoted by excessive levels of estrogen relative to progesterone (estrogen dominance), which is primarily seen in women and accounts for the fact that the incidence of Hashimoto's disease is five times greater in women. Estrogen dominance is fostered by an increase in body fat and the increased consumption of animal products high in saturated fat and of all processed, refined sugar products.

Reducing the impact of stress and healing the intestine and the immune system are absolutely critical for endocrine support and long-term weight regulation. The combination of healthy whole-plant nutrition, detoxification programs, and stress-response management tools can help you restore the appropriate balance of intestinal flora, balance the function of the hormonal system, reduce inflammation, and heal the intestine to promote significant weight and fat loss over time.

Strategies for Hormonal Recovery

To promote the recovery of the thyroid and adrenal glands, it is essential to:

- Eliminate all stimulants, especially caffeine in all its forms, i.e., coffee, sodas, chocolate, "energy" drinks, some over-the-counter medications (often for headaches), etc.

- Eat only plant-exclusive foods containing high-quality plant protein, including nuts; whole grains; legumes (lentils and beans); fresh, juicy fruit; a large volume of greens that keep your blood sugar stable (e.g., collards, mustard greens, dandelion greens, arugula, spinach, kale); and higher-sodium plants including tomatoes, Swiss chard, celery, and zucchini, while avoiding animal-food products and processed foods high in refined sugar and in saturated and trans fats. If your thyroid has been compromised, remember that cooking/steaming these cruciferous greens will reduce the negative effects of the goitrogens they contain and promote better thyroid hormone production and function. The addition of sea greens/seaweed (including dulse and vegan nori) to the diet provides calcium, magnesium, and iodine that promote better mineral balance, further supporting thyroid and adrenal function.

- Maintain adequate hydration.

- Engage in moderate, rather than excessive, activity.

- Avoid, or at least minimize, the stressful circumstances in your life and engage in daily stress-management practices that improve your stress response.

- Increase your rest/sleep in order to significantly enhance the healing of your endocrine organs.

Perception, Stress, and Mind-Body Balance

The general adaptation response is so important to human function that Hans Selye, the Canadian physician who unraveled its three steps, came a hair away from winning the Nobel Prize in medicine. However, in my opinion, he also did us a bit of a disservice.

I think you can appreciate that the GAR's steps (homeostasis, alarm, response, exhaustion) are not directed by our conscious control and choice. They occur subconsciously as part of our autonomic nervous system. You don't consciously make the physiological and biological choices involved in alarm and resistance. The body doesn't want to depend on your ability to do the right thing if your life is threatened, so it takes that task out of your hands, so to speak, and makes it part of your ingrained, automatic survival response and action.

Since there are automatic subconscious features to the GAR, it leaves you with the impression that when it comes to the stress response, there's not much you can actively do about it. In a way, you feel like you have no choice but to be enslaved by the automatic functions and reactions of your own nervous system. It is therefore incredibly important to realize that while there are subconscious features of the stress response, there is still a great deal that you can do consciously and proactively for stress management, resilience, and mind-body balance.

Every second of every day, millions of bits and bytes of information in your experience and environment are being filtered by the highest level of your brain, the cerebral cortex, into the thoughts, ideas, and language that are unique to you. No two people process this information in exactly the same way. Each of us has a specific, personal history, background, and set of experiences that have served to create what Albert Einstein liked to call a personal frame of reference through which your individual perception interprets and constructs your particular, unique, "real world."

So, it is safe to say there is no one real world, but rather as many real worlds as there are people perceiving them. In fact, quantum physics suggests that the world of experience you think you see is shaped and changed by the very act of your looking at it. It is only when the fields of energy in the external world collide and interact with your brain and consciousness that you can perceive the sights, colors, sounds, and objects of your life. As Dr. Robert Lanza has stated, "Nothing can be perceived that is not already interacting with your consciousness."[14] So as remarkable as it may sound, the outside world is actually located within your own brain and/or mind. What you think you see is the result of your brain organizing the energy of the environment into the substance and objects of your experience.

This filtering process also shapes and defines your individual beliefs, behaviors, and experience. What you come to believe leads to specific behaviors that shape and create experiences that often reinforce your beliefs like a self-fulfilling prophecy. Unfortunately, as a result, you can commonly get into the rut of thinking that what you believe is all there is. Therefore, you can be trapped, your thinking imprisoned by a limited view of the world that is etched inside your own mind. Fortunately, any time you so choose, you can also break out of the prison of your own mind and open yourself up to a more diverse and expansive world of possibility.

Imagine that you're watching a goldfish swimming around in a watery bowl. To the goldfish, its whole world is confined to the small environment of the bowl. However, as you know, there is a huge universe outside the fish bowl that the fish has no idea about. What is the fish bowl that you have chosen that restricts your world of possibility? It is a limitation of your own making. Your beliefs can change, your behavior can be modified in a supportive, healthy direction, and you can open up to a new and varied set of experiences. Understand the power of your own perception, because stress is truly not in the events of your life, but in the perception of the events. This suggests that the most important major component of stress management is using the tool of your own perception to alter how you look at, construct, and react to the events of your life. You have the power to change the impact of the events of your life by simply delaying your reactive responses while looking at and reframing the events in a different way. As the poet Maya Angelou stated, "If you don't like something, change it. If you can't change it, change your attitude." Looking at things differently, in a more open-minded manner, can often make all the difference and reduce your stress significantly. Never, never forget it is you and only you who decides who or what gets to use or abuse your power.

Also, because of the remarkable capability of the higher cortex of the brain, you have the capacity, any time you so choose, to make pro-active choices through your own free will. Your choices can modify the automatic, reactive survival responses of the lower, more primitive, limbic parts of the brain and directly affect the function of the nervous, immune, muscular, and endocrine systems of the body. This brain-body interaction is what is referred to as the mind-body connection, a term that suggests that because of the information that is channeled through the brain and nervous system, every thought and emotion you have will have some impact on or connection with every other system and function of the body.

When you first learn anything, whether it's playing a musical instrument, dancing, playing a sport, driving a car, or whatever, all the elements feel disjointed, fragmented. However, as you stick with it over time, any learned act becomes what Alexander Luria (one of the foremost brain scientists) called a "kinetic melody." It becomes a smooth-flowing act in the fabric of the brain and nervous system. But it always requires what I call the three Ps: practice, patience, and perseverance. Lifestyle choice and change is no different. When you make certain choices and execute particular behaviors repeatedly over time, specific pathways within the nervous system are established so that it becomes easier for information to travel over those old, familiar paths in the nervous system. This results in a tendency to repeat and further reinforce those behaviors. Negative choices, negative mindsets, and even addictions can be reinforced by this process. However, as you make healthier, more positive choices with practice, patience, and perseverance, new pathways can be established by the neuroplasticity of the brain, thereby accessing, facilitating, and manifesting these choices and behaviors more easily over time. In this way, new, constructive choices can be woven into the behavioral tapestry of your brain and nervous system by the repetitive forward-feed of information from the brain to the body and the feedback of information from body to brain, coursing through the neurological pathways of the mind-body connection. This process allows new healthy choices of not only diet and lifestyle, but also empathy, compassion, gratefulness, forgiveness, and love, all of which support physical health, mental health, stress reduction, and weight regulation to become habitual parts of your behavioral repertoire.

As you bring your attention into more present-time awareness, you can become more conscious of how you are using your own mind-body connection for your benefit or detriment and become more successful at resolving the stressful circumstances of your life. For example, because of constant mind-body communication, if you are experiencing body or muscle pain, this discomfort will be associated and intimately connected with the pattern of your thoughts and emotions. By resolving negative emotional patterns like chronic fear, anxiety, anger, and hostility, you can release musculoskeletal tension and pain. Similarly, by addressing, releasing, and dissolving your muscular patterns of restriction and pain via activities and meditative techniques such as yoga, tai chi, and qi gong, you will be more able to access and potentially dissolve the deeper layers of emotional trauma and dysfunction that are associated with your physical pain and dysfunction.

Another thing to keep in mind is that whenever the body can perform a function, it also has the ability to perform the opposite function. For example, blood pressure and heart rate can be increased or decreased based on the demands that the body perceives. So, if you have the inborn ability to create a fight-or-flight response, you also have the ability to produce a relaxation response. Unfortunately, while we have become unknowing, unconscious prisoners of a chronic, debilitating stress response, most of us have never been properly introduced to our relaxation response.

The relaxation response and healthy support of your mind-body connection require what I like to call focused awareness, or what the Buddhists call mindfulness. In our hectic culture, so many of us labor under the delusion that because we are running around frantically with our eyes open, we are actually conscious and awake. If I were to put electrodes on your head and measure the brain waves coming off your skull while you're reading this book, those of you who haven't fallen asleep yet would be producing the beta waves of the normal waking state. These are the waves produced when we are in the typical state of evaluation, information processing, and analyzing this or that, a state dominated by our usual concerns and worries and the constant judgments demanded by life. However, when brain waves slow down, as they do in relaxation and meditation, you move into what's called an alpha level. The alpha level is more of an egoless state, devoid of judgment and associated with more present-time awareness. In fact, it is more of a state of pure, present time.

For example, if you're in a yoga class and you're trying to get your body into the shape of a pretzel, you're probably not going to get lost in your shopping list at that moment. To ground yourself in this present-time awareness, it is in your best interest to take some time each day, at least 10–15 minutes, to incorporate some yoga, tai chi, or another relaxation or meditation technique. This is the most constructive way for you to step back from the chatter of your life and to journey into the private sanctuary of your own inner space to encounter what one of the great family therapists, Virginia Satir, called the "sacred place," where you discover the treasure that is called by your name. Simple meditation and relaxation techniques can be done using a mantra (as does transcendental meditation); simple breathing or progressive relaxation; alternating tension and relaxation in the eyes, neck, arms, hands, legs, and feet; or creative visualization. There are a variety of relaxation programs you can purchase or download online to use for your relaxation process. Or, you can take some time to just sit still or lie down and listen to quiet, peaceful music at the end of your busy day to promote a relaxed state of mind. This quiet time alone and these constructive practices are essential parts of any stress-response management program, and therefore critical for any long-term weight-loss program.

Following is a simple progressive relaxation exercise that you can use to enhance your body awareness and mindfulness. Initially, until you become comfortable with the process, you can record this in your own voice on any recording device (laptop, phone, tablet, etc.). Then whenever you're ready, you can play it back and follow the directives of your own voice.

Progressive Relaxation and Visualization

- Sit or recline quietly in a comfortable chair in a quiet room or space where you will not be disturbed.

- Take a long, slow, deep breath, exhale as slowly as you can, and close your eyes. With your eyes closed, you cut out the visual sensory input that is always demanding your attention, distracting you, constantly pulling you outside yourself, and you can begin to go inside and become more aware of who and what you truly are and to become more aware of the different parts of your body.

- Turn your attention first to your eyes, the beautiful organs of sight always on the job helping you see, appreciate, and create the world around you. Become completely aware of your eyes and any tension that you may be holding there. Then, as you inhale, increase the tension and tighten it as much as you can. As you exhale, let the tension completely go, feeling your eyes relax and the wave of relaxation move down from the eyes throughout the entire body. This feels very, very good, and you feel wonderful as your body becomes more and more comfortable, at ease, and relaxed, breathing deeper and deeper.

- Move your attention down now into the base of your skull and neck, areas that are tense and tight for so many of us. Again, become completely aware of these areas and any tension that you may be holding here. Then, as you inhale, increase the tension, tighten it, and while slowly exhaling, let the tension completely go, feeling the neck relax and the wave of relaxation move down from the neck throughout the entire body. This feels very, very good, and you feel wonderful as every muscle of your body becomes more and more at ease, comfortable, and relaxed, breathing deeper and deeper.

- Move your attention now into your shoulders and upper back, places where you hold so much of your daily tension and anxiety. Become completely aware of these areas and any tension that you may be holding here. Then increase the tension, tighten it, and exhale, let it completely go, feeling the wave of relaxation move from these areas throughout the entire body. This feels very, very good, and you feel wonderful as every muscle of your body becomes more and more at ease, comfortable, and relaxed, breathing deeper and deeper.

- Turn your attention to your belly and stomach area, a place where daily life typically binds us and ties us in knots. Picture this area as a tight ball of rubber bands all knotted and twisted together. Then, direct the area to relax, with a relaxed slow breathing pattern; feel the bands begin to unravel and become loose, flexible, falling apart, relaxed. Feel the wave of relaxation move from this area throughout the entire body. This feels very, very good, and you feel wonderful as every muscle of your body is more and more at ease, comfortable, and relaxed, breathing deeper and deeper.

- With each breath, feel your body, your being-ness completely in this moment, totally and completely relaxed. As you breathe slowly and deeply, tell yourself, "Each and every day I am getting better and better, better able to appreciate the world and people around me and better able to appreciate the light and love that moves within me, organizing, maintaining, and supporting the supreme value of conscious life. I am ready to go on about my day expressing this light and love in my communication, contacts, and relationships."

On the count of three, slowly open your eyes. Your eyes will be clear, your head will be clear, and you'll feel like you've just had a comfortable rest. One, slowly coming back; two, coming back more and more; and three, eyes opening, toes and fingers wiggling, ready to go about your day.

Breathing, Biofeedback, and Relaxation

The way that you breathe has a major impact on your stress-management process. Breathing is the most primal survival function of life. You can go a long time without food and a short time without water, but you can't go more than a few minutes without oxygen. Consistent with the well-established mind-body connection, your breathing pattern is directly linked with your emotional state and mental health status. In fact, your breathing pattern will dictate your emotional state; you can't simultaneously have a relaxed pattern of breathing and an anxious state of emotion, nor can you maintain a breathing pattern of anxiety and tension and expect to feel relaxed and calm. That's why, in the practice of yoga, tai chi, and qi gong, breathing techniques are taught to foster a relaxed and balanced physical and emotional state. In our stressed-out culture, since so many of us are breathing in the pattern of tension and anxiety, we ultimately create and reinforce anxiety whether we have anything to be anxious about or not.

Because of the intimate relationship between breathing and mind-body balance, I want to share the following breathing exercise with you. It is a combination of breathing, relaxation, and biofeedback. It is a simple and easy process that can be done anywhere.

- Sit comfortably in a chair with your hands resting low down on your belly.

- Take in a long, slow breath only through your nose.

- Let the breath take an elevator ride down into your lower belly and hands. In a normal healthy breath, the muscle that separates your chest and abdomen (the diaphragm) typically drops down, expanding the space to allow a sufficient volume of air to fill the lungs. As the diaphragm drops, it pushes the abdomen out so that as your lungs fill with air, your belly should also push outward.

- Therefore, as the breath fills your belly, your hands that are resting on your belly will be pushed out from your body. This is the biofeedback part of the exercise. If the hands aren't moving, you're not taking a full breath. My recommendation is then to lie flat on your back on the floor instead of sitting. Some of us have difficulty dealing with the force of gravity when we're more upright, but most people can breathe more efficiently and abdominally in this position.

- As you breathe in and the belly moves, slowly count the number one.

- Exhale slowly through the nose and mouth. In exhalation, there is an activation of the parasympathetic nervous system that produces maximum relaxation. Eventually, you'll make both phases of breathing as long and slow as possible, but initially, try to make the exhalation process slower and longer.

- Repeat the process, counting higher each time you exhale to lengthen exhalation time. By the time most people get to between 5 and 10, most anxieties and tensions of the moment are reduced.

This only takes minutes of your life and can be done right in the moment when you are dealing with stress and tension. It works great for cigarette-craving and craving in general. For smokers, the peak craving for a cigarette usually lasts about three to four minutes, and if you can do anything in that period of time to take the edge off, you can get past the urge to smoke. It also will work for other cravings, including those for food, and it is especially useful in the workplace. If you're at work, and you're hassling with your boss or a coworker, you can't usually say, "You're really pissing me off. I need to go meditate for a half hour." However, you can take a few minutes at your desk or in the bathroom and do this simple breathing exercise to relax.

Meditation is a time-honored relaxation and centering technique, but it is also true that even short periods of consistent, daily meditation can confer many other profound health benefits. Just 10-15 minutes of daily meditation significantly decreases cortisol release, increases heart rate variability indicating decreased stress, decreases stimulation of the brain's fear center (amygdala) that codes the fear response preceding fight or flight, increases the activity of the command and control center of the brain (prefrontal cortex) to help you become more consciously proactive rather than destructively reactive, increases weight loss, decreases cravings, and significantly improves sleep quality, energy, and mood.

To illustrate how your view of the world establishes stress and negative attitudes, I am wrapping up this chapter on stress with my favorite stress anecdote. This is the story of a young man who worked on Wall Street in New York City. After the economic upheaval that occurred in the banking institutions and financial field a few years ago, this young man, who had saved enough money to be comfortable, decided that he was fed up with the whole thing, and he was going to retire from life. He heard about a monastery up in the mountains of New York and decided he was going to spend the rest of his days living the quiet, monastic life.

He met with the head monk, who cautioned him, "I have no problem with you coming to live here, but we take this very seriously. If you come here, you have to take a complete vow of silence, except each year you can say two words."

The young man agreed, and went into the woods to meditate. At the end of the year, he met with the head monk, who asked him if he had anything to say.

"*Hard bed,*" the young man said. And he returned to the woods to meditate.

A year passed, and the young man again met with the head monk, who asked him if he had anything to say.

"*Bad food,*" he said. And he returned to the woods to meditate.

Another year of meditation passed, and the young man met again with the head monk, who asked him if he had anything to say.

"*I quit,*" he said.

"Well, it doesn't surprise me," the head monk said. "You've done nothing but complain since you got here."

Have *you* been complaining since you got here, or are you taking taking proactive steps to alter how you look at the world and how you reframe your experience to alleviate your stress? Remember, you don't have to be a slave to the automatic, reactive patterns of your own nervous system. You have the power to exert your own free will and make proactive choices that can help you resolve the stressful events of your life. Make no mistake: managing stress is as important as the food you eat and the exercise you do for maintaining a healthy lifestyle that supports weight control.

I don't know anyone in our crazy, hectic culture who would not benefit from taking some private practice time each day to step back from the chatter of life. So make this commitment to yourself. In fact, if it is possible in your home, I recommend creating a private space that you designate just for your meditation/relaxation, a place where you are not disturbed. It can be anywhere that works for you. There was a time when I was living in a house, raising five kids, and caring for about 10 different animals. I lived on Noah's ark. Sometimes, the only place I could find privacy and sanctuary was in the walk-in closet, with the dog scratching at the door. It didn't matter. I found as much refuge there as if I were in some quiet chapel or monastery.

Eliminating the conditions and stimulants that program relentless exhaustion, eliminating the toxic chemical environment promoted by eating animal and processed food products, and participating in routine stress-management practices like mindful breathing, meditation, relaxation, yoga, tai chi, and qi gong are critical, absolutely essential, for helping you achieve mind-body balance and long-term successful weight loss.

CHAPTER 19

SLEEP DEFICIENCY AND WEIGHT GAIN

W hen we talk about resolving the problem of exhaustion, the really important good news is that there is only one biological activity, easily within your reach, that is the real and powerful solution—sleep! I think that most everyone can appreciate the health value of a good night's sleep. Yet as much as the need for adequate sleep is generally recognized, it is something we do quite poorly. In fact, I'll go a big step further and state that, in my experience, sleep is pretty much the only biological activity that we constantly feel compelled to apologize for.

When's the last time you had dinner with others, got just enough to eat, got up from the table, and apologized to your host or friends for getting enough? It's an absurd notion. You wouldn't even consider it. However, it's not uncommon that if you were napping and someone awakened you with a call, realized they'd disturbed your rest and asked, "Were you sleeping?" that you would reply, "Who me? No, not at all. I wasn't sleeping," as if it's a badge of honor to avoid this most important biological activity, a sign of weakness to surrender to the most primal need of all living things—deep physiological rest and repair. Recognize this: it is incredibly important to heed and surrender to the whispers and seduction of Morpheus.

Many countries of the world urge their people to make time in their busy days for siestas and rest periods. It's so civilized. Unfortunately, the U.S. and other Western nations just don't get it, always promoting a pressured pace that makes rest a guilty pleasure and coerces people to feel apologetic for replenishing themselves. Even worse is the inherent suggestion that they need stimulant abuse to tap dance around their exhaustion, instead of addressing it head-on with nature's only real remedy. Instead of a deep respect for rest and sleep, you're working to exhaustion, then stimulating yourself chemically to the point of reactive chronic fatigue, sleeping less and less, and swelling our streets with the over-fat living dead that can barely make it through the day.

In 1998, 35% of Americans were getting eight hours of sleep per night, but by 2005, it dropped to 26%.[1] How important is this lack of sleep? Some of the greatest catastrophes of recent memory, including the Exxon Valdez oil spill, nuclear reactor accidents like Chernobyl, and multiple vehicular and air accidents have occurred because people fell asleep on the job, creating health and environmental burdens tolling in the billions of dollars. By some government estimates, the price tag for insomnia is more than $63 billion each year![2]

The normal sleep cycle includes two basic phases of sleep, the REM (rapid eye movement) phase and the non-REM phase. The non-REM phase occurs in four stages, starting with light sleep in stage one, as we transition from wakefulness to sleep, and progressing to the deepest sleep in stages three and four, characterized by slow delta-wave brain activity. During the deepest stages of sleep, the body repairs and regenerates cells, builds bone and muscle while decreasing body fat percentage, and strengthens the immune system. The REM phase is characterized by dreaming, increased brain activity, and paralysis of voluntary muscles.

In a normal sleep pattern, we cycle through all the stages of sleep several times through the night. I will discuss this in greater detail shortly, but understand that stimulants, sleep medications, poor diets, alcohol, and stress can disturb the deep regenerative phases of sleep that promote weight regulation, potentially interfering with weight loss. In fact, the burgeoning body of evidence strongly suggests that sleep deficiency may be one of the most important risk factors for the current pandemic of obesity and weight gain.[3]

Impact of Adult Sleep Patterns on Weight

To understand the impact of sleep deficiency on weight gain, it is essential to have some understanding of the basic need for sleep in adults and children. From the collective data, we know that the need for sleep in adults is six to eight hours per night.

In one of the most extensive longitudinal studies on adult sleep habits and weight, almost 70,000 women were followed over a 16-year period. Women who slept five hours per night gained significantly more weight and were more likely to become obese than women who slept seven hours per night.[4] Other studies on sleep habits done in the U.S., Canada, the United Kingdom, and other parts of Europe also have found consistent links between short sleep duration and obesity in young adults.[5] Sleep deficiency in young adults also results in a constellation of metabolic and endocrine changes, including insulin resistance, elevated evening cortisol levels, and hormonally driven increases in appetite that are all also associated with obesity and weight gain.[6]

To look at it another way, past studies have indicated an association between sleep deficiency and increased body mass index (BMI).[7,8] People who only slept two to four hours per night were 73% more likely to be obese than people with more normal sleeping patterns.[9] This is consistent with data that indicate that adults who consistently get less than six hours of sleep per night are two and one-half times more likely to develop diabetes.[10] In addition to obesity and diabetes, a variety of additional studies have shown that sleep deficiency is linked to a significantly increased risk of high blood pressure, heart disease, stroke, depression, and substance abuse.[11] Even joint and muscle pain is exacerbated by sleep deficiency.

Impact of Children's Sleep Patterns on Weight

The data on sleep deficiency and weight gain is even stronger for children. According to the Cleveland Clinic, preschoolers aged 3 to 5 years require 10 to 13 hours of sleep, children aged 6 to 12 years require 9 to 12 hours, and teenagers from 13 to 18 years require 8 to 10 hours.[12]

Multiple studies done across many countries of the world have shown a convincing link between sleep deficiency and childhood obesity.[3,13,14] In a large population of British children, children who slept fewer than 10.5 hrs per night at age three had a 45% increased risk of obesity by age seven.[13] Interestingly, the sleeping habits of children can have a long-term impact on weight well into adulthood. More than 1,000 children were followed from birth until age 32. Parents provided information about the average number of hours their children slept at five, seven, nine, and eleven years of age. Every hour of sleep reduction during childhood was associated with significantly higher risks of obesity at age 32.[15]

Another reason for the increased need for sleep in children is the fact that they are growing. Growth hormone release is at its peak in the early growing years up to and including early adulthood (ages 16–25), and it declines significantly with age (ages 36–50).[16] This hormone is primarily released in the sleep phase, and it peaks in the deep, slow-wave, delta phase of sleep about 90 minutes after sleep onset.[17] So in addition to promoting weight gain, sleep deficiency in children can interfere with the normal body development driven by growth hormone.

In my experience and opinion, this has become a significant problem in our overly competitive culture, affecting the children from many of the families I have worked with. There are so many intense pressures to succeed earlier and earlier in the lives of children today. They are so frequently overloaded with homework and extracurricular activities that they often seem to have no time to just be children, and they end up stressed-out and sleep-deprived.

I know that life has gotten more competitive in many more ways than when I was a child working my way toward college and pro-fessional training. And I believe that it is important for children to be held accountable for the work and projects they are asked to do. Teaching them what a diligent work ethic is all about and what kind of real effort it takes to be truly successful is an important responsibil-ity of parents and teachers. However, it also is important to help your children find a healthy balance between hard work and play, teaching them healthy sleep habits and stress-response management behaviors and strategies with which they can ground and stabilize themselves psychologically.

Although growth hormone is significantly and naturally reduced as we age, it still plays an important supportive role in adults, especially for achieving optimal recovery and results from your weight training and workout programs. Even as an adult, there is a direct, positive correla-tion between the amount of time you spend in deep delta-wave sleep and the amount of growth hormone that is released.[16]

I have worked with athletes, bodybuilders, and other people doing heavy resistance training. There were times when they were working very intensely but not getting the results they felt they should have based on their effort. Many times, the solution was not to get them to work out more but to get them to rest and sleep more. With more sleep, before they knew it, muscle mass increased, and more progress toward their goals was achieved. While sleep may seem like doing nothing, we need to under-stand the impact of this profound biological process and embrace the mentality of just how important sleep is for recovery and performance.

The million-dollar question is "How does sleep deficiency promote weight gain?" Sleep deficiency is defined as less than six hours per night for adults and less than nine to ten hours per night for children and adolescents. When you are sleep-deprived, there are four factors that can have significant impact on reactive weight gain. While this is the best science that we know at this point, more studies are ongoing that will elaborate on these factors and answer more questions on the mechanisms behind sleep-related weight gain. The four factors affecting weight gain are:

• Increased release of cortisol

Sleep deficiency increases the release of the stress hormone cortisol. While the lack of sleep may seem like a non-issue to you, the body responds to sleep deficiency like it's being attacked by a tiger. The body sees it as a major stressful event. Also, sleep deprivation is often accompanied by caffeine use to make it through the exhaustion of your day, triggering the release of cortisol and overstimulating the adrenal glands.[18] This cycle of continuous assault on the adrenal glands promotes adrenal exhaustion and potential energy dissipation and weight gain. Remember, too, that excessive cortisol can increase the deposition of abdominal belly fat, reinforcing this risky pattern of weight gain.

In addition, higher cortisol levels increase inflammation and decrease the level of antioxidants in the body, resulting in more inflammation and oxidative damage throughout the body. As a reminder, oxidative stress occurs when free radicals—the scavenger molecules produced by exposure to oxygen—destabilize and damage the organs and tissues of the body. Antioxidants in the diet, as well as those produced naturally by the mitochondria of all cells, eliminate free radicals. Since sleep deficiency reduces antioxidant production in the body, it is an important factor for promoting disease and aging.

• Increased insulin resistance

Now that you are familiar with the function of insulin, you can appreciate how important it is that sleep deficiency provokes insulin resistance. Since insulin resistance is a major aspect of obesity and type 2 diabetes, this suggests that sleep deficiency may significantly increase the risk of these devastating conditions. Remember, insulin resistance means that glucose cannot enter cells, and the body protects itself against the toxic impact of elevated blood glucose by converting the excess into fat, hence weight gain. In addition, the cells become starved for glucose, leading to a craving for all kinds of refined carbohydrates and sugar. So, sleep deficiency is another factor behind increased craving for all the foods you're trying to avoid when you want to lose weight.

The next point will even more emphatically highlight the powerful impact of sleep deficiency on weight gain.

• Increased ghrelin, decreased leptin

Ghrelin is a short-acting hormone produced in the gut that is the body's natural appetite stimulant. When you need food, the body releases ghrelin, which travels to the brain, stimulates the appetite centers in the brain, and drives us to eat. But if all you had was appetite stimulation, you would overeat until you exploded, and that's not going to work. So there has to be something that helps you put the brakes on and control appetite: leptin. Leptin is a long-acting hormone released from fat cells that provides information about our metabolic reserves and calorie needs. When it increases, it gives the brain the signal that you have had enough to eat. The combination of and balance between ghrelin and leptin stabilize food consumption.

Sleep deficiency causes a significant increase in the release of ghrelin that stimulates appetite and a significant decrease in the release of leptin that gives you the signal to stop eating. In extensive research done at Stanford University and the University of Wisconsin, people who only slept five hours per night had an almost 15% increase in ghrelin and a 15.5% decrease in leptin compared with people who slept eight hours per night.[9] These researchers also reported that those three hours of sleep deficiency, from eight down to five hours per night, increased body mass index (BMI) by 3.6%.

In a smaller study, young men who were sleep-deprived had higher levels of ghrelin and lower levels of satiety-inducing leptin, resulting in increased hunger and an appetite for foods high in fat and refined carbohydrates.[8] Consistent with this result, a study of Japanese workers found that workers who slept less than six hours per night had more irregular meal patterns and gravitated to more refined-food snacking behavior than those who slept more than six hours per night.[19]

It is important to realize that both inflammation and increased cortisol also can hinder the release and activity of leptin and interfere with our experience of satiety, revealing additional ways these two conditions can interfere with the crucial feedback and communication between the body and brain, leading to overeating, compulsive food use, and weight gain. In addition, sleep deficiency, along with the consumption of processed foods containing sugar, salt, and oil, can also promote leptin resistance. As a result, the body ignores or is unable to recognize the information from burgeoning fat cells, and the signals for satiety and fullness can be absent or short-circuited, driving compulsive food use and overeating.

• Decreased physical activity

People who don't get enough sleep are more tired during the day and may reduce their physical activity as a result.[4] This is pretty obvious to all of us. Think about it: when you're short of sleep, is the first thing you want to do to suit up, get in your car, and head to the gym for a vigorous workout? I thought not. I think most of us know that sleep deprivation interferes with any desire to exercise, or even to perform the necessary tasks of the day.

To summarize, in any successful weight-loss program the element of sleep is as important as the food you're eating, the exercise you're doing, and the stress-response management you are performing. In fact, sleep may be the best stress-management tool you have! And that begs the question: how can we improve our sleep patterns?

Factors Improving the Quality of Sleep

Nighttime—sleep time—is really a time for winding down. Too many of us are winding up at bedtime and taking the stress of the day to bed with us, which is definitely not conducive to quality sleep. It is in your best interest to respect the natural circadian rhythm of the body by increasing activity and eating behavior during the day while minimizing stress, physical activity, and eating at night.

Beneficial sleep preparation and sleep can be effectively organized in three categories: optimal mindset, optimal environment, and optimal physical conditions.

Create an Optimal Mindset

I would never want to come across as glib or thoughtless about the circumstances that you are dealing with in your life. I have the greatest respect for you and the severity and intensity of your life situations. Yet, it is also important to engage in nighttime behaviors that help you minimize any ongoing stress, including the stress of your day, so you can comfortably wind down as you prepare for and attempt to fall asleep. Even if there is no complete resolution in the moment for you, ideally the burden of the situational stressors of your life, including illness, financial concerns, the tribulations of family members, work, etc., need to be lightened and let go as much as possible using the behaviors of stress-response management and present-time awareness techniques that we discussed previously. Gentle meditation, leisure reading before bed, watching inspirational movies and/or lighthearted comedies earlier in the evening, listening or playing soothing music, journaling your thoughts and ideas from the day, and even listing in a quiet moment the things you need to handle the following day(s) to stop perseverating on these tasks can all help you create the stillness and peace of mind needed to step back from the chatter of your day.

In addition, research studies have shown that people actively practicing gratitude—the art and act of acknowledging and appreciating the positives in your life—have less stress, increased happiness, and a significant decrease in depressive symptoms. Research has shown that individuals writing gratitude letters were liberated from negative emotions and thoughts and experienced positive lasting effects in the brain.[20] Journaling and expressing gratitude are fantastic practices to participate in at the end of your day to promote a happier, more peaceful state of mind so as to improve your sleep habits.

Performing some slow, deep abdominal breathing close to bedtime will relax the body and promote an easier transition into sleep, and if you wake up during the night, it is a helpful way to fall back asleep. Attention to your breath is a powerful and simple approach to create a parasympathetic relaxation response that can help you quiet what the Buddhists call "monkey mind," the frenetic thoughts of the day that keep running around in your head like a group of wild monkeys, preventing you from falling asleep. Make the exhalation as long and slow as you can. This fosters an even deeper level of relaxation, and it will be much easier for you to fall asleep again.

Create an Optimal Environment

Keep your sleeping room as dark and cool as possible. If there is any light in your room it should never be the blue and green screens of computers, TVs, and phones. Blue and green lights signal creative, wake-up time for the brain. If there is any light in your bedroom, it should be red light that triggers melatonin release and a state of rest and repose. Bedtime is not the best time to watch the late-night news that is replete with trauma and violence. That's certainly not going to help you relax and settle into a good night's sleep.

Create Optimal Physical Conditions

Taking the hottest bath you can tolerate before bed will create a reactive cooling effect in the body after the bath that allows you to fall asleep more effectively. Consider making this an Epsom salt bath, as the magnesium from the salts will relax muscle tension, promoting an additional relaxation effect.

Build a consistent bedtime routine close to the same time each the evening, including cleaning your teeth, removing make-up, bathing, dressing for bed, etc., to provide repeated patterns that foster rest for the body and mind.

The more you create consistent daily times for sleeping and waking, the greater is your potential for quality, restful sleep that supports fat and weight loss. Consistent with this idea, a study of young, college-age women showed that the women who had consistent bedtimes, slept between 8 and 8.5 hours per night, and, most importantly, had consistent similar daily wake-up patterns, had the lowest levels of body fat.[21]

Finally, engage in some intimate sexual behavior. Yes, you heard me correctly. Sex will reduce cortisol levels; raise opiate, oxytocin, and dopamine levels; and promote a deep feeling of relaxation. In fact, the bedroom is best used for just two things: sex and sleep. By earmarking the bedroom in this way, the association of the bedroom with sleep is strengthened, further guiding the transition into quality rest.

Additional Lifestyle Considerations and Choices

Eliminate Stimulants in Your Day

A variety of other lifestyle choices can also help improve the quality and duration of your sleep. Foremost among them is reducing or eliminating the many stimulants that abound in modern life. Let's take a look at how caffeine, foods, and medications can play a role in the quality of your sleep.

The neurotransmitter adenosine is released in the brain to ease you into sleep. Since caffeine antagonizes the effects of adenosine, it interferes with normal, healthy sleep cycles. And since caffeine has a long half-life in your system, it can take many hours for the caffeine that you consumed at any time in your day to be eliminated from the body. People receiving moderate doses of caffeine at bedtime and at three and six hours before bedtime had significant sleep disturbances, suggesting that if you do consume any caffeine products, you should refrain from doing so a minimum of six hours before bedtime.[22] In addition, since caffeine provokes the release of the stress chemicals cortisol and adrenaline, it establishes and maintains a fight-or-flight stress response that will compound the stress of your day, making it impossible for your brain to quiet down at bedtime and achieve the peace and relaxation it needs to ease into restful sleep. Caffeine also can interfere with the action of another neurotransmitter of sleep, serotonin, to compromise your ability to achieve adequate rest.

So, when you are having difficulty falling or staying asleep, I recommend the elimination of all caffeine-containing products, including coffee, tea, chocolate, sodas, and over-the-counter medications for a period of at least several months and potentially forever. In my own experience, for example, if I have any chocolate in the evening, I can fall asleep, but my rest is disturbed during the night; I will often wake up in the night or too early in the morning before I have gotten a full night's sleep.

Even non-caffeinated stimulants like sugar and nicotine need to be avoided, because they also can play into your sleep cycle and disrupt good-quality sleep. As you get healthier, you will be even more sensitive and able to recognize the effects of stimulants.

Increase Regular Physical Activity

Since routine exercise can enhance the production of serotonin and promote natural opiate release, regular activity during the day will improve your ability to sleep more effectively at night. People who consistently move more typically sleep better at night. Because evening time is a time for winding down, I don't recommend heavy exercise and training at night. Instead, focus on gentle, more meditative and low-intensity activity, like a gentle evening walk, to help the body make an easier transition to sleep.

Increase Healthy, Fruit-Based Snacks at Bedtime

Sometimes having a little something sweet, preferably fresh fruit, close to bedtime may extend sleep through the night. This may occur for two reasons. Depending on your personal history of stress, poor diet, and adrenal exhaustion, there may be some disturbance of blood-sugar regulation and the possibility of episodes of hypoglycemia during the sleep cycle. If blood sugar drops too much during sleep, you will be awakened. Fruit at bedtime can help stabilize blood sugar during the sleep cycle and extend sleep time.

In addition, a fruit snack close to bedtime may improve the production of serotonin to enhance a more effective, healthy sleep cycle. Previously, I discussed the role of insulin in blood-sugar regulation. Insulin not only drives glucose into cells, it also promotes the delivery of amino acids—the building blocks of protein—into cells.[23] One of these essential amino acids, tryptophan, is used by the brain to make serotonin, which is essential to the onset and maintenance of sleep. A carbohydrate meal or snack has been shown to enhance the movement of tryptophan more than other amino acids across the blood-brain barrier, increasing its concentration in the brain.[24,25] So, fruit at night induces the release of insulin, which supports the movement of amino acids from the proteins you consumed in the day, especially tryptophan, to be absorbed more effectively into brain cells, potentially increasing serotonin production and improving sleep.

Connecting with the Earth

As I mentioned previously, the human body is electromagnetic in nature. Although it is a controversial idea, it is becoming increasingly more accepted that there is a vital electrical connection between the Earth and everything that lives on it, and that our contact with the Earth is essential for maintaining and restoring the natural, healthy, electrical state of the body.[26] Unfortunately, as our cities have evolved into the concrete jungles that they are and our hectic lifestyles disconnect us from outdoor earth-bound activity, we have become more and more separated from the Earth.

It has been suggested that spending more time "earthing," or grounding ourselves, i.e., lying, sitting, standing, and walking barefoot on the ground, can restore and maintain the body's most natural electrical state and promote optimal function.[26] Consistent with this idea, ancient systems like the Taoist energy arts, such as the outdoor practice of tai chi and qi gong in grassy parks or at the beach, teach techniques of rooting and grounding in the Earth's energy as a way to promote balance and health. Walking, sitting, and standing barefoot on the earth for even 30 minutes per day can have some significant health benefits.

In addition, the Earth itself appears to be a major sleep booster and anti-inflammatory agent. Earthing during sleep has been shown to reduce sleep disturbances and affect the regulation of the hormonal system of the body, including the synchronization of the natural circadian release of cortisol. Since we spend so much time disconnected from the Earth in our day-to-day experience, extending the earthing process for the eight hours or so of sleep can significantly enhance its beneficial effects. To promote earthing during sleep, earthing sheets are available that can be attached directly to the ground plug of the electrical sockets of your home. These sheets can be purchased from earthing.com or radiantlife.com.

When to Sleep

The best hours for sleep are thought to be between 10:00 p.m. and 5:00–6:00 a.m. So many people I've met claim to be "night people," but there are no vampires in the human population—although there seems to be a growing group of people who think they are. They're really not. There are no night people.

The truth is that we are diurnal animals. We have evolved and are genetically programmed to go to sleep when it gets dark and to wake up with the light. Night-shift workers and others who consistently disrupt this natural cycle often pay a price with compromised health. Yet, so many of us like to push the envelope and stay up well past 10:00. I confess that I'm definitely one of those thieves of the night, trying to steal as many hours as I can get. Back in the days when I was raising my children, after making breakfasts and lunches, homeschooling several kids, working all day, and then doing my homework and pleasurable activities at night when everyone else was finally down for the night, it was "Frank time" for me, and I tried to stay up as long as possible. I knew I would have to get up early in the morning and start the whole trip all over again, but I was willing to pay the price. So, I do understand. But for your health, my recommendation is that if you have been going to bed very late, try to back it up an hour or two to get closer to the window between 10:00 p.m. and 5:00–6:00 a.m. A good guideline to follow is to go to bed at night in the same day you woke up.

Sleep Medications, Supplements, and Alcohol

As I discussed, the phases and duration of sleep and accompanying growth-hormone release are critical for enhancing lean muscle mass and reducing body fat. This is where the prevalent use of sleep medications and the consumption of alcohol may create some significant problems. The chronic use of sleep medications—over-the-counter sleep aids and prescription sleep medications, including the benzodiazepines (Ativan, Xanax, and Valium) and benzodiazepine-like drugs (Ambien, Lunesta, and Sonata)—tend to interfere with the quality and patterns of sleep, while also potentially promoting debilitating withdrawal symptoms, a rebound decrease in REM sleep, and rebound insomnia.[27] While benzodiazepines are still some of the most prescribed drugs for anxiety and insomnia, decades of scientific research in the U.S. and England have clearly shown that the repeated long-term use of these drugs and the withdrawal from them can increase the risk of brain damage, addiction, anxiety, and depression.[28] Unfortunately, the medical idea is that if you're having a difficult time sleeping, getting any sleep at all is better than getting no sleep, regardless of whether there are any adverse rebound effects, so they continue to be prescribed.

There is a legitimate concern that the long-term use of sleep medication, including the sedatives and hypnotics that are often prescribed for insomnia, may actually exacerbate sleep problems by adversely affecting the natural progression from one sleep phase to another.[29] The drugs may induce sleep, but they do not promote the fully restorative, regenerative sleep that is so critical for tissue repair, hormonal balance, increased metabolic efficiency, and long-term weight regulation. Therefore, if you are dealing with chronic sleep deficiency, it is truly in your best interest to unravel the causes of your problem and seek lifestyle solutions that support your greatest opportunity for consistent restorative sleep rather than rely on sleep medications.

These concerns also apply to some degree to the use of amino acids, hormones, and herbal sleep aids that are commonly used to treat insomnia. The supplementation of the serotonin precursor L-tryptophan and/or the mineral magnesium, the hormone melatonin, and herbal products containing some combination of valerian, passion flower, and chamomile may promote better sleep. However, while these supplements may provide some temporary relief from insomnia and are not typically disruptive like the aforementioned medications, they can still promote some hormonal disruption and can distract you from addressing the nutrition and lifestyle factors that are at the root of your sleeplessness.

The routine use of melatonin is an example of how supplementation can go wrong and provoke critical hormone imbalance. Melatonin should not be used as a routine sleep aid. It is a hormone released by the pineal gland in the brain when night falls and is the chemical expression of darkness. Your brain's awareness of the darkness of night is not what directly leads to sleepiness. Instead, the brain reacts by releasing melatonin to signal that it is nighttime and time for sleep. Melatonin plays a major role in setting the daily light-dark cycle and is best used when you travel across different time zones and need to establish a new diurnal rhythm to reduce jet lag. However, when you take melatonin routinely, it leads to negative feedback inhibition in which it signals the brain to make less of its own melatonin, creating a significant deficiency over time that reinforces sleep disturbances.

Alcohol will also disrupt the quality and efficiency of sleep, so drinking alcohol at night is not a good idea.[29] Yet, when is most alcohol consumed? At night. It may feel good. Alcohol can increase the release of natural opiates and the neurotransmitter gamma-aminobutyric acid (GABA), which promotes a relaxing, anti-anxiety effect that may even knock you out enough to fall asleep (or even pass out), but it creates a disturbed sleep pattern that only reinforces fatigue. That's one of the reasons why, when you wake up after a night of drinking, you can still feel exhausted even though you may have slept 10 hours or more. In addition, alcohol promotes fluid retention, disturbances of sugar metabolism, and weight gain and may interfere with your ability to lose weight.

There is no doubt that insomnia has become a significant problem in our hectic culture. It is estimated that transient insomnia affects 80% of the population, while 15% of us suffer with chronic insomnia.[31] The field of sleep medicine has improved and can now pinpoint specific physiological causes of sleep deficiency like sleep apnea, but the typical medical approach is shortsighted and often treats just the outcomes and symptoms of sleeplessness without regard for the causes of this dysfunction.

It is so important, whenever possible, to address and eliminate the constellation of factors that contribute to your symptoms and not sidestep the issues that are the root cause of your sleep problems. Know that a variety of natural, non-drug approaches, e.g., stress-response management techniques, relaxation training, and cognitive therapies, have been shown to be remarkably beneficial in the treatment of insomnia.[31]

In conclusion, it is apparent that one of the most overlooked and misunderstood factors in the weight-loss story is the need for sleep. Sleep is a major biological activity that demands your full respect and consideration, and when you utilize nutrition and other lifestyle factors to improve the dynamics of your sleep process and get adequate, quality sleep, you are taking a giant step toward successful long-term weight loss. Hold on to your vision and goals of healthy weight loss and body image, and in your actions embrace the immortal words of the bard, Billy Shakespeare, "To sleep, perchance to dream."

CHAPTER 20

ENVIRONMENTAL TOXINS, OBESOGENS, AND WEIGHT GAIN

My holistic vision and program for successful, healthy weight loss would be incomplete if I did not discuss the negative impact of environmental toxicity on weight regulation. Remarkable research in England, Canada, and the United States suggests that the most overweight people are found in cities and areas with the greatest amount of industrial and environmental pollution.[1]

In the United Kingdom, where, like many other countries of the world, they are dealing with their own piece of the global pandemic of obesity, a demographic map showing the location of the greatest number of overweight people significantly matched a map of the major industrial waste centers in England. Consistent with this observation, in the U.S., the 10 cities with the greatest number of overweight/overfat people are in the industrial South.[1] They are connected either to the Mississippi River, the most polluted river in the U.S. or, in the cases of West Virginia, Texas, Alabama, Louisiana, and Georgia, to some of the top 20 mercury-polluting power plants in the nation.

In an attempt to understand these data, it has been suggested that disease-promoting lifestyle factors associated with these areas could be the cause of the increase in weight gain. However, while these industrial waste areas may promote lifestyles that support poor eating habits and sedentary behavior, it appears that it is the increased level of industrial pollutants that may be contributing to the obesity observed in these populations.

When toxic products like pesticides are produced by factories and refineries for commercial sale and use, other toxic chemicals that are by-products of these operations are released into the environment. A number of these toxic products are derived from fossil fuels, i.e., the same gas and oil reserves that are used to generate energy in our country and others. Fossil fuels, as the name implies, are made from a combination of the bones of ancient dead animals, decaying earth, and vegetation laid down over time. Since these toxic compounds are formed in part from the bodies of animals long gone, they are capable of affecting bodily functions, especially the hormonal systems of a variety of mammals, including humans. As a result, they are often referred to as "endocrine disruptors" that can negatively affect key biological hormones. This disruption can compromise fertility and the reproductive cycle of mammals, compromise adrenal and thyroid function, and invoke changes that may influence the creation of fat cells and, hence, the outcomes of obesity and reactive weight gain.[2,3] In Table 5, you can see three classes of these chemical toxins on the left, with examples of common toxins in each class on the right.

Organochlorines Used in pesticides, dyes	PCBs and insecticides DDT, DDE, and DDD
Phthalates Used as plasticizers in plastics production, metal and medical tubing, food packaging, and infant toys	DEHP, DBP, BBP, and DEP
Nonsteroid synthetics Used in food containers, water bottles, and metal casings of canned foods	Bisphenol A (BPA), Bisphenol F (BPF), and Bisphenol S (BPS)

Table 5. Major classifications of environmental toxins and their common names and sources.

Environmental Toxins and Common Sources
Organochlorines

Organochlorines include the pesticides DDT, DDE, and DDD and poly-chlorinated biphenyls (PCBs) found in the dye used to color farm-raised salmon and the feathery insulation in the attics of homes. They can decrease the levels of thyroid hormones, slow down the metabolism, and interfere with weight loss.[4] These toxic chemicals can act directly on the sympathetic nervous system to interfere with weight-regulating hormones and the receptors on fat cells that may be involved in reactive weight gain.[1] This is another reason why the consumption of farm-raised fish is not in your best interest when you're trying to lose weight. The use of farm-raised fish—especially salmon, which is high in PCBs—should be avoided.

Phthalates

Phthalates such as DEHP, DBP, BBP, and DEP are plasticizers used to increase the flexibility of plastics. They are found in soft vinyl products and personal-care products. The effects of phthalates are similar to those of organochlorines and bisphenols; they can act as hormone disruptors that promote problems with reproductive, developmental, and endocrine health.

Unfortunately, phthalates can also make their way into our food supply when they leach from food-processing equipment, food packaging, and food-preparation materials. Milk can be a significant food source of phthalates. Robin Whyatt, a professor of environmental health sciences at Columbia University, has described the commercial processing and packaging of milk to explain how phthalates get into the milk supply.[5] Typically, milk passes sthrough plastic tubes of milking machines on its way from cow to bottles or containers. These plastic tubes leach DEHP, a dangerous phthalate that is fat-soluble and can dissolve easily in the high fat content of milk. Significant, excessive levels of DEHP, measured as metabolites of DEHP in the urine of human subjects, were found in commercial organic spices and milk and suggest the need for better regulatory approaches for minimizing food sources of phthalates.[6]

Non-Steroid Synthetics

Bisphenols are widely used in any number of products and are found in our homes, schools, workplaces, and even indoor dust and supermarket foods.[7] Bisphenol A (BPA) is the most well-known of these toxins. It's found in many plastic bottles, baby bottles, and juice containers and in the epoxy resins that line the inside of most food cans. It is also used in thermal paper (such as store receipts), in dental sealants and polymers, and to make hard reusable plastic products and flame retardants. The effect of BPA on estrogen function has been studied for more than a decade; it mimics the structure of estrogen and promotes effects similar to that of excess estrogen. Repeated exposure can dangerously affect the reproductive cycle and potentially trigger the abnormal growth of cells and tumors in the breast, ovaries, and uterus.[8] Thus, it is in your best interest to use only BPA-free plastic bottles, cans, and containers whenever possible; choose glass bottles rather than cans or plastic containers whenever you can. Bisphenol F (BPF) and bisphenol S (BPS) are chemically similar to BPA and are being increasingly used as replacements for BPA.

Industrial Toxicity and Weight Gain

It is important to understand the unique impact these chemicals can have on weight gain. Since these industrial toxins are derived from fossil-fuel oil reserves, they are oily in nature and are therefore fat-soluble (capable of dissolving in fat and oil). When the body is exposed to these chemicals, they can be dissolved and stored in oily fat cells and tissue. Storing these chemicals removes the toxins from the general blood circulation and reduces potential toxic effects on the brain, the heart, the liver, and the rest of the body. Since the body can protect itself by storing this toxicity in its fat tissue, it may enhance protection by overproducing fat cells in response to an increased toxic load. Consistent with this idea, it has been suggested that environmental toxins can signal and trigger dormant baby-fat cells (pre-adipocytes) to grow into mature fat cells. For this reason, these environmental and industrial chemicals are referred to as "obesogens," chemicals that promote an increase in body fat. The term obesogen originated within the last few decades to define molecules that inappropriately regulate the metabolism of fat and the creation of fat cells to promote obesity.[9]

As fat cells grow in response to toxic chemical exposure, it is harder to keep weight down. To make things worse, an increase in weight gain can slow down the detoxifying systems of the body, so that more and more toxins may be stored in the growing mass of available fat, resulting in the body becoming increasingly fatter and more toxic. In some cases, these chemicals may also elicit inflammatory responses and have additional toxic effects on brain, liver, and kidneys.[1] The additional toxic load may eventually overwhelm the body's detoxification pathways. Under this pressure, the body continues to try to dilute these fat-soluble toxins by making even more fat cells in which to store them, thereby reinforcing an ongoing cycle of toxicity, fat cell production, and weight gain.

Research has shown very specific connections between these toxic chemicals and specific health and weight-related conditions. In a national evaluation of men in the U.S., increased levels of phthalates in the urine were associated with increased waist size, abdominal obesity, and insulin resistance, emphasizing the impact of this chemistry on weight gain and insulin function.[10] While these results do not indicate that chemical toxicity is a direct cause of the problem, they do suggest that exposure to phthalates may contribute to the population burden of obesity and insulin resistance.

In another national health survey, increased serum levels of toxic, organic pollutants had a direct relationship on the increased risk of diabetes.[11] In this evaluation of six different organic pollutants that are typically found in at least 80% of the population, the prevalence of diabetes correlated significantly with the extent of the exposure to organic pollutants.

Importantly, exposure to chemical obesogens early in life may affect your health, hormonal integrity, and weight gain later in life. The pubertal growth and development of boys and girls was significantly affected by their prenatal and lactational exposure to organochlorines, PCBs, and dichlorodiphenyldichloroethane (DDD).[12] In this study of almost 600 children, boys with the greatest prenatal exposure to DDD from their mothers' placentas were 2½ inches taller and 14 pounds heavier at puberty than boys with the lowest exposure. Girls with the highest prenatal/placental exposure to PCBs were almost 12 pounds heavier at puberty than girls of similar height with the lowest exposure.

Furthermore, even low doses of BPA during prenatal development and early infancy can activate genetic mechanisms that promote fat-cell production and activity that can last a lifetime.[10] Based on this information, it's hard not to think about the impact these toxins may have on the widespread, damaging outcome of childhood and teenage obesity.

The possible role of environmental toxins in weight gain is especially important when you consider how prevalent pesticides are in the conventional foods that are now available. While the benefits of eating plant-exclusive foods far outweigh the risks of not eating them, the Environmental Working Group (EWG), a research and advocacy group focused on toxic chemicals, drinking-water pollutants, and agribusiness subsidies, reported that recent government tests showed significant pesticide contamination of conventionally grown fruits, vegetables, and tap water. In government tests analyzed by the EWG, pesticide residues were detected on 67% of produce samples even after they had been washed or peeled. Even more upsetting was the fact that government scientists found that pears and green beans in three popular brands of baby food were contaminated with fungicides and bug killers.[13]

The EWG reported striking differences in pesticide contamination between what they call the *Dirty Dozen* and the *Clean 15* foods. If you are going to eat food that is not always organic, you can reduce your pesticide exposure by limiting or always choosing organically grown versions of the fruit and vegetables in the Dirty Dozen while being more liberal with the Clean 15.

The Dirty Dozen for 2024 were:

1. Strawberries
2. Spinach
3. Kale, collard, and mustard greens
4. Grapes
5. Peaches
6. Pears
7. Nectarines
8. Apples
9. Bell and hot peppers
10. Cherries
11. Blueberries
12. Green beans

The Clean 15 for 2024 were:

1. Avocados
2. Sweet corn
3. Pineapples
4. Onions
5. Papayas
6. Sweet peas
7. Asparagus
8. Honeydew melons
9. Kiwi
10. Cabbage
11. Mushrooms
12. Mangos
13. Sweet potatoes
14. Watermelon
15. Carrots

Genetically Modified Foods

Although the jury is still out on the long-term biological impact of genetically modified (GMO) produce and grains on health and weight loss, I recommend avoiding these foods. Preliminary controversial animal studies have shown that the consumption of GMO corn significantly increased weight gain in female rats while also increasing serum triglyceride levels and the risk of liver and kidney toxicity.[14] Typically, the nutrient value of GMO foods is lower than that of non-GMO foods, because GMO crops are bred for higher yield by increasing their resistance to environmental threats like drought and bugs rather than for better nutrient value. Because of their nutrient deficiencies, animals, including humans, may overeat these foods to compensate for the lack of nutrients.

Only a small fraction of commercial sweet corn—the corn that is sold on the cob, canned, and frozen for direct consumption—is genetically modified, but field corn is one of the most genetically modified crops used for human and animal consumption in America. Field corn is produced from GMO seeds and is used to make tortillas, chips, high-fructose corn syrup, animal feed, and biofuels.

All products with corn additives, especially everything containing high-fructose corn syrup and the additive maltodextrin, should be completely avoided.

There is no way to know at this time what impact genetically modified feed has on the meat and dairy products that you may be consuming, but I am personally wary and concerned about potential negative health consequences. Remember, too, that because of biological magnification, the bodies of animals that eat plants treated with pesticides harbor a concentration that is 10 times higher than in the plants themselves. Therefore, the potential obesogen exposure is much greater when you eat animal foods—another reason why eating animal products may significantly increase the risk of weight gain. If you feel compelled to eat these animal-based foods, I recommend getting them from animals that have been raised in a more organic manner.

Clearly, avoiding and/or eliminating toxic obesogens is truly in our best interest for health in general and for weight loss in particular. Since organic foods are not sprayed with pesticides and are not genetically modified, eating in a more organic manner eliminates the need to be concerned with whether food is clean, dirty, or genetically changed and is ideal for long-term, successful weight loss. The good news is that organic produce is widely available now at more reasonable prices than in the past in most large conventional supermarkets, including Publix, Costco, Winn-Dixie, Kroger, and even Walmart, as well as in smaller, health-focused food stores such as Whole Foods, Sprouts, and Natural Grocers.

It is also important that your home cleaning products and beauty products be as green, clean, and devoid of these toxic chemicals as possible. Constant exposure to obesogens in cleaning and beauty products may be an additional significant factor interfering with your weight-loss success. As with organic produce, the market for eco-green products is growing, and they are becoming widely available. The Environmental Working Group's website and app include ratings on 130,000 personal care, cleaning, and food products that will help you choose the cleanest products to minimize these toxins and support your ongoing weight-loss program.

In conclusion, there is no question that for long-term successful weight loss, implementing the full array of lifestyle choices we discussed earlier is critical. However, environmental toxins—the toxic chemicals spewed into our environment by business and industry as well as the chemicals in our foods, home, and beauty products—may contribute significantly to our problems with weight gain. Some of this toxicity is out of your control, and you have no choice but to live with it to a certain extent. It doesn't pay to get overly stressed and obsessed about the things you can't change, however, you should take as many positive, proactive steps as possible to change what you can. Your lifestyle choices should include, wherever possible, food, cleaning, and personal products that are the least toxic and the most supportive of your health.[xxiv]

[xxiv] I believe that businesses, corporations, and industries must take more responsibility for the toxicity they are producing. They must be made more accountable for their actions, and legally pressured, if necessary, to realize they can't keep poisoning people and the environment for profit. It is also up to governments to shoulder some of the responsibility and take action to address the toxic by-products of the industrialization and urbanization of modern society. Governmental action needs to pressure these industries and corporations to reduce environmental toxicity, make human health and safety a priority, and potentially also protect people globally from the disabling consequences of excess weight and body fat.

PART
5

PROMOTING
OPTIMAL WEIGHT
AND HUMAN POTENTIAL

CHAPTER 21

PSYCHO-EMOTIONAL FACTORS: DISCARDING OLD PROGRAMS

I have described the relationship and impact of stress on weight gain and the role of perception in shaping stressful responses to your real world. However, to fully appreciate how these concerns establish poor food choices, compulsive eating, and even the foundation of food addiction, it is necessary to go into culturally conditioned factors of stress and body image and plunge deeper into the emotional and psychological parts of the weight-loss story. The obsessions, preoccupations, and pressures common to your personal history can establish conditioned programs of response that may compromise your potential for long-term weight loss. These need to be addressed and discarded.

In a culture that continues to grow increasingly fatter, there are conflicting developments in mindset that promote confusing and potentially dangerous behaviors. On one hand, there is a pervasive obsession with thinness, and on the other, there is a rebellion against it and an embrace of risky fat and weight gain.

On the thinness side, an unrealistic model of thinness has been incorporated into the psyche of our culture by the fashion and entertainment industries. The obsessive preoccupation with unnatural models of body image has created a dangerous situation where for many the end of thinness justifies any means of getting there. You can vomit your way to thinness. You can amphetamine your way to thinness. You can nicotine and diuretic your way to thinness. There was a show on national television a few years back about the disturbing, burgeoning epidemic of bulimic, purging/vomiting behavior for weight loss in girls under the age of 10, and even a fair number of girls under the age of five. It's hard to imagine children at these ages already so psychologically disturbed and obsessed, but it doesn't stop there. I'm not a psychologist, but if you sat in my office over the past 30 years and listened to the litany of people, including doctors, lawyers, and other highly educated professionals, who have participated in bizarre, life-threatening behaviors to lose weight, it would blow your mind. I have known a judge who, in her private chambers in between cases, would consistently vomit her brains out, and a surgeon who, in between surgical procedures, consistently purged herself. These dysfunctional behaviors occur more commonly in women, but women have not cornered the market on such compulsive disorders; there is a growing population of men participating in bulimic behavior. Sadly, men have also vigorously entered the arena of body dysmorphia and decided that they should adopt this nasty strategy for weight-loss.

The problem is that you can end up chasing unrealistic goals and unreasonable expectations that are often divorced from any real consideration of health or healthy behavior. You're buying into standards and goals that are close to impossible to achieve. I'm never going to look like Mark Wahlberg or some other entertainment icon. That's not my body type, facial structure, or genetic background. As a woman, you're probably not going to look like a movie star or a supermodel. Even they don't look like that; I love the line by the supermodel Cindy Crawford, who was quoted in an interview, "When I get up in the morning, I don't even look like Cindy Crawford." Professional makeup, hair styling, clothes, and photo-enhancing create images that aren't based in reality at all.

As a result of this distorted cultural mindset and the perceived pressure it bestows, people with weight issues are bullied in schools, shamed online, passed over for jobs, and routinely judged in everyday social interactions, causing untold pain, psychological damage, unhealthy behaviors, and negative self-judgment. The bottom line is that we have adopted images and ideals in our minds that are totally unrealistic and inconsistent with who we actually are, what we are truly capable of achieving, and, most importantly, the health goals we should be trying to achieve.

Unfortunately, as a backlash to a painful history of this shaming and prejudice, there is a burgeoning "body positivity" movement in which people are adamantly and proudly embracing their fatness. Everyone deserves respect, compassion, and love regardless of the labels and conditions that have been used to describe them. I strongly support people feeling comfortable about themselves. However, this movement to accept risk factors like extra weight and body fat ignores, sidesteps, or even condemns the strong evidence and practices of natural hygienic living and lifestyle medicine that support optimal health. Powerful evidence clearly shows that excessive weight and body fat are associated with the most devastating medical conditions of modern times, including heart disease, type 2 diabetes, stroke, and cancer. You no more want to celebrate increased weight and fat than you want to celebrate and defend high blood pressure, high blood sugar, high cholesterol, or increased inflammation.

Typically, it is still more common for people with excessive weight and body fat to seek quick-fix diets, drugs, and surgeries that often reinforce failure over time and develop into an endless quest to buy hope wherever it can be found. The checkout stands in nearly every store offer promises of help with their racks of popular magazines and journals full of miracle diets, celebrity endorsements, and supposed success stories. What these reports fail to tell you is that those calorie-restricted diets and exaggerated-nutrient diets (high-protein, high-fat) are doomed to fail

over time because they do not address the full range of hormonal, metabolic, and lifestyle factors associated with fat and weight gain. That's
why the glaring truth is that the multibillion-dollar dieting industry has
more than a 90–95% failure rate.

Follow these restricted diets, and you are not only going to put that
weight back on, but you're going to put it back on with a vengeance.
Eventually, you'll try again with another unsustainable approach that
leads to more extreme deprivation, drives your starvation response,
increases insulin resistance, and escalates craving, compelling you to eat
(and overeat) the very refined, calorie-dense foods you're trying to avoid,
often secretly so as to avoid the judgment of others but still filling you
with guilt and despair. Overwhelming feelings of hopelessness and helplessness follow, driving you to seek comfort anywhere you can find it.
Unfortunately, the only real comfort you may ever have found is in the
overeating and compulsive food use at the root of the entire cycle.

This cycle of deprivation-hunger/craving-overeating-guilt-hope-
lessness-failure is a very common program playing in the heads of so
many dieters, compulsive eaters, and food addicts. My goal is to help you
replace this disheartening and ultimately futile program with the new
program that has been presented in this book emphasizing awareness,
responsibility, and self-esteem.

For decades, you have been inundated with and addicted to hyperpalatable, processed foods and animal products loaded with salt, oil, and
refined sugar that have distracted you away from the taste and value of
the whole plant food that is in your best interest. These processed foods
have distorted the brain's pleasure-reward system and assaulted and
compromised our instinctive awareness of what and when to eat. Combined with how we have been conditioned to view food use in our families
and cultures, they have promoted ingrained lifetime habits around how
we use foods for a variety of psychological reasons, including boredom,
stress, discomfort, and pain, that are inevitable parts of life and truly
have nothing to do with the biological reason for food consumption.

Watching young children eat provides a remarkable example of instinctive awareness. When children are full, they usually simply quit eating and start playing with their food; the peas and carrots become planes, trains, and automobiles and start flying around the house, so you know they're done.

As little children grow and change, they unknowingly become some of the best psychologists on the planet. They recognize all of your schticks (a perfect Yiddish word for the games and behaviors people often employ to get by) from a mile away, and they can pull all of your chains before you even walk in the room as they look to see how far they can stretch the rules before you rope them in. This testing of the limits, this give-and-take, is part of normal growth and development. However, as these little ones whine, disobey, misbehave, and generally noisily push the envelope, a parent or grandparent can get frustrated to a point where they don't want to deal with it any longer, and they'll use food as a comfort, a bribe, or a reward. These little ones are being taught to use food to deal with their anger, sadness, and boredom, but this has nothing to do with their real, basic needs. In this way, the seeds are planted for distorted behavior that uses food for reward, distraction, and problem-solving they will inevitably encounter throughout their lives.

If you were brought up like I was, you may have a lot more work to do, as you have likely gone deeper into the twilight zone. Why? Because families tend to perpetuate the same food patterns. So you may have been taught to deal with your stress by finding comfort and distraction in food from the earliest moments of your life, probably even when you emerged from your mother's womb.

My personal experience serves as a classic example of how dysfunctional food use can occur around family and cultural patterns to establish a distorted relationship with food and eating. In my Italian household, on holidays like Christmas and Easter, we would sit down for the big meal at about two o'clock in the afternoon. Guess where we were many hours later? That's right, still at the dinner table. Guess what went on during those hours? I would fall asleep several times (right at the dinner table!), head dropping down, banging on the table, bouncing back up, eyes springing open, eating more of whatever was still on the table, because empty bowls just got refilled with another course, keeping that table full. Food and overeating unequivocally became equated with love, family, and all the comfort and well-being of hearth and home.

And when you can eat that way in my Italian household (and for many others in their own other ethnic and cultural settings), surely there could not be any other problems in the universe—no deep-rooted issues and emotional trauma seething under the surface (molestation, emotional abuse, relationship problems, etc.). Just eat something, everything will be just fine. There's no problem that a good meal and/or overeating can't fix. So, the small dysfunctional child becomes the big dysfunctional adult. And the big adult has a tough day at work, so what does he do? Well, he eats. If he's sexually frustrated or deprived of intimacy, what does he do? He eats. If he needs emotional and spiritual nourishment in his life that he is not satisfying in constructive ways, what does he do? He eats. And if he marries someone who was brought up the same way, they will stare across the table at each other and eat, and no one will get any closer to their personal truth, either individually or as a couple.

It is essential to become more aware of the situations and emotional conditions that are attached to your compulsive food use. Discovering and imbuing the experiences of our lives with some meaning and purpose is a powerful way to handle and survive the inevitable pain and suffering of life. It is imperative to embrace the moments of your life and feel the feelings, connect to the feelings, that come up as you process the traumas of your life. This will help you generate and build an awareness of the deep-rooted issues prompting your compulsive food use and other lifestyle and relationship choices that may be sabotaging your health and weight loss goals instead of consistently using food to escape your feelings of discomfort and pain. Awareness, connection to the magic and mystery of the moments of your life, purposeful meaning, and love are essential for you to heal the trauma of your life, discard old programs of compulsion and addiction, and establish new programs in your behavioral repertoire for optimal health and weight regulation.

It is crucial to extinguish your conditioned patterns of reactive, compulsive food use if you are ever going to develop a balanced, positive relationship with healthy food and eating. A mindful awareness of the role food plays in your life, especially in times of stress and discomfort, is critical for discovering alternative, healthy ways to satisfy your basic needs. It is the most effective way to stop using mindless, compulsive food consumption to sidestep the psychological, emotional, and even spiritual issues that need your attention and resolution. Committing to healthy choices will establish and reinforce the responsible actions that promote long-term weight loss. In addition, by dedicating yourself to maintaining responsible, healthy action, you are making a strong commitment to your best self. As a result, you can build the self-esteem that comes from honoring and supporting your true value, your true self. This is extremely valuable and necessary for successful weight regulation. In the next few chapters, we will dive deeper into the process of addiction while further emphasizing and expanding on the important roles of responsibility, self-worth, self-love, and self-esteem in establishing healthy body image and succeeding at fat and weight loss.

CHAPTER 22

FOOD ADDICTION, MINDFULNESS, AND SELF-CARE: WHAT'S EATING YOU?

The ways you think about food and integrate it into your life can lead to addictive and compulsive behavior and potential problems with body weight. Therefore, having some understanding of the addictive process and how our awareness and choices can modify this process can remarkably improve your chance for successful weight loss.

Because the definition of addiction can be confusing, I emphasize a simple definition adopted from Dr. Jay Holder and the American College of Addictionology and Compulsive Disorders to clarify the distinctions between addiction, abuse, compulsive behavior, and other excessive lifestyle activities. For practical purposes, addiction is defined as the the continued or compulsive use of any mood-altering substance or behavior without regard for negative consequences.[1] The component of disregard of negative consequences is the most crucial part of this definition. That means the individual knows their behavior is either causing them harm directly or is hurting family members or others in their community, but they continue the behavior anyway. It also means that they cannot fulfill normal, routine, social-, family-, and work-related responsibilities without the substances and behaviors of abuse, compromising their entire sphere of psychosocial behavior and function.

The mindless disregard, and especially the denial, of the dangers and consequences of addiction is fundamental to the addictive process. For example, the addictive use of food can promote excessive weight gain and an increased risk of diabetes, heart attacks, strokes, and cancers. An obese person with health problems or a diabetic who knowingly disregards and denies the potential harm of their overconsumption of refined, junk food would satisfy this definition. People who continue to drive drunk even though they know they're putting their own life and the lives of others at risk would satisfy this definition. However, the person who more occasionally uses alcohol or other drugs or overeats or gambles without negative consequences to themselves or others is an abuser, not an addict.

Even essential behaviors can become addictive. People who overexercise but do not create harm would not satisfy the definition of addiction. However, I have worked with exercise anorexics who push their bodies to such a dangerous degree of exhaustion, debilitation, and disease that they definitely exhibit an exercise addiction. Disregard for negative consequences and denial are the hallmark signs of true addiction.

Brain-Reward Cascade

A model has emerged from the science of addictionology that is fundamental to our experience of pleasure and our understanding of addiction. It is called the brain-reward cascade.[2] I love the word cascade. It is a waterfall of chemistry—neurotransmitters and neuropeptides—flowing in specific pathways and locations in the brain that is associated with our ability to experience pleasure, joy, and reward from the simple acts of life.

We are all creatures capable of feeling satisfied and at peace with ourselves while experiencing a high degree of pleasure from simple, basic life situations, such as the hug of a mate, the laughter of a child, a walk in the park, the exhilaration of a sunrise or sunset, a good meal, and a sensual kiss. The chemistry in the brain associated with the brain-reward cascade provides the chemical environment and foundation for the experience of pleasure and satisfaction and involves the activation and release of key neuropeptides (like neuropeptide-Y) and neurotransmitters (serotonin, opiates, norepinephrine, and GABA), culminating in the release of dopamine, the ultimate pleasure transmitter. The pleasure cascade has evolved specifically to ensure both individual and species survival by associating significant pleasure with food that supports individual survival and with sex that promotes the propagation of our species. Furthermore, to enhance survival potential, there are multiple dopamine pathways in the brain that enhance our memories of these pleasures and our motivation to experience them again.

Neurotransmitters are made in specialized nerve cells in the brain and nervous system; following the electrical stimulation of these nerve cells, the neurotransmitters are released from nerve endings in the brain. When this happens, they travel across a small space—the synapse—before they attach to special receptors in the membranes of adjacent nerves, muscles, or organs. This electrochemical connection is manifested in waves of chemical and electrical events in billions of nerve cells every second of every day, controlling every function of the body by transmitting and translating the endless field of electromagnetic frequencies around us into the objects and experiences of day-to-day reality. All of our joys, pleasures, ups, downs, and the emotional value we give to them occur as a result of the integration, balance, dynamic communication, and feedback of the pulsing, shimmering chemistry of the brain, nervous system, and the brain-reward cascade.

If I asked you why you continue to do what you do and why you make the choices that you do, you may say that some of these choices were influenced by your parents at an early stage of life, by influential people you may have met along the way, or by your own personal experiences and challenges over time. The truth is that you continue to make the choices you do because, on a very basic level, you have associated these choices with pleasure, reward, and survival. This truth holds even for people in the throes of addiction. I have worked with many drug and food abusers, including myself, and addicts dealing with just about every form of addiction through the years. I have yet to find even one addict for whom, at least in the early stages, their addiction was not a friend in the night. It was how that person created some pleasure and survival value, because they did not have the inborn capability, personal resources, or cognitive tools to do it in a more supportive, healthy way. Unfortunately, because of a specific genetic modification and/or a variety of negative lifestyle factors, some people experience a deficiency and dysfunction of this brain reward that is viewed as the common denominator in all forms of addiction, the reward deficiency syndrome (RDS).[3,4]

The Impact of Reward Deficiency

There is a well-recognized genetic defect that is present in a large segment of the human population that is a major cause and predisposing factor for the breakdown of natural brain reward and the disease of addiction. This genetic defect of the dopamine receptor in the brain's limbic system interferes with the production, attachment, and action of dopamine. In addition, this genetic defect can compromise the production and function of other brain neurotransmitters essential to normal reward and pleasure and alter metabolic pathways in the brain to produce highly addictive, toxic chemicals that dramatically boost the addictive process. In addition to this potential genetic modification, factors of poor nutrition, chronic stress, sleep deficiency, and loss of neurological function due to physical, emotional, and chemical trauma can compromise and deplete the brain chemistry involved in brain-reward activity, reducing the amount of dopamine that is released at the brain-reward sites in the mesolimbic part of the brain and creating reward deficiency.

Reward deficiency syndrome makes it no longer possible to effectively experience pleasure from the simple acts and joys of life. When you can't experience pleasure and joy, feelings of emptiness, need, and craving will result. As the breakdown of the reward cascade continues and the RDS is maintained, feelings of isolation, loneliness, depression, and anxiety will ensue.

The self-centeredness and isolation so typical of addicts are classic examples of this distress. Guess what? No person wants to experience discomfort, emptiness, and isolation. No person wants to experience that. In fact, I'll go on record and state that the brain naturally wants to get high. It wants to feel good, happy, and well. If you can't feel good from the routine physical, emotional, and spiritual activities and experiences of your life, you're going to seek out any substance or behavior that will stimulate the normal feel-good pathways of the brain-reward system in order to relieve the discomfort of your own craving, emptiness, and need. As a result, you will tend to self-medicate the problems of the RDS with any one of the five major forms of addiction: food, drugs (including alcohol), sex, risk taking/gambling, and compulsive behaviors (called process addictions) including work, shopping, Internet use, video games, and porn. While a variety of personal and lifestyle factors contribute to your personal addiction, there is a suggestion that other unique modifications of the genetic machinery can also urge you to choose a particular substance or behavior of abuse over another.

What do these addictive behaviors have in common? They can create an illusion of well-being, even sociability and function, by chemically or behaviorally stimulating the brain-reward cascade. It is a false sense of feeling good and at peace with yourself. It's not that the feelings are not real, but they are an illusion, because over time the pleasure of the initial high becomes harder to come by as you "chase the first high," seeking the initial euphoric feeling but never quite getting there. With repeated use, the person becomes more tolerant and needs more and more of the substance or behavior to get the desired result. Ultimately, you get very little pleasure, and you're "using" now just to quiet your discomfort and pain, just to get out of bed in the morning, just to get by and create some degree of functionality. At this point, you are in the throes of dependency as the more primitive, limbic, survival part of the brain hijacks the intellectual part of the brain and screams the message that without this food, this substance, or this behavior, you cannot survive.[5] This makes resolving addiction an extremely difficult task unless you address the physical, cognitive, emotional, spiritual, and metabolic factors that are at the foundation of the addictive behaviors and relearn how to truly satisfy your unfulfilled needs for comfort, healthy sociability, and balanced function.

Compulsive Eating and Food Addiction

Food addiction is unique because it is so directly involved with your survival needs. Eating is directly and intimately involved with nurturing ourselves on every level. We don't really need to shoot heroin, but we do have to eat several times per day. So, food addicts are confronting that monkey constantly, meal in and meal out.

Because of our need for carbohydrates for energy production, our brains perceive them as necessary for survival and sweet foods as especially ideal. In the distant past, when food scarcity was common, the dopamine surge and pleasure response caused by sugar-laden plants and calorie-dense foods drove our desire to obtain these foods. While this primitive characteristic once ensured survival, the inborn drive to eat these foods is no longer vital in the modern Western world because calorie-dense foods are available everywhere. Refined, concentrated sugar especially promotes a huge surge in dopamine release, and the brain can be tricked into believing that processed food is necessary for survival, tempting us to overeat and potentially leading us into compulsive use.

However, the continued consumption of processed food loaded with sugar eventually reduces the amount of dopamine produced in the brain as well as the number and function of dopamine receptors, so that tolerance, withdrawal, and craving will result when sugar is removed from the diet. Since sugar alters reward processing in the brain and can cause a surge of dopamine, even people with other addictions like alcohol or other drugs can exhibit intense sugar cravings during their recovery process to compensate for the alcohol or drug withdrawal's reward deficiency.

Unfortunately, the brain-reward cascade has been manipulated by food conglomerates and the food-processing industry to drive compulsive food use and food addiction, pushing their food-as-drug agenda for profit while maliciously promoting pandemics of obesity, addiction, and chronic disease.

Many years ago, the food-processing industry discovered that the trio of sugar, salt, and fat could produce a state of satiety and exaggerated pleasure that is mediated by dopamine and the brain-reward system. They worked with market researchers and psychophysicists like Howard Moscowitz, who coined the term "bliss point" for that point where saltiness, sweetness, and richness was perceived by consumers as "just right." They then took it further and added crunchiness to the bliss-point formula. Food manufacturers now use these elements extensively to create an assortment of highly processed products, including chips, sweetened cereals, candies, cookies, fried foods, and even tomato sauces.[6] These hyperpalatable, craveable foods drive their profits through the roof, but they can dysregulate the brain's food-reward system to increase dopamine production, increasing the addictive nature of these foods.[7] This makes it truly necessary to adopt an SOS-free, plant-exclusive eating plan to free yourself from the pleasure prison that has been etched into the consciousness and the habits of our population and give yourself the best opportunity to lose weight and body fat.

What's Eating You?

From an awareness/cognitive standpoint, it is essential to deeply understand and become more mindful of both the context of your food use as well as the content of what you're eating. What are you using food for? What are you really hungry for? Are you attempting to satisfy all your physical, emotional, and spiritual needs with food? As wonderful as it can be, food was not designed for that purpose. What can you do individually, along with counseling and group support if necessary, to become more aware of the deeper issues that are driving your compulsive food use? How can you develop the physical, emotional, and spiritual tools needed to address and resolve these issues, create more balance in your life, and nurture yourself without compulsive, obsessive food use? As you do the much-needed personal introspective work to answer these questions, you will understand the importance of your own mindfulness and the need for ongoing support.

Some experts in the addiction field assert that people resolving addictions need a month of treatment for every year of addiction, and that is care on every level: physical, emotional, and spiritual. The point is that it is not an instantaneous process. It takes major attention to detail over time, especially if you are one of the many people dealing with the genetic defect I already explained that is always lurking to foster relapse into addictive behavior. That's also why, when people go into 30-day or extended rehabilitation programs, these are not "treatment" programs per se. They are stabilization programs that allow the individual to stabilize their use so they can complete the mind-body work that needs to be done. The limited days of short rehab programs are not enough to satisfy the ongoing need for emotional and spiritual support to prevent relapse and the reinstatement of addictive, destructive behavior. Because isolation is such a major part of the dis-ease of addiction, recovery is very much about connection—connecting in healthy relationships with others and yourself. However, when people do recovery work, it is often recommended that they avoid getting involved in new love relationships for some period of time because until you have resolved the major causes of your addiction, the new relationship can become the new addiction.

It is imperative to understand what is at the core of your addiction's craving urges. For some short period of time, keep a journal of the things that are going on when your craving is at its worst. Look more closely at the kinds of foods that are of greatest interest. Whenever you can, delay your responses and examine how the routine events of your life make you feel in the moments that you are experiencing them. Examine the pattern of your lifestyle activities, including work, exercise, sleep, family, and outside stresses around the times that you find yourself losing your way and going off-track.

How can you more mindfully address your function and your choices on physical, emotional, and spiritual levels? If your eating pattern is truly a repeat pattern of addiction with abnormal, negative health consequences, I urge you to get involved with an addiction support program. You will have a sponsor, group interaction and support, fellowship to resolve your isolation and self-centeredness, and possibly even a 12-step program that encourages you to seek outside help, to trust in some thing or process bigger than yourself, to metaphorically clean house, and to help others.

Remember, these things are not just happening *to* you. *You* are the actor. *You* write the script. It is *your* brain that perceives the infinite number of wave forms within and around you and translates them into the data of personal experience. If you have the same problems with food over and over again or if you have been on the same roller coaster of weight loss and reactive weight gain over years of your life, I can guarantee you one thing—food is not your problem. Your brain is the problem; food is the symptom. Addiction is the dis-ease. Until that is addressed, you will not get any closer to resolving your addictive or compulsive food use or to the deep healing that needs to be done.

All of our past physical and emotional traumas and experiences concretize as layers of constrictions, blockages, and restrictions that become etched and sculpted into the behavioral tapestry of our neurological systems and expressed in both body and mind. It is important, then, that on a basic level you go into what some people have referred to as the "pain body" in order to process, dissolve, and heal these layers of change. Attaining health and balance is not always comfortable. It is not a straight stairway to heaven, because the symptoms and actions of recovery can be downright painful. It may involve, to some degree, what I call going to hell and back as you deal with the pain of recovery. But you know what? The reward is absolutely worth it when you get to the heart of your own desire and experience the sublime freedom and pleasure of recovery that comes from confronting and unraveling the drives, triggers, and blockages that are promoting your repeated rounds of failure.

Too often you may opt for a deceptive level of simplicity and take the more mindless path of blaming your problems on the food that you're eating or the substances or the behaviors or even the people you're involved with. Unfortunately, this allows you to sidestep the causative conditions at hand and avoid addressing the real issues that need to be resolved. The chocolate, the candy, the cake, the cookies, or the cheese are not the problem. There is no doubt that these food items have their own addictive quality and that removing them from your life is a necessary, supportive step on the road to recovery and success. However, these food items are the symptoms of your dis-ease of addiction. You have met the enemy—and it is *you*. It is way past time to get real. This is a huge piece of the recovery and weight-loss story.

Employing lifestyle practices that promote the balancing of brain chemistry and function is critical for dealing with the addictive process. By engaging in the behaviors of whole-plant-exclusive eating, consistent activity, stress management, adequate sleep, and other natural, supportive lifestyle factors, you will promote the health of the body in general and the balance and function of the brain in particular. In addition, in cases of long-term addiction where there is an extensive imbalance of brain chemistry (or even a genetic defect), supportive therapeutic approaches, including chiropractic care, amino-acid supplementation, cranial nerve augmentation, counseling, and even 12-step programs have been discovered that have helped people deal with the craving, depression, and withdrawal associated with the reward deficiency syndrome.

Supportive Supplementation for Escaping Addiction

As I mentioned previously, the key neurotransmitters of the brain-reward cascade are serotonin, opiates, GABA, norepinephrine, and dopamine. These transmitters are made by specific biochemical reactions that combine amino acids (protein's building blocks) with some key vitamins and minerals. These nutrients are provided by properly balanced nutrition, but since they may be chronically depleted in long-term addiction, a period of supplementation over several months and sometimes even much longer may also have some value in increasing the production of these important neurotransmitters and balancing brain chemistry over time.

Amino Acids

Some supplemental amino acids can block the action of a specific enzyme, enkephalinase, that ultimately inhibits the release of the plea-sure neurotransmitter dopamine. As a result, these amino acids promote an increase in the release of dopamine and its healthy, normal brain reward so that the simple pleasures of being alive and well can be sup-ported, maintained, and fully experienced. This is especially important for people who have the underlying genetic defect in the dopamine receptor, since they need all the help they can get to keep dopamine levels as consistently high as possible. Importantly, these amino acids also can help you stay on a healthy track of recovery when the pain of withdrawal threatens to promote relapse.

Following is a modified list of the key amino acids, vitamins, and minerals typically used in a treatment protocol that has been shown to have the most significant positive impact on brain-reward activity in a variety of addiction treatment programs.[4] I only share this with you as part of this general discussion, not as a prescription. *These supplements should not be taken without the consent, care, and evaluation of your primary physician and other health-care providers.*

• L-Glutamine

This amino acid is critical for the production of the neurotransmitter GABA, which helps reduce anxiety and overstimulation of dopamine. It can also improve the integrity of a damaged gut, e.g., leaky gut, that may occur as a result of alcohol toxicity, long-term relentless stress, and/ or long-term use of animal products and refined, processed foods low in fiber content.

• DL-Phenylalanine

This amino acid is essential in the production of the neurotransmitters norepinephrine and dopamine. Due to the stimulatory effects of dopamine, it should not be taken if there is any history of anxiety or panic attacks. This also should not be taken by nursing mothers, since some infants may not process this amino acid effectively and may be predisposed to develop a condition called phenylketonuria (PKU), leading to a form of ketosis that can damage the bodies and brains of infants.

• L-Tyrosine

The amino acid L-tyrosine is also directly involved in the production of the neurotransmitters norepinephrine and dopamine. Tyrosine is a major component of the enzyme tyrosine hydroxylase that is a rate-limiting enzyme and major catalyst in the pathway that converts phenylalanine to dopamine. It is also key in the production of thyroid hormones.

• L-Tryptophan

This is the amino acid that is essential for serotonin production. As I mentioned previously, serotonin is critical for emotional stability and well-being, and it is the initiator of the brain-reward cascade that can be significantly reduced in reward deficiency syndrome (RDS). Also, when you remove the substances and behaviors of addiction, some feelings of depression may rear their ugly heads. Tryptophan supplementation may be helpful in reducing the feelings of depression associated with RDS and withdrawal. Its role in promoting healthy sleep may also be very beneficial and significant for promoting healthy sleep during the early phases of withdrawal when sleep can be extremely disturbed.

Consistent with the brain changes associated with reward deficiency syndrome, some people with addictions may be given a dual diagnosis of addiction and anxiety and/or depression, and so they are often put on antidepressant and/or anti-anxiety medication. This can be a huge mistake. Very often, the depression may be related to the withdrawal of the substances or behaviors of abuse, not a psychiatric problem of true depression or anxiety. These medications can compound and even intensify the problems of addiction. Keep this in mind. All of the systems of the body, including the regulation and production of hormones and enzymes, are subject to a potential consequence called negative feedback inhibition. As you may remember, that means that if the body makes a chemical or hormone normally and you put a similar chemical into the body, the body believes that it has already made enough of it and shuts down its own natural production. This also applies to the use of antidepressant medication. As we have mentioned, the reward deficiency syndrome can lead to a depletion, a true deficiency, of neurotransmitters that affect mood and emotions, promoting feelings of depression. To truly improve this circumstance, it is necessary to improve the body's ability to make more of its own natural neurotransmitters. Medication for depression does not do this.

The body exerts even more sophisticated modulation of mood and emotion by controlling how neurotransmitters linger in the synaptic space. Not only can neurotransmitters be released from the ends of nerve cells, but these same nerve endings can take these transmitters back up and break them down to smooth and shape behavior more effectively. Many antidepressant medications (Prozac, Paxil, Zoloft, and others) are reuptake inhibitors that block the body's ability to resorb and process the neurotransmitters serotonin and norepinephrine that it has already released, causing them to linger longer in the synapse, which helps to maintain an uplifting effect. Remember, there may already be a deficiency of these neurotransmitters; but when the medications cause them to linger longer in the synapse, it sends the brain the signal that it has made enough of these messengers, and the brain will decrease its own natural production of them, making the deficiency even worse. So, although antidepressants may promote temporary mood elevation, it is an illusion. They may be dangerously depleting an already existing deficiency. This is why, as we have already discussed, so many people on antidepressant medication are still depressed. It's the reason why, when you abruptly stop these drugs, there can be a dangerous reactive crash of depression and even suicidal tendencies.

Vitamins and Minerals

The amino-acid program can be further bolstered by a diverse WFPE diet to provide adequate overall nutrition, especially high-quality micro-nutrients from whole foods. Targeted vitamin and mineral supplementation, including vitamin C, zinc, and pyridoxal-5-phosphate (the activated form of vitamin B6), may potentially be helpful to provide the body with the raw materials needed to make more of its own neurotransmitters, resulting in a true resolution of the underlying deficiency without confusing the body's feedback system. Consult your healthcare provider for specific recommendations regarding whether and how much of these vitamins and minerals are appropriate.

Targeted Chiropractic Care for Addiction and Weight Loss

Healthy brain function and relapse prevention have been significantly improved by combining vitamin and mineral supplementation with chiropractic care and auriculotherapy, the treatment of reflex points in the ear with low-intensity, microcurrent electrical stimulation of variable frequencies. In two separate studies done three years apart at the Exodus drug treatment facility in Miami Beach, FL, torque-release chiropractic care and auriculotherapy were significantly effective for reducing the pain and craving of withdrawal, while promoting a 100% retention rate of people staying in the rehab program to complete treatment.[8] This result was remarkable and even revolutionary, especially when you consider that typically a high percentage of people drop out of drug rehab programs in the early days of treatment when the pain of withdrawal tends to promote relapse. It's also important to mention that in these studies, chiropractic care helped resolve the depression and anxiety in the addicted population faster and better than the conventional drug treatments typically utilized for these psychological disturbances, providing additional evidence for the significant and profound impact of chiropractic care on improved state of well-being and the full expression of human potential. I have had consistent success in helping people with compulsive food use and other addictions (to nicotine, caffeine, and even harder drugs and alcohol) by utilizing this program of treatment and supplementation.

It is worth emphasizing that the positive benefits of chiropractic care on brain-reward systems and general state of well-being also make it an invaluable tool in any health and weight-loss program. Typically, the stressors that you encounter in your day-to-day experience occur in three categories that I previously referred to as the three Ts:

- physical *trauma* due to sports injuries and other accidents;

- *toxic* chemical stress from poor nutrition, drug abuses, and exposure to food additives and preservatives, pesticides, and environmental toxins; and

- *thoughts*, psychological stress, and emotional traumas and abuses.

As different as these stressors are, they have one thing in common: they can compromise your brain and nervous system. Since the brain and nervous system exert a controlling influence over the entire body, neurological insult can interfere with the healthy function, communication, and regulation of all cells, organs, and systems of the body, promoting dysfunction and disease. In the chiropractic profession, the primary insult to and interference with the nervous system is called a subluxation, a neurodystrophic process that can be corrected by specific adjustments to the spinal column and interactive neuromuscular system. Because of the widespread influence of the nervous system on the function of the body, the elimination of neurological interference through chiropractic care can increase healthy neuroplasticity of the brain and enhance the function of the hormonal and immune systems, as well as your performance and general state of well-being. It's no mystery why the biggest groups of people participating in chiropractic care are people in pain, people suffering from traumatic accidents and injuries, and high-performance athletes. Balancing the function of your brain and nervous system will improve performance in all your activities while also improving digestive function and metabolic efficiency. In addition, the correction of aberrant neurological and proprioceptive information from the spine associated with subluxations can activate brain areas that help you manage stress more effectively and also elicit a calming effect in the parasympathetic nervous system to potentially promote more restful sleep. So, when you are experiencing physical, chemical, and emotional stress, it is in your best interest to eliminate neurological interference with more regular chiropractic care. Also, keep in mind that addiction and/or compulsive behavior is a multifactorial problem that includes physical, psychological, spiritual, genetic, and metabolic components. Eliminating neurological interference can help restore the integrity of all mind-body interaction and function.

While my program, supported by some adjunctive care, can help stabilize dysfunctional biochemistry, neurological dysfunction, and some of the emotional ups and downs associated with addictive and compulsive food use, it is still essential to get in touch with the underlying motivations of your abnormal desire for food and the context of your craving and food use. This awareness can help you clarify the choices that are in your best interest and markedly increase your motivation to implement them in your life. The consequences of these positive choices inspire personal empowerment and a powerful, deep-rooted experience and expression of self-worth, self-love, and self-esteem, naturally reinforcing a lifestyle that is in your best interest and critical for optimal health, weight, and body fat.

CHAPTER 23

BEYOND THE PHYSICAL: BODY IMAGE AND EMOTIONAL CARE

Body Image and Self-Judgment

I have emphasized the importance of promoting healthy, realistic goals of weight and body fat and being acutely aware of the negative consequences associated with the addictive consumption of animal and processed foods that drive weight gain and chronic disease. These factors play a significant role in establishing not only your physical appearance but also the psychological construct of body image that is a combination of how you see yourself and how you believe the world sees you. Your perception of yourself is psychologically etched in your brain by a variety of factors including societal ideals, media biases, and input from family members, friends, voices of authority, and others, and it often originates in our early years and sticks with us for life. We judge ourselves, fairly or unfairly, against not just the many standards of the world around us, but also against our own sometimes-skewed perception of the ideal, which is often unrealistic. This can contribute to negativity and destructive, unhealthy beliefs about yourself that generate stress, anguish, and personal trauma.

In our quest to achieve the perfection we imagine for ourselves, many people seek dangerous, quick-fix, extreme fad diets; medication programs; or risky cosmetic procedures that provide short-lived reductions in weight or body fat but rarely have any lasting effect. It seems there's always more that can (and should) be done. As a result, you can be disengaged from a healthy perception of your true, inherent beauty and self-worth. At the extreme, this can lead to extremely dangerous conditions such as anorexia, bulimia, or addiction to cosmetic surgery that compels you to repeatedly inject, nip, tuck, and obliterate every line, wrinkle, and sign of living you have earned in your dance of life, behaviors requiring psychological as well as physical intervention. But for most, it leads to dissatisfaction, regrets, unhappiness, insecurity, and a sense of defeat as they pursue some fleeting, arbitrary, superficial ideal of beauty that always seems to be just a little bit out of reach.

As a result of these emotional and psychological disturbances, we can be so hard on ourselves, and unfortunately, women are often the most brutal in their self-judgment. There is typically a big difference in the perception of body image between men and women in our culture. Very often, a man in his 50s, 60s, or older gets that protruding beer-belly look, with love handles at the waist dripping over his belt, and he is grey-haired, balding, and scruffy; yet when he looks in the mirror, he will say to himself, "Yesss, I don't look too bad—actually, I'm looking good!" You will rarely find a woman at any size or weight who does that and doesn't judge herself as flawed in some way. So it is true for all of us, and especially for women; you have got to lighten up and have more compassion and love for yourself where you are, even when you look in the mirror and say, "Who the heck is that?"

You Are More than Your Body

While this book has primarily focused on our physical selves as I've shared my vegan, WFPE program to guide you to the healthiest, happiest, strongest you possible, it is also necessary to acknowledge, explore, and celebrate our larger selves. Never forget that you are so much more than the words, labels, and dysfunctions that have been used to describe you. No matter what your appearance or physical condition is, you are a masterpiece of creation and evolution, full of mystery and wonder that defies any attempts to portray you with the shortcomings of words and definitions. You are love, compassion, and empathy in connection with all that is.

The body is your temple. It is a magnificent, miraculous endowment. It is a wise, intelligent ecosystem capable of distilling the ocean of energy waves and the chaos around you into the order and manifestation of creative life, including love, sex, music, art, and dance, everything from the sacred to the profane. You are intrinsically divine and perfect at any size or weight. Imagine holding an infant in your arms. See this incredible creature gurgling, cooing, and laughing. See and feel the innocence, the purity, the egoless surrender staring back at you. That's how we all arrived on this planet—pure, innocent, perfect, the essence and expression of divine love. That is who you still are right now and who you will always be, regardless of the negative life experiences that have tried to separate you from that understanding. Now, see your own face on the baby in your arms, looking back at you and embracing and loving yourself unconditionally. Recognize and experience this respect and love for yourself.

We all spend so much time and energy in love affairs with people outside of ourselves— girlfriends, boyfriends, husbands, wives, and children. Yet everything we know about love actually springs from what is going on inside each of us deep down at the cellular level. If you damage any part of the body or even lose an organ, everything that is left behind attempts to compensate for that damage and loss. Nurturing, love, integration, and connection are biological and cellular imperatives. Yet in the face of this loving organismic directive, it's amazing to me how, when we go off track—however we interpret that—we are so willing to become our own whipping post, beat ourselves up, and then go to hell in a handbasket, making choices that only continue to foster breakdown, damage, and disease. We do this to ourselves even though we would never do that to someone we loved.

Imagine it's a slick, rainy night and you need to run an errand, but your car is out of commission, so you go to your best friend and ask to borrow his brand-new car. With some trepidation he gives you the keys, expressing concerns about the inclement night and fears about damage to his car. You assure him that you will be safe, but an accident occurs, and the car is totalled. When you call to tell him, he initially derides you and is irate that you could possibly have been so careless. However, in the midst of his tirade, he realizes that you could be injured; he catches himself and comes from a more compassionate, spiritual place, a place of unconditional forgiveness and concern, and asks, "Are you okay?" "What can I do to help?" It's interesting to me that in some ways the body comes from the "What can I do to help?" perspective every time.

Over the years, I have counseled numerous people who have diseases that can take many years to develop, but by making positive lifestyle choices over the course of several months to a year or two, they experience a significant recovery. It is as if mercy and forgiveness are built into the genetic machinery of the body, an inborn program of compassion intimately woven and expressed in the magnificent healing power of the body. So, when you find yourself going off track, instead of beating yourself up and reinforcing your self-loathing and lack of worth, ask yourself the question, "What can I do to help?" just like you would for anyone you truly cared about and loved.

Ask yourself what you can do to get back on track; forgive and love yourself. True forgiveness for your parents, others, and especially yourself will dissolve your greatest burdens, including guilt, shame, and trauma, and open up a world of your greatest possibility, compassion, love, and success. Forgiveness and self-love are two of your greatest sources of strength; they help facilitate peace of mind and the ability to promote the habits essential for health and long-term weight loss.

It is essential to have goals for change, but these goals should be realistic and consistently promote the greatest expression of your health, value, and self-worth. It is supremely important to pass beyond the illusion of physical appearance as you open, identify with, and inhabit the sacred space deep within yourself where you encounter "the perfect treasure that is called by your name."

Self-Esteem, Commitment, and Change

Nurturing self-esteem is critical for maintaining a healthy perception of yourself, as well as eliminating addictive behavior and promoting optimal weight and body fat. Self-esteem is built by keeping commitments and agreements with yourself and with others with the little things of life and routine activities of daily living, in addition to creating success in the bigger arenas of your personal and professional life including education, business, athletic events, etc. When you can consistently depend on yourself, first for the little things like being on time for appointments or sticking to a variety of routine scheduling demands, you generate a trust in yourself that gradually bolsters your self-esteem. You begin to believe and trust in yourself. As this continues, you build momentum for bigger commitments like making positive choices for your health and well-being, and your self-esteem grows further. You can then acknowledge the victories, small and large, that occur in your life as a consequence of your commitments and responsible actions, and you can push yourself to limits you may not have thought possible.

That's easy enough to state, but it can be much harder to do, especially with making positive choices for diet and lifestyle. We disappoint ourselves on so many occasions. Today is the day you're going to start your diet. So, you get the prepackaged bird seed out of the closet, put it in your dish, eat it, and flit off to work. Then about 10:30 in the morning, here comes break time, and you head to the employee lounge, where the coffee and donuts are on full display. And you say to yourself, "You know what, I want coffee and a donut." In the big picture, what's a coffee and a donut? Not a whole lot. However, once you break your diet commitment and bite into that donut, your disappointment in yourself deepens. Often, this failure goes on day in and day out, sabotaging your goals.

While the coffee and donut may not be that big a deal, constantly breaking agreements with yourself is. When you consistently disregard the agreements you've made with yourself, you are making a subliminal statement that you are not worthy of your own respect and commitment. You are making a subtle, subconscious statement of the lack of your own self-worth. I guarantee you that this is far worse than any coffee and donut you will ever have.

Instead, remember this: even successful people all go off track now and then, but truly successful people get back on track in some reasonable period of time. Don't shoot for perfection and sainthood; that's going to take three miracles and a good resumé, and no one's going to make it. Just commit to some percentage of the diet and lifestyle I'm recommending. In a sense, it doesn't matter if you start with 10% or 90%, but if you have health and weight issues, you may not have much leeway for error, and a more immediate, more extensive commitment will be a lifesaver. At the very least, make some commitment to yourself and stick to it. See what these positive choices can do for you, and let them lead you into more extensive change and commitment over time.

Believe in yourself. Love yourself. The power and capacity for positive change, optimal health, and healthy weight loss resides within you every second of every day. Make changes you can live with, be patient with the process, and embrace the remarkable opportunity that is within your reach. Know, deep within the very fabric of your being, that you are so worth it, and allow yourself to experience the rewards of joy, health, and happiness that are truly your legacy.

CHAPTER 24

KEYS TO SUCCESSFUL LIFESTYLE CHANGE

W e are constantly surrounded by and inundated with a plethora of information on mainstream media and the Internet that is often in conflict with the powerful and successful plant-exclusive nutrition and lifestyle choices I have shared with you. This information often creates confusion and resistance to the very choices that can ensure your optimal health, body-fat levels, and weight. But let's face it: it's not rocket science to truly understand what it takes to produce the optimal results that are well within your reach. Intuitively, I think we can all agree that if we eat better, move more, sleep more, drink more water, reduce stress, have gratitude, create healthy relationships, etc., we would all enjoy better health and weight control. However, in my experience, there is often a big gap between the intellectual understanding of healthy lifestyle choices and our ability to practically apply and implement these choices in our day-to-day experiences. Following are some key elements, ideas, and strategies that can help you achieve and sustain a successful health and weight-loss program over time.

One thing that is safe to say is that whenever you make a choice, there's another one immediately lurking around the corner. So don't get lost in the last one you made. You always have an opportunity to use the consequences of your actions from moment to moment to transform your future choices. This is the alchemy of mindfulness and consciousness: the ability to transform pain, dysfunction, and failure into an opportunity for success and optimal function. So don't get lost in guilt and the perceived failure of your last choice, but use the consequences of that choice to change what happens next. Make choices you can live with, not ones that make your life unbearable.

Creative Strategies to Foster Success

Change can be hard; but taking advantage of the creative strategies presented below can make even significant, challenging changes more bearable and doable.

• Make it much more difficult and energy-demanding to do the wrong thing than to do the right thing.
There is one fact common to all mammals and especially humans: we like to use the least amount of energy to experience the greatest amount of pleasure. So, if you're trying to make a change in your life, make the option that you're trying to change a complete pain in the ass to do. For example, take better control of your food options by keeping healthy, plant-exclusive options near at hand—at your desk, in your car, in your bra if you have to—so that when it comes time to reach for something to eat, you don't have to walk to the vending machines or drive around looking for fast-food joints for some processed crap. Make it easier, less work, to be successful. Give yourself what I like to call the "opportunity to win." First, box up and give away all of the off-plan, unhealthy foods that tempt you to make unhealthy choices. If these trigger foods are in your house, you will eventually be drawn into their seductive trap. Make sure you fill your refrigerator and kitchen cabinets with healthy options you enjoy so that in the middle of the night you don't have to take that zombie-like journey in your pajamas down to the 7-11 for some conventional ice cream, potato chips, or other junk food.

• **Practice patience and avoidance.**

Remember, these changes will not occur overnight. If you recall, many of the processed and animal foods that you're used to have an addictive quality that makes it difficult to stop eating them, so being patient with yourself and respecting the time factor for change is very important for a successful transition to healthier choices.

To reiterate what I said in the addiction chapter, remember that addiction rehabilitation centers typically offer a range of programs from 21-30 days because, while it only takes a week to detox, it takes additional time for new choices and strategies to begin to become a part of you and your regular routine. This is the case with all long-term change. Be patient with yourself and keep moving forward.

• **Don't try to manage use of addictive substances. The only people who think they can are addicts, and you know how well they do it.**

Let me ask you a question. Do you have an addiction to or compulsion to eat chocolate and/or sugar? A substantial number of people do. There are people who can open up a chocolate bar, take a small piece off the corner, wrap it up, and put it away. Can you? Most chocolate addicts would small-piece that chocolate bar to death. How many times have you cut just a "tiny" slice of cake or pie to eat? And then you cut another "tiny" slice, and another, eyeing the cake from all angles like Frank Lloyd Wright studying architectural blueprints, making sure that you achieve some elusive cake symmetry so that you will be safe from its weight-enhancing effect. And what about when you break off all those tiny cookie pieces, as if eating a plethora of tiny pieces instead of a whole cookie is some magical, calorie-restricting, weight-loss strategy?

When trying to change a long-ingrained habit or addiction, it is necessary to practice some degree of avoidance while incorporating creative distraction tactics in order to create some separation between what you were doing and the new things you're trying to do now. For instance, if you have a problem with sugar, then sugar can't be in your house. Even a little is too much, too tempting. You wouldn't go up to a heroin addict and say, "I'd like you to shoot a $3 bag rather than a $5 bag." Yes, it is less heroin, but it is still the same problem, and indulging even a little bit will continue to reinforce the addiction. That's why 12-step programs for addiction recovery promote abstinence.

• Make small changes consistently over time.
Understand that the things that you're doing right now have had a long history of being part of your routine behavior. Regardless of what I say or how much sense I make, there's a part of your brain that just can't believe that you can become any different than you are right now. These old choices and addictive habits have been like old friends in the night providing you with that false sense of pleasure and well-being. However, as you make even small changes consistently over time, you will gradually get to a place where, when you look back, you'll have a hard time believing that you were once where you started. If you stop and think about it for a moment, you'll realize that you have probably done this with other things in your life before. Lifestyle change is no different.

Initially, make changes you can live with, but tackle others as you become more focused and committed over time. This will allow new choices an opportunity to weave their way into your behavioral tapestry and become an integral part of your brain/neurological system as you move forward to new challenges.

• Center your life more around your personal passion and interests rather than around food.
Doesn't it often seem like all you ever do to socialize is go out and eat? "Hey, haven't seen you in a while, let's get together for dinner." "Hey, bro, how you been, let's grab a sandwich!" Let's eat, eat, eat! Don't get me wrong. I love to eat. I love socializing around great food. But it is

necessary to find other, more creative ways to spend leisure time and express yourself. You are a creature with a big brain that demands creative expression. It has become apparent that people who express themselves more creatively, whether it be with hobbies or work, tend to create a deeper level of pleasure, purpose, satisfaction, and well-being while aging better with fewer chronic degenerative diseases.

However, let's face it. A great many of us have jobs that enable us to put food on the table and take care of our families' financial needs but don't allow us to express ourselves most creatively. If you have a job or a profession that allows you to do both, it is a blessing. I contend, however, that if you don't have some creative outlet, at some point you will be tempted by a variety of compulsive or addictive behaviors, including eating, drinking, etc., that may take the edge off but will only provide unhealthy distraction and pleasure and an illusion of well-being.

Therefore, I urge you, in the quiet of your meditation, to get in touch with your personal passion, that thing that gives you the greatest pleasure, what has been referred to in the Neo-Tech movement as your Friday-night essence. What would be the thing that you would choose to do when you're tired on a Friday night after a busy 40-hour work week? What is your greatest interest and gives you a profound feeling of pleasure, the behavior that makes you feel the most timeless and inspires you to lose all track of time?

Losing yourself in the moment allows you to be truly open to the spontaneous, unknown wonder that unfolds moment to moment in all our lives. This is the essence and true art of living. How can you make this behavior a hobby, or even reinvent yourself to change your direction later in life, adopting a livelihood more in line with your deepest drives and passions? This may take you back to your teenage years or even your childhood, to remember your greatest passion. Explore ways to incorporate this interest or passion into your life. Maybe all you can do right now is read a book on the subject or research related local options online, like a club, a meet-up group, a facility that houses what you need for working out, firing pottery, or taking music lessons. Even if you can't start right now, doing *something* and knowing the available options is a valuable first step.

I have sons who are musicians, writers, and artists. I recognized their passions very early in their lives. I even homeschooled them through some of the middle and high school years when music and art were being phased out of the public school system due to budget cuts. I wanted them to be able to devote more of their time to their passionate pursuits. I spent 25 years in school getting two doctorates, but my boys didn't even want to see the side wall of an educational facility. They certainly had no interest in going to conventional colleges. As a father, I agonized over it at times, with the worries and concerns any parent would have. My children, mein Kinder—are they going to be able to take care of themselves? Are they going to be able to get jobs and survive? Heck, there are PhDs driving cabs in our major cities, and we can't know how life will play out. Certainly nothing about any future is ever guaranteed. It wasn't easy, but I had to let it go in my mind and heart. I'll tell you what I told them: "Go for your first choice." There's always going to be a second, third, and fourth choice. You're always better off succeeding or failing with your greatest passion as the bull's-eye of the target. I have counseled some of the wealthiest, apparently successful people in the world who were the sickest, most depressed, and anxious individuals I have ever met. They had followed paths that they thought they should or that some authority figure told them they should, but they never got truly in touch with or truly expressed their personal passion. Too many of us live lives of regret about the things we didn't do but wished we did (and probably should have), and that path creates craving, emptiness, unrest, depression, and gaping holes in our psyche.

Addressing this idea of passion, I read an interview with the renowned singer Tony Bennett in *The New York Times Magazine* that was published around the time of his 80th birthday. The interviewer asked

Bennett why he seemed so happy and content a lot of the time. Tony said two things that really stuck out for me.

He said that he discovered his personal passions when he was very young, and he pursued them for the rest of his life. For him, it was singing and painting. He said that when he is walking down the street or on vacation, he's singing to himself. That's who he is. His second point was even more telling. Not only did he choose to embody his personal passions, but he dedicated himself to sticking to his ideals to make them a reality in his life, even when the pressures of life conspired to drive him off course.

This is the harder part of pursuing our life goals, because there always seem to be pressures and people trying to dissuade us from going for and achieving our dreams. Keep in mind that many of the people who voice discouragement, discontent, and unhappiness, the people who feel compelled to rain on our parade, are those coming from a sense of failure to stay the course and succeed in their own dreams. It is easy to let the adversities of life cause you to give up and settle for less than what you truly love and want to do. Don't give up. Persevere!

Tony's experience is a great example. In the 1970s there were three major shifts in popular music: the development of punk rock, the evolution of Latin music into salsa, and the beginnings of hip-hop in the Bronx that put Tony, this renowned crooner from the past, on the back burner and made him persona non grata with record companies. Those were lean times for Tony, and I'm sure there were some incredible adversities that would have driven many of us to give up our dreams and settle for some much smaller vision. However, Tony stood his ground, reinvented himself, and, in the 1990s and 2000s, ended up performing with rap stars and other current, younger artists, even winning Grammys in duets with, of all people, Lady Gaga and Amy Winehouse.

Furthermore, you can discover and use your personal passion and creativity as an important resource and support for healthy lifestyle change. Participating in activities that express your greatest interests can be a major supportive tool for reinforcing the choices that ensure optimal health and weight over time. Do not underestimate the power of passionate, creative expression as a tool to keep you on the right track. Even when you are evolving in a healthier direction, understand that it is a process. You're not going to transform in one quantum leap. There will be times, under stress and adversity, when the voices of old demons and addictions will rise up and try to pull you back into old patterns of behavior. Remember, these choices, compulsions, and perhaps addictions of the past were how you formerly dealt with things in an effort to create some sense of survival and well-being. They were your old friends in the night. However, if you are passionate about a creative outlet or ideal, you can more easily divert your attention from the momentary temptation and focus instead on a constructive option that will help you stay on track.

There was a time in my own life when I went through a period of excessive drug use. I grew up as a teenager in the 1960s on the streets of New York City. It was a time of fermentation and revolution. By the time I was in my late teenage years, I already had taken the flight of the eagle with Krishnamurti, embraced the sanity of Korzybski's non-Aristotelian world view, wrestled with David Bohm's enfolded universe, and tripped the light fantastic with Procol Harum at the Fillmore East in Greenwich Village.

I had been exposed early in my life to the principles of natural hygiene, vegan nutrition, the importance of a healthy lifestyle, new challenging philosophies and psychological frameworks, and the investigation of a variety of spiritual paths, but I also was a product of my time. Not only was I sampling and experimenting with new ways of thinking, I was sampling and experimenting with each new high I could find on the streets of the city. Everything was fair game on my path of self-realization.

I was definitely getting by and high with a little help from my friends, but I also started experiencing a sense of aimlessness. Life was beginning to feel bleak and pointless. As a result, there was even a time in my life, around the ages of 19 or 20, when heroin became an additional drug of choice. One time, I found myself shooting heroin in a run-down apartment in an old tenement building in the Bronx in New York City with good friends just back from the Vietnam war. I can remember it like it was yesterday. I sat in a stupor on the floor of a naked, dark room bordered by cracked walls with peeling paint, listening to Janis Joplin crying "Ball and Chain" from a cheap turntable. In that moment, time seemed to stand still in a place so dark that I just couldn't find the light. I spiraled down deeper and darker in the quicksand of despair. At one point, I contemplated taking my own life with such emotional intensity that my body trembled. Inexplicably, Janis's voice pulled me back into a momentary desire to go on. Somehow, I got up and wandered out, weaving through the city streets, inhabiting a place without space or time, still clinging to precious life.

Thankfully, by the grace of something seemingly bigger than me and an intrinsic realization of my own self-worth, I eventually decided I needed to make a change. I began the hard work of recovering and refocusing my efforts and interest, and I found the light that led me toward health and wellness.

You can question and challenge my judgment, and I certainly am glad that I made the decision to choose life. But I have no regrets, and I urge you to avoid regrets in your own life. It's all about the yin and the yang. There is always an up to your down. There's always some light lurking in every heart of darkness. Everything I've ever done has contributed to the best that I am today. It has helped me understand myself and the process of addiction, which helps me to be more empathetic and compassionate for the people I work with clinically.

My old experiences seem like several lifetimes ago, and in some ways they are. However, more recently, as I raised my children, there were times when the stresses and demands of work and family life were so overwhelming, I felt like nothing I did was good enough. These were times of hopelessness, anxiety, and depression when the idea of smoking, shooting, or snorting something sounded like a pretty good idea, the old patterns promising an illusion of comfort and escape. Ultimately, it's not your temptations that are the most important consideration, but rather what you choose to pay attention to and focus on. Doing the things that I do—music, writing, tai chi, and qi gong (the specifics really don't matter, you might do different things)—helped me shift my focus from those seductive, addictive voices of the past that would rise up like demons in the night calling me into old ways and helped me maintain my direction and focus on healthier ways of being. Do not underestimate the power of your own passion and creativity as a tool for transformation, recovery, and change.

• Cultivate friends and environments of support for your new, healthier lifestyle choices.
Have you ever had some success with a healthy vacation retreat or a home diet and lifestyle program and then met up with friends who said things like, "You're not going to keep doing that/going back there/ eating that way, are you?" They're thinking (and maybe even hoping) that you're going to put the weight back on. They may say, "Come on, you look great, you can celebrate this once! Let's go out to our favorite burger/pizza/ice cream joint." Unfortunately, misery does truly love company. These friends—who may have had a difficult time maintaining any success themselves—just seem compelled to minimize or disregard your success to keep you in the failure club with them. You don't need that misery in your life.

The healthy changes you are making are probably new to you and not entirely ingrained in your life and behavior yet. As a result, you're more vulnerable to being drawn off track because there is a part of you that still finds these old choices attractive and compelling. Over time, as you make your healthy choices more consistently, they will become more and more a part of your new behavior, and you'll eventually become an old curmudgeon like me, not caring what anybody says or thinks. But initially, it matters a lot, because as much as we need the same biological necessities as other mammals (food, water, shelter, warmth, etc.), there is something we crave perhaps even more than other creatures: we crave the acceptance of others.

In our distant past, we survived by living in supportive social groups or tribes that helped us procure our basic needs and minimize dangerous environmental pressures. As a result, on a deep-rooted level, social rejection triggers a fear response and is perceived as a threat to the survival of the individual. Although we may no longer need to depend on small clans or tribes for survival, the current fascination with and dependence on social media and the way people reach out into the dim, dark corners of cyberspace to connect with anybody who's out there is an extension of our ancient need for social survival.

There are psychological studies that indicate that humans will make choices that they know are wrong, and even threatening or dangerous, just so they fit in with the majority of other people who are making similar choices. You may not need to get rid of your old friends, but you must find a way to cultivate some new major relationships, find new communities, and engage in activities of support at home. Perhaps you can find a walking or exercise group that will help you stay on track. Perhaps you can find some health-promoting groups, organizations, online courses or programs, a lecture series, websites, podcasts, or a vegan cooking program online or near your home. An important lesson learned from observing the various long-lived Blue Zone cultures is that community involvement and social interaction are essential to longevity and healthspan. This need for sharing and interaction is in our DNA and is a fundamental requirement of health. I can remember back to the days of my childhood in the 1950s and '60s in the old neighborhoods in the Bronx. In the summer evenings, the friends and neighbors from my tenement building would spread their folding chairs in front of the stoops of the building and sit in a circle to just hang out and share the stuff of their days and lives. The friendship, laughter, camaraderie, and intimate sharing of the ups and downs of their lives was truly the best medicine.

Through my own work, I have at times established phone and online health-at-home programs by which I stay in contact with the people I've worked with to provide ongoing support and information for healthy living and weight loss. For you, the idea is to actively seek out a new or ongoing nucleus of people and activities that will promote and support the new food, exercise, and lifestyle choices you need to maintain for healthy, successful weight loss.

Evolution, Growth, and Change

We have all been conditioned to look at choices from a very limited perspective that is often shaped by the duality of our Judeo-Christian culture. A mentality of sin and religious retribution can skew the process and benefits of healthy choice and change, diverting your attention from the true task at hand. As a result, you become more preoccupied by, or even lost in, whether a choice is good or bad rather than considering its impact on the bigger picture of your life and the true consequences of health.

What's more important to me is what it means to you. The search for meaning in all life pressures and situations provides a bigger context to the stress, pain, and uncertainty of life and supports freedom and well-being. Every choice you make has a consequence. As I have said before, it is futile to get lost in the last choice you made because there is always another one immediately lurking around the corner. It is critical to take advantage of the unique opportunity always available to you and use the consequences of your actions to transform your future choices into health and weight-loss success.

Socrates was absolutely correct when he said a life that is not examined is not worth living. That may sound harsh, but it addresses an incredibly important point. Any time you so choose, you have the remarkable ability to examine your life, to consciously and mindfully evaluate the consequences of your actions, and to decide whether your choices are consistent with the goals you have established for yourself. This moves your choices from the simplistic discussion of good, bad, or evil into a larger consideration of where your choices fit on the path of your own evolution, growth, and change.

As absurd as it may sound, if you tell me that your goal is to be fatter than you've ever been, sicker and more disabled than ever, and every choice you're making is moving you in that direction, I applaud you. You are achieving your goal. On the other hand, if you tell me you want to be healthier, more fit, and have less fat and weight on you, and your choices are not congruent with that outcome, then I would suggest that you need to take a closer look at your life and actions and make the appropriate adjustments. It's time to put the "big-boy" and "big-girl" pants on. Only *you* can make the decisions to fully participate in responsible actions that delineate and shape the positive, successful outcomes of your own life. Every choice you make then affords you a unique opportunity to develop a deep-rooted consciousness of health grounded in self-care and self-love. As Rumi, the famous Sufi poet, wrote: "When you truly become a lover, duties become inspirations." With all due respect to Rumi, I have modified this in the following way: "When you truly love yourself as all life and connection, the duties of responsible action become inspirations."

As you truly embrace your evolution towards goals of health and weight loss, you will learn to love yourself enough to naturally gravitate toward and implement the choices that are in your best interest. You will continue to recognize that these healthy choices are clearly associated with your greatest vitality, function, and performance, and, as a result, you will implement them with less pressure and drudgery, ensuring that they become a consistent part of your life and a fundamental source of inspiration. This fosters not only a healthy life, but an inspired life—and that is your legacy. It is your requisite natural inclination born of a deep connection to the rhythms and cycles of the natural world around and within you. It is the direct extension of body wisdom and the creative value of conscious life.

But it is not common. The pressures and pursuits of our mindless, frantic culture continue to disturb and distort our connection to what is natural and beneficial. I urge you—I implore you—to listen to the deep, primal, proactive beat of your personal drummer pounding a divine cadence for an inspired dance on a road less traveled. Only you can utilize your personal dynamic dance of action, reaction, evaluation, and transformation to foster physical, emotional, and spiritual balance and to promote optimal health and weight loss.

EPILOGUE

Creating a healthy body image and achieving optimal weight is within the reach of everyone. There is every reason for you to be hopeful, especially when your behavior is grounded in whole-food, plant-exclusive nutrition without added salt, oil, and sugar and in the greatest force of all, love, supported by mindfulness, passion, and creativity. Your love can inspire a commitment to lifestyle choices that are in your best interest, choices that most successfully address and incorporate the essential factors of whole-plant nutrition, activity, hormonal balance, stress management, sleep, awareness, self-esteem, and the reduction of environmental toxicity. It is never too late.

No matter how much trauma, pain, and failure you may have experienced in your life, as Winston Churchill said, "This is the lesson: never give in, never, never, never, never—in nothing great or small, large or petty—never give in except to convictions of honor and good sense." Any time you so choose, any time you so desire, you can make proactive choices that program and shape your mind-body connection to promote health in general and the body image and weight you would love to have in particular, not only in this moment, but for years to come. It is only by embracing the constellation of lifestyle factors we have discussed that you can transcend the abysmal failures of the dieting industry and the quicksand of dangerous, quick-fix, fad approaches to create and inspire long-term success without mortgaging your health future in the process. Give yourself this incredible opportunity.

REFERENCES

Introduction

1. Thomas P. The big fat fix. *Ecologist.* 2006 Nov;36(9):33-43.

2. O'Neill P. Office of Health Economics. Shedding the pounds: obesity management, NICE guidance and bariatric surgery in England. 2010.

3. Campbell, D. Cost of being overweight in the UK now 98 billion pounds, study finds. *The Guardian.* Dec 4, 2023.

4. Flegal KM, Carroll MD, Kit BK, Ogden CL. Prevalence of obesity and trends in the distribution of body mass index among US adults, 1999-2010. *JAMA.* 2012;307(5):491-497. doi:10.1001/jama.2012.39.

5. Center for Disease Control and Prevention. Overweight and obesity. http://www.cdc.gov/obesity/index.html. Accessed December 12,2013.

6. World Cancer Research Fund, American Institute for Cancer Research, *Food, Nutrition, Physical Activity, and the Prevention of Cancer: A Global Perspective.* Washington, DC: AICR; 2007.

7. 100 million dieters, $20 billion: The weight-loss industry by the numbers. https://abcnews.go.com/Health/100-million-dieters-20-billion-weight-loss-industry/story?id=16297197. Published May 7, 2012.

Chapter 1: Why Weight? The Need for Changing Focus

1. Cheung L, Hahn TN. *Savor: Mindful Eating, Mindful Life*. New York, NY: Harper Collins; 2010.

2. Xu H, Cupples LA, Stokes A, Liu CT. Association of Obesity With Mortality Over 24 Years of Weight History: Findings From the Framingham Heart Study [published correction appears in JAMA Netw Open. 2018 Dec 7;1(8):e186657]. *JAMA Netw Open*. 2018;1(7):e184587. Published 2018 Nov 2. doi:10.1001/jamanetworkopen.2018.4587

3. Scully T, Ettela A, LeRoith D, Gallagher EJ. Obesity, Type 2 Diabetes, and Cancer Risk. *Front Oncol*. 2021;10:615375. Published 2021 Feb 2. doi:10.3389/fonc.2020.615375

4. Bhaskaran K, Dos-Santos-Silva I, Leon DA, Douglas IJ, Smeeth L. Association of BMI with overall and cause-specific mortality: a population-based cohort study of 3·6 million adults in the UK. *Lancet Diabetes Endocrinol*. 2018;6(12):944-953. doi:10.1016/S2213-8587(18)30288-2

5. Spieker EA, Pyzocha N. Economic Impact of Obesity. *Prim Care*. 2016;43(1):83-ix. doi:10.1016/j.pop.2015.08.013

6. Dor A, Ferguson C, Langwith C, Tan E. A heavy burden: the individual costs of being overweight and obese in the United States. Washington, DC: The George Washington University Department of Health Policy; 2010.

7. Newbold RR, Padilla-Banks E, Jefferson WN, Heindel JJ. Effects of endocrine disruptors on obesity. *Int J Androl*. 2008;31(2):201-208. doi:10.1111/j.1365-2605.2007.00858.x

8. Coppack SW. Pro-inflammatory cytokines and adipose tissue. *Proc Nutr Soc*. 2001;60(3):349-356. doi:10.1079/pns2001110

9. World Cancer Research Fund, American Institute for Cancer Research. Food, Nutrition, Physical Activity and the Prevention of Cancer: A Global Perspective. (Washington, DC. AICR, 2007).

10. Calle EE, Rodriguez C, Walker-Thurmond K, Thun MJ. Overweight, obesity, and mortality from cancer in a pro-spectively studied cohort of U.S. adults. *N Engl J Med.* 2003;348(17):1625-1638. doi:10.1056/NEJMoa021423

11. Männistö S, Harald K, Kontto J, et al. Dietary and lifestyle characteristics associated with normal-weight obesity: the National FINRISK 2007 Study. *Br J Nutr.* 2014;111(5):887-894. doi:10.1017/S0007114513002742

12. St-Onge MP. Are normal-weight Americans over-fat?. *Obesity (Silver Spring).* 2010;18(11):2067-2068. doi:10.1038/oby.2010.103

13. Fryar CD, Gu Q, Ogden CL. Anthropometric reference data for children and adults: United States, 2007-2010. *Vital Health Stat 11.* 2012;(252):1-48.

14. Pollock ML, Wilmore JH. *Exercise in Health and Disease: Evaluation and Prescription for Prevention and Rehabilitation.* Philadelphia, PA: WB Saunders Company; 1990.

Chapter 2: Diet and Nutrition: The Vegan Plant-Exclusive Solution

1. CDC Natonal Center for Chronic Disease Prevention and Health Promotion; Division of Nutrition, Physical Activity and Obesity; Research to Practice Series, No. 5. https://www.cdc.gov/nccdphp/dnpa/nutrition/pdf/r2p_energy_density.pdf.

2. Novick J. Calorie Density: A common sense approach to sound nutrition. *Health Science.* 2014;37(2):20-23.

Chapter 3: The Basic Truth About Protein

1. Campbell TC. *The China Study*. Dallas, TX: BenBella Books; 2004.

2. Smit E, Nieto FJ, Crespo CJ, Mitchell P. Estimates of animal and plant protein intake in US adults: results from the Third National Health and Nutrition Examination Survey, 1988-1991. *J Am Diet Assoc*. 1999;99(7):813-820. doi:10.1016/S0002-8223(99)00193-5

3. Bauer J, Biolo G, Cederholm T, et al. Evidence-based recommendations for optimal dietary protein intake in older people: a position paper from the PROT-AGE Study Group. *J Am Med Dir Assoc*. 2013;14(8):542-559. doi:10.1016/j.jamda.2013.05.021

4. Houston DK, Nicklas BJ, Ding J, et al. Dietary protein intake is associated with lean mass change in older, community-dwelling adults: the Health, Aging, and Body Composition (Health ABC) Study. *Am J Clin Nutr*. 2008;87(1):150-155. doi:10.1093/ajcn/87.1.150

5. Pasiakos SM, Lieberman HR, Fulgoni VL 3rd. Higher-protein diets are associated with higher HDL cholesterol and lower BMI and waist circumference in US adults. *J Nutr*. 2015;145(3):605-614. doi:10.3945/jn.114.20520

6. USDA Agricultural Research Service. *Composition of Foods: Raw, Processed, Prepared. USDA National Nutrient Database for Standard Reference, Release 26*, Aug 2013.

7. Davis B, Melina V, and Davis D. *Plant Powered Protein*. Summertown, TN: Healthy Living Productions; 2023:35-39.

8. Burros M. Chicken with Arsenic? Is That O.K.? *New York Times*. April 5, 2006. www.nytimes.com/2006/04/05/dining/05well.html/?_r=0.

9. Campbell TC. *The China Study*. Dallas, TX: BenBella Books; 2004.

10. Oda M, Satta Y, Takenaka O, Takahata N. Loss of urate oxidase activity in hominoids and its evolutionary implications. *Mol Biol Evol*. 2002;19(5):640-653. doi:10.1093/oxfordjournals. molbev.a004123

11. Fleming RM. The effect of high-protein diets on coronary blood flow. *Angiology*. 2000;51(10):817-826. doi:10.1177/000331970005101003

Chapter 4: The Pros and Cons of Fats and Oil

1. Campbell TC. *The China Study*. Dallas, TX: BenBella Books; 2004.

2. Esselstyn CB Jr, Ellis SG, Medendorp SV, Crowe TD. A strategy to arrest and reverse coronary artery disease: a 5-year longitudinal study of a single physician's practice. *J Fam Pract*. 1995;41(6):560-568.

3. Ornish D, Brown SE, Scherwitz LW, et al. Can lifestyle changes reverse coronary heart disease? The Lifestyle Heart Trial. *Lancet*. 1990;336(8708):129-133. doi:10.1016/0140-6736(90)91656-u

4. Halliwell B, Gutteridge JMC. *Free Radicals in Biology and Medicine*. New York, NY: Oxford University Press; 1989.

5. Golomb BA, Evans MA, White HL, Dimsdale JE. Trans fat consumption and aggression. *PLoS One*. 2012;7(3):e32175. doi:10.1371/journal.pone.0032175

6. Ochiai M, Fujii K, Takeuchi H, Matsuo T. Effects of dietary trans fatty acids on fat accumulation and metabolic rate in rat. *J Oleo Sci*. 2013;62(2):57-64. doi:10.5650/jos.62.57

7. Kochan Z, Karbowska J, Babicz-Zielińska E. Trans-kwasy tłuszczowe w diecie--rola w rozwoju zespołu metabolicznego [Dietary trans-fatty acids and metabolic syndrome]. *Postepy Hig Med Dosw (Online)*. 2010;64:650-658. Published 2010 Dec 27.

8. Micha R, Mozaffarian D. Trans fatty acids: effects on metabolic syndrome, heart disease and diabetes. *Nat Rev Endocrinol.* 2009;5(6):335-344. doi:10.1038/nrendo.2009.79

9. Lopez-Garcia E, Schulze MB, Meigs JB, et al. Consumption of trans fatty acids is related to plasma biomarkers of inflammation and endothelial dysfunction. *J Nutr.* 2005;135(3):562-566. doi:10.1093/jn/135.3.562

10. Scher JU, Pillinger MH. The anti-inflammatory effects of prostaglandins. *J Investig Med.* 2009;57(6):703-708. doi:10.2310/JIM.0b013e31819aaa76

11. Simopoulos AP. The importance of the ratio of omega-6/omega-3 essential fatty acids. *Biomed Pharmacother.* 2002;56(8):365-379. doi:10.1016/s0753-3322(02)00253-6

12. Rizzo NS, Jaceldo-Siegl K, Sabate J, Fraser GE. Nutrient profiles of vegetarian and nonvegetarian dietary patterns. *J Acad Nutr Diet.* 2013;113(12):1610-1619. doi:10.1016/j.jand.2013.06.349

13. Sarter B, Kelsey KS, Schwartz TA, Harris WS. Blood docosahexaenoic acid and eicosapentaenoic acid in vegans: Associations with age and gender and effects of an algal-derived omega-3 fatty acid supplement. *Clin Nutr.* 2015;34(2):212-218. doi:10.1016/j.clnu.2014.03.003

14. Rosell MS, Lloyd-Wright Z, Appleby PN, Sanders TA, Allen NE, Key TJ. Long-chain n-3 polyunsaturated fatty acids in plasma in British meat-eating, vegetarian, and vegan men. *Am J Clin Nutr.* 2005;82(2):327-334. doi:10.1093/ajcn.82.2.327

15. Brasky TM, Darke AK, Song X, et al. Plasma phospholipid fatty acids and prostate cancer risk in the SELECT trial. *J Natl Cancer Inst.* 2013;105(15):1132-1141. doi:10.1093/jnci/djt174

Chapter 5: The Carbohydrate and Sugar Story: Fundamentals and Concerns

1. Davidson EA. Carbohydrate. Encyclopaedia Britannica. https://www.britannica.com/science/carbohydrate. Accessed February 11, 2024.

2. Cherney K. Simple carbohydrates vs. complex carbohydrates. https://www.healthline.com/health/food-nutrition/simple-carbohydrates-complex-carbohydrates#what-are-carbs. Accessed October 10, 2023.

3. Buettner, D. *The Blue Zones: Lessons for Living Longer from the People Who've Lived the Longest.* National Geographic Society. National Geographic Books, 2008.

4. U.S. Department of Agriculture, Economic Research Service. Food Availability (Per Capita) Data System. http://www.ers.usda.gov/Data/food consumption/datasystems.asp. Accessed May 11, 2004.

5. Cleave TL. *The Saccharine Disease.* Bristol, UK: John Wright and Sons, Ltd; 1974:6-27.

6. Monsivais P, Drewnowski A. Lower-energy-density diets are associated with higher monetary costs per kilocalorie and are consumed by women of higher socioeconomic status [published correction appears in J Am Diet Assoc. 2009 Jul;109(7):1296]. *J Am Diet Assoc.* 2009;109(5):814-822. doi:10.1016/j.jada.2009.02.002

Chapter 6: Hormones, Glycemic Index, and Weight Control

1. Björntorp P, Brodoff BN. *Obesity.* Philadelphia, PA: JB Lippincott Co.; 1992: Chapter 40.

2. DeFronzo RA, Ferrannini E, Hendler R, Felig P, Wahren J. Regulation of splanchnic and peripheral glucose uptake by insulin and hyperglycemia in man. *Diabetes*. 1983;32(1):35-45. doi:10.2337/diab.32.1.35

3. Björntorp P, Sjöström L. Carbohydrate storage in man: speculations and some quantitative considerations. *Metabolism*. 1978;27(12 Suppl 2):1853-1865. doi:10.1016/s0026-0495(78)80004-3

4. Jackson RA, Roshania RD, Hawa MI, Sim BM, DiSilvio L. Impact of glucose ingestion on hepatic and peripheral glucose metabolism in man: an analysis based on simultaneous use of the forearm and double isotope techniques. *J Clin Endocrinol Metab*. 1986;63(3):541-549. doi:10.1210/jcem-63-3-541

5. Foley JE, Thuillez P, Lillioja S, Zawadzki J, Bogardus C. Insulin sensitivity in adipocytes from subjects with varying degrees of glucose tolerance. *Am J Physiol*. 1986;251(3 Pt 1):E306-E310. doi:10.1152/ajpendo.1986.251.3.E306

6. Rodin J. Insulin levels, hunger, and food intake: an example of feedback loops in body weight regulation. *Health Psychol*. 1985;4(1):1-24. doi:10.1037//0278-6133.4.1.1

7. Davis W. *Wheat Belly*. New York, NY: Rodale Books; 2011.

8. Shivakoti R, Biggs ML, Djoussé L, et al. Intake and Sources of Dietary Fiber, Inflammation, and Cardiovascular Disease in Older US Adults. *JAMA Netw Open*. 2022;5(3):e225012. Published 2022 Mar 1. doi:10.1001/jamanetworkopen.2022.5012

Chapter 7: Fiber and Water and Salt, Oh My!

1. Juste C, Gérard P. Cholesterol-to-Coprostanol Conversion by the Gut Microbiota: What We Know, Suspect, and Ignore. *Microorganisms*. 2021;9(9):1881. Published 2021 Sep 5. doi:10.3390/microorganisms9091881

2. Bernaud FS, Rodrigues TC. Fibra alimentar--ingestão adequada e efeitos sobre a saúde do metabolismo [Dietary fiber--adequate intake and effects on metabolism health]. *Arq Bras Endocrinol Metabol.* 2013;57(6):397-405. doi:10.1590/ s0004-27302013000600001

3. Levings J, Cogswell M, Curtis CJ, Gunn J, Neiman A, Angell SY. Progress toward sodium reduction in the United States. *Rev Panam Salud Publica.* 2012;32(4):301-306. doi:10.1590/ s1020-49892012001000009

4. Appel LJ, Angell SY, Cobb LK, et al. Population-wide sodium reduction: the bumpy road from evidence to policy. *Ann Epidemiol.* 2012;22(6):417-425. doi:10.1016/j. annepidem.2012.04.003

Chapter 8: Limited Supplementation, Not Substitution

1. Campbell TC, Jacobson H. *Whole.* Dallas, TX: BenBella Books; 2013.

2. Medical News Today. Link Between Successful Weight Loss and Vitamin D Levels. AAAS. http://www.medicalnewstoday. com/releases/153669.php

3. Zimmermann MB. Iodine deficiency. *Endocr Rev.* 2009;30(4): 376-408. doi:10.1210/er.2009-0011

4. Rizzo NS, Jaceldo-Siegl K, Sabate J, Fraser GE. Nutrient profiles of vegetarian and nonvegetarian dietary patterns. *J Acad Nutr Diet.* 2013;113(12):1610-1619. doi:10.1016/j.jand.2013.06.349

5. Zamroziewicz MK, Paul EJ, Zwilling CE, Barbey AK. Determinants of fluid intelligence in healthy aging: Omega-3 polyunsaturated fatty acid status and frontoparietal cortex structure. *Nutr Neurosci.* 2018;21(8):570-579. doi:10.1080/10284 15X.2017.1324357

6. Conquer JA, Tierney MC, Zecevic J, Bettger WJ, Fisher RH. Fatty acid analysis of blood plasma of patients with Alzheimer's disease, other types of dementia, and cognitive impairment. *Lipids*. 2000;35(12):1305-1312. doi:10.1007/s11745-000-0646-3

7. Söderberg M, Edlund C, Kristensson K, Dallner G. Fatty acid composition of brain phospholipids in aging and in Alzheimer's disease. *Lipids*. 1991;26(6):421-425. doi:10.1007/BF02536067

8. Harris WS. The omega-3 index as a risk factor for coronary heart disease. *Am J Clin Nutr*. 2008;87(6):1997S-2002S. doi:10.1093/ajcn/87.6.1997S

9. Lukaschek K, von Schacky C, Kruse J, Ladwig KH. Cognitive Impairment Is Associated with a Low Omega-3 Index in the Elderly: Results from the KORA-Age Study. *Dement Geriatr Cogn Disord*. 2016;42(3-4):236-245. doi:10.1159/000448805

Chapter 9: Fads, Fixes, and Magic Bullets: The Dangers of Paleo and Keto Diets, Surgery, and Off-Label Drugs

1. Gibbons, A. The Evolution of Diet. *National Geographic*. September 2014.

2. Alalwan AA, Friedman J, Park H, Segal R, Brumback BA, Hartzema AG. US national trends in bariatric surgery: A decade of study. *Surgery*. 2021;170(1):13-17. doi:10.1016/j.surg.2021.02.002

3. Tomb, D. "You might go through hell for your post-Ozempic body." *New York Magazine*. 15 Nov 2022.

Chapter 10: Water-Only Fasting: Detoxification and Weight Loss

1. Lee C, Longo VD. Fasting vs dietary restriction in cellular protection and cancer treatment: from model organisms to patients. *Oncogene*. 2011;30(30):3305-3316. doi:10.1038/onc.2011.91

2. Shelton H. *Fasting Can Save Your Life*. Tampa, FL: National Health Association; 1981.

3. de Duve C. The lysosome turns fifty. *Nat Cell Biol*. 2005;7(9):847-849. doi:10.1038/ncb0905-847

4. Saftig P, Klumperman J. Lysosome biogenesis and lysosomal membrane proteins: trafficking meets function. *Nat Rev Mol Cell Biol*. 2009;10(9):623-635. doi:10.1038/nrm2745

5. Cahill GF Jr. Starvation in man. *N Engl J Med*. 1970;282(12):668-675. doi:10.1056/NEJM197003192821209

6. Cahill GF Jr. Fuel metabolism in starvation. *Annu Rev Nutr*. 2006;26:1-22. doi:10.1146/annurev.nutr.26.061505.111258

7. Cahill G Jr, Felig P, Owen O, Wahren J. Metabolic adaptation to prolonged starvation in man. *Nord Med*. 1970;83(3):89.

8. Saudek CD, Felig P. The metabolic events of starvation. *Am J Med*. 1976;60(1):117-126. doi:10.1016/0002-9343(76)90540-4

9. Goldhamer A, Lisle D, Parpia B, Anderson SV, Campbell TC. Medically supervised water-only fasting in the treatment of hypertension. *J Manipulative Physiol Ther*. 2001;24(5):335-339. doi:10.1067/mmt.2001.115263

10. Kerndt PR, Naughton JL, Driscoll CE, Loxterkamp DA. Fasting: the history, pathophysiology and complications. *West J Med*. 1982;137(5):379-399.

11. Mosley M, Spencer M. *The Fast Diet: The Simple Secret of Intermittent Fasting*. Great Britain: Short Books; 2013.

12. Kjeldsen-Kragh J, Haugen M, Borchgrevink CF, et al. Controlled trial of fasting and one-year vegetarian diet in rheumatoid arthritis. *Lancet*. 1991;338(8772):899-902. doi:10.1016/0140-6736(91)91770-u

Chapter 11: Compassionate Eating for Environmental Balance, Animal Rights, and Weight Loss

1. Benoff M. Animals Are Not "Things": Happy the Elephant and Personhood. *Psychology Today*. https://www.psychologytoday.com/us/blog/animal-emotions/202306/animals-are-not-things-happy-the-elephant-and-personhood.

2. Machado S, Machado C, Wise S. *Thing: Inside the struggle for animal personhood*. Washington DC: Island Press; 2023.

3. Williams L. *Environmental Science Demystified*. New York, NY: McGraw-Hill; 2005.

4. Hartman T. *The Last Hours of Ancient Sunlight*. Northfield, VT: Mythical Books; 1998.

5. Rao S. Animal Agriculture is the Leading Cause of Climate Change—A Position Paper. *Journal of Ecological Society*. 2020-2021;(32-33):155-168.

6. Steinfeld H, et al. *Livestock's Long Shadow: Environmental Issues and Options*. United Nations Food and Agricultural Organization, 2006. https://www.fao.org/3/a0701e/a0701e.pdf

7. Fiala N. The Greenhouse Hamburger. *Scientific American*, 2009300(2):72-75.

8. Thomas M. The Road to Vegetopia, (Re)imagining the Future of Food. *VegNews.* 2009;March+April.

9. Fiala N. Meeting the demand: an estimation of potential future greenhouse gas emissions from meat production. *Ecological Economics* 2008; 67(3):412-419.

10. Cheung L, Hanh TN. *Savor: Mindful Eating, Mindful Life.* New York, NY: Harper Collins; 2010.

11. Olafsson B. What farm subsidies are and why they matter, explained. https://sentientmedia.org/why-are-farmers-subsidized/. Published August 11, 2023.

12. Simon D. *Meatonomics.* Miami, FL: Conari Press/Mango Publishing; 2013.

Chapter 12: Practical Nutritional Strategies

1. Roza JM, Xian-Liu Z, Guthrie N. Effect of citrus flavonoids and tocotrienols on serum cholesterol levels in hypercholesterolemic subjects. *Altern Ther Health Med.* 2007;13(6):44-48.

2. Zou J, Huang Y, Chen Q, Wei E, Cao K, Wu JM. Effects of resveratrol on oxidative modification of human low-density lipoprotein. *Chin Med J (Engl).* 2000;113(2):99-102.

3. Gliemann L, Schmidt JF, Olesen J, et al. Resveratrol blunts the positive effects of exercise training on cardiovascular health in aged men. *J Physiol.* 2013;591(20):5047-5059. doi:10.1113/jphysiol.2013.258061

4. Jinsmaa Y, Yoshikawa M. Enzymatic release of neocasomorphin and beta-casomorphin from bovine beta-casein. *Peptides.* 1999;20(8):957-962. doi:10.1016/s0196-9781(99)00088-1

5. Kurek M, Przybilla B, Hermann K, Ring J. A naturally occurring opioid peptide from cow's milk, beta-casomorphine-7,

is a direct histamine releaser in man. *Int Arch Allergy Immunol.* 1992;97(2):115-120. doi:10.1159/000236106

6. Lisle DJ, Goldhamer A. *The Pleasure Trap.* Summertown, TN: Healthy Living Publications; 2006.

7. Levings J, Cogswell M, Curtis CJ, Gunn J, Neiman A, Angell SY. Progress toward sodium reduction in the United States. *Rev Panam Salud Publica.* 2012;32(4):301-306. doi:10.1590/s1020-49892012001000009

Chapter 13: Simple Meal Plans

1. Funk K. *Breasts: The Owner's Manual.* Nashville, TN: Thomas Nelson; 2018.

2. Kellis JT Jr, Vickery LE. Inhibition of human estrogen synthetase (aromatase) by flavones. *Science.* 1984;225(4666):1032-1034. doi:10.1126/science.6474163

3. Fioravanti L, Cappelletti V, Miodini P, Ronchi E, Brivio M, Di Fronzo G. Genistein in the control of breast cancer cell growth: insights into the mechanism of action in vitro. *Cancer Lett.* 1998;130(1-2):143-152. doi:10.1016/s0304-3835(98)00130-x

4. Rice S, Mason HD, Whitehead SA. Phytoestrogens and their low dose combinations inhibit mRNA expression and activity of aromatase in human granulosa-luteal cells. *J Steroid Biochem Mol Biol.* 2006;101(4-5):216-225. doi:10.1016/j.jsbmb.2006.06.021

5. Greger M. Who shouldn't eat soy? https://nutritionfacts.org/video/who-shouldnt-eat-soy/ Published November 25, 2016.

6. Zhang FF, Haslam DE, Terry MB, et al. Dietary isoflavone intake and all-cause mortality in breast cancer survivors: The Breast Cancer Family Registry. *Cancer.* 2017;123(11):2070-2079. doi:10.1002/cncr.30615

7. Shu XO, Zheng Y, Cai H, et al. Soy food intake and breast cancer survival. *JAMA*. 2009;302(22):2437-2443. doi:10.1001/jama.2009.1783

8. Chi F, Wu R, Zeng YC, Xing R, Liu Y, Xu ZG. Post-diagnosis soy food intake and breast cancer survival: a meta-analysis of cohort studies. *Asian Pac J Cancer Prev*. 2013;14(4):2407-2412. doi:10.7314/apjcp.2013.14.4.2407

9. Greger M. How to block breast cancer's estrogen producing enzymes. https://nutritionfacts.org/video/how-to-block-breast-cancers-estrogen-producing-enzymes/ Published April 17, 2007.

10. Pisani P, Bray F, Parkin DM. Estimates of the world-wide prevalence of cancer for 25 sites in the adult population. *Int J Cancer*. 2002;97(1):72-81. doi:10.1002/ijc.1571

11. Lee HP, Gourley L, Duffy SW, Estéve J, Lee J, Day NE. Dietary effects on breast-cancer risk in Singapore. *Lancet*. 1991;337 (8751):1197-1200. doi:10.1016/0140-6736(91)92867-2

12. Otun J, Sahebkar A, Östlundh L, Atkin SL, Sathyapalan T. Systematic Review and Meta-analysis on the Effect of Soy on Thyroid Function. *Sci Rep*. 2019;9(1):3964. Published 2019 Mar 8. doi:10.1038/s41598-019-40647-x

13. Messina M, Redmond G. Effects of soy protein and soybean isoflavones on thyroid function in healthy adults and hypothyroid patients: a review of the relevant literature. *Thyroid*. 2006;16(3):249-258. doi:10.1089/thy.2006.16.249

14. Doerge DR, Sheehan DM. Goitrogenic and estrogenic activity of soy isoflavones. *Environ Health Perspect*. 2002;110 Suppl 3(Suppl 3):349-353. doi:10.1289/ehp.02110s3349

Chapter 14: Recipes for Success
No References

Chapter 15: Jump-Start Weight/Fat Loss Programs
No References

Chapter 16: Eating Out in the Real World

1. Campbell TC. *The China Study*. Dallas, TX: BenBella Books; 2004.

Chapter 17: The Role of Exercise and Activity: Move It and Lose It

1. Pollack ML, Wilmore JH. *Exercise in Health and Disease*. Philadelphia, PA: WB Saunders Company; 1990.

2. Russell AP, Foletta VC, Snow RJ, Wadley GD. Skeletal muscle mitochondria: a major player in exercise, health and disease. *Biochim Biophys Acta*. 2014;1840(4):1276-1284. doi:10.1016/j.bbagen.2013.11.016

3. Romieu I, Touillaud M, Ferrari P, et al. Activité physique et survie après cancer [Physical activity and cancer survival]. *Bull Cancer*. 2012;99(10):979-994. doi:10.1684/bdc.2012.1648

4. Schreuder TH, Maessen MF, Tack CJ, Thijssen DH, Hopman MT. Life-long physical activity restores metabolic and cardiovascular function in type 2 diabetes. Eur J *Appl Physiol*. 2014;114(3):619-627. doi:10.1007/s00421-013-2794-5

5. Orio F, Muscogiuri G, Ascione A, et al. Effects of physical exercise on the female reproductive system. *Minerva Endocrinol*. 2013;38(3):305-319.

6. Wroblewski AP, Amati F, Smiley MA, Goodpaster B, Wright V. Chronic exercise preserves lean muscle mass in masters athletes. *Phys Sportsmed*. 2011;39(3):172-178. doi:10.3810/psm.2011.09.1933

7. Bailey SP, Davis JM, Ahlborn EN. Neuroendocrine and substrate responses to altered brain 5-HT activity during prolonged exercise to fatigue. *J Appl Physiol* (1985). 1993;74(6):3006-3012. doi:10.1152/jappl.1993.74.6.3006

8. de Castro JM, Duncan G. Operantly conditioned running: effects on brain catecholamine concentrations and receptor densities in the rat. *Pharmacol Biochem Behav*. 1985;23(4):495-500. doi:10.1016/0091-3057(85)90407-1

9. Dey S, Singh RH, Dey PK. Exercise training: significance of regional alterations in serotonin metabolism of rat brain in relation to antidepressant effect of exercise. *Physiol Behav*. 1992;52(6):1095-1099. doi:10.1016/0031-9384(92)90465-e

10. Whitaker R. *Anatomy of an Epidemic*. New York, NY: Broadway Books; 2010.

11. Asmundson GJ, Fetzner MG, Deboer LB, Powers MB, Otto MW, Smits JA. Let's get physical: a contemporary review of the anxiolytic effects of exercise for anxiety and its disorders. *Depress Anxiety*. 2013;30(4):362-373. doi:10.1002/da.22043

12. McCann IL, Holmes DS. Influence of aerobic exercise on depression. *J Pers Soc Psychol*. 1984;46(5):1142-1147. doi:10.1037//0022-3514.46.5.1142

13. Blumenthal JA, Babyak MA, Doraiswamy PM, et al. Exercise and pharmacotherapy in the treatment of major depressive disorder. Psychosom Med. 2007;69(7):587-596. doi:10.1097/PSY.0b013e318148c19a

Chapter 18: Stress and Weight Gain: Kissing Stress Good-bye

1. Segerstrom SC, Miller GE. Psychological stress and the human immune system: a meta-analytic study of 30 years of inquiry. *Psychol Bull.* 2004;130(4):601-630. doi:10.1037/0033-2909.130.4.601

2. Felten SY, Felten DL. Neural-immune interactions. *Prog Brain Res.* 1994;100:157-162.

3. Anstead MI, Hunt TA, Carlson SL, Burki NK. Variability of peripheral blood lymphocyte beta-2-adrenergic receptor density in humans. *Am J Respir Crit Care Med.* 1998;157(3 Pt 1):990-992. doi:10.1164/ajrccm.157.3.9704071

4. Herbert TB, Cohen S. Stress and immunity in humans: a meta-analytic review. *Psychosom Med.* 1993;55(4):364-379. doi:10.1097/00006842-199307000-00004

5. Ader R, Cohen N, Felten D. Psychoneuroimmunology: interactions between the nervous system and the immune system. *Lancet.* 1995;345(8942):99-103. doi:10.1016/s0140-6736(95)90066-7

6. Epel ES, Blackburn EH, Lin J, et al. Accelerated telomere shortening in response to life stress. *Proc Natl Acad Sci USA.* 2004;101(49):17312-17315. doi:10.1073/pnas.0407162101

7. Yao BC, Meng LB, Hao ML, Zhang YM, Gong T, Guo ZG. Chronic stress: a critical risk factor for atherosclerosis. *J Int Med Res.* 2019;47(4):1429-1440. doi:10.1177/030 0060519826820Segerstrom SC, Miller GE. Psychological stress and the human immune system: a meta-analytic study of 30 years of inquiry. *Psychol Bull.* 2004;130(4):601-630. doi:10.1037/0033-2909.130.4.601

8. Sapolsky RM. *Why Zebras Don't Get Ulcers; An Updated Guide to Stress, Stress Related Diseases, and Coping.* New York, NY: W. H. Freeman; 1998.

9. Selye H. Stress and the general adaptation syndrome. *Br Med J.* 1950 Jun 17;1(4667):1383-92. doi: 10.1136/bmj.1.4667.1383. PMID: 15426759; PMCID: PMC2038162.

10. Talbott S, Kraemer W. *The Cortisol Connection: Why Stress Makes You Fat and Ruins Your Health—And What You Can Do About It.* (Alameda, CA: Hunter House; 2007, 2002.

11. Bjorntorp P, Brodoff BN. *Obesity.* Philadelphia, PA. Lippincott Williams & Wilkins; 1992).

12. Ip CK, Rezitis J, Qi Y, et al. Critical role of lateral habenula circuits in the control of stress-induced palatable food consumption. *Neuron.* 2023;111(16):2583-2600.e6. doi:10.1016/j.neuron.2023.05.010

13. Hayakawa H, Iwata T, Yata J, Kobayashi N. Primary immunodeficiency syndrome in Japan. I. Overview of a nationwide survey on primary immunodeficiency syndrome. *J Clin Immunol.* 1981;1(1):31-39. doi:10.1007/BF00915474

14. Lanza R. *Biocentrism: How Life and Consciousness Are the Keys to the True Nature of the Universe.* Dallas, TX: BenBella Books; 2009.

Chapter 19: Sleep Deficiency and Weight Gain

1. National Sleep Foundation. 2005 Sleep in America Poll, Summary of Findings. https://www.thensf.org/wp-content/uploads/2021/03/2005_summary_of_findings.pdf

2. Science Daily: American Academy of Sleep Medicine. Insomnia costing US workforce $63.2 billion a year in lost productivity, study shows. https://www.sciencedaily.com/

releases/2011/09/110901093653.htm. Published September 2, 2011.

3. Patel SR, Hu FB. Short sleep duration and weight gain: a systematic review. *Obesity (Silver Spring)*. 2008;16(3):643-653. doi:10.1038/oby.2007.118

4. Patel SR, Malhotra A, White DP, Gottlieb DJ, Hu FB. Association between reduced sleep and weight gain in women. *Am J Epidemiol*. 2006;164(10):947-954. doi:10.1093/aje/kwj280

5. Nielsen LS, Danielsen KV, Sørensen TI. Short sleep duration as a possible cause of obesity: critical analysis of the epidemiological evidence. *Obes Rev*. 2011;12(2):78-92. doi:10.1111/j.1467-789X.2010.00724.x

6. Van Cauter E, Knutson KL. Sleep and the epidemic of obesity in children and adults. *Eur J Endocrinol*. 2008;159 Suppl 1(S1):S59-S66. doi:10.1530/EJE-08-0298

7. Hasler G, Buysse DJ, Klaghofer R, et al. The association between short sleep duration and obesity in young adults: a 13-year prospective study. *Sleep*. 2004;27(4):661-666. doi:10.1093/sleep/27.4.661

8. Taheri S, Lin L, Austin D, Young T, Mignot E. Short sleep duration is associated with reduced leptin, elevated ghrelin, and increased body mass index. *PLoS Med*. 2004;1(3):e62. doi:10.1371/journal.pmed.0010062

9. Mignot E. Stanford study links obesity to hormonal changes from lack of sleep. https://med.stanford.edu/news/all-news/2004/stanford-study-links-obesity-to-hormonal-changes-from-lack-of-sleep.html.

10. Gottlieb DJ, Punjabi NM, Newman AB, et al. Association of sleep time with diabetes mellitus and impaired glucose

tolerance. *Arch Intern Med*. 2005;165(8):863-867. doi:10.1001/archinte.165.8.863

11. Colten HR, Altevogt BM, Institute of Medicine (US) Committee on Sleep Medicine and Research, eds. *Sleep Disorders and Sleep Deprivation: An Unmet Public Health Problem*. Washington (DC): National Academies Press (US); 2006.

12. The Cleveland Clinic. How Much Sleep Your Kids Need: Recommendations by Age. https://health.clevelandclinic.org/recommended-amount-of-sleep-for-children. Published September 15, 2022.

13. Reilly JJ, Armstrong J, Dorosty AR, et al. Early life risk factors for obesity in childhood: cohort study. *BMJ*. 2005;330(7504):1357. doi:10.1136/bmj.38470.670903.E0

14. Agras WS, Hammer LD, McNicholas F, Kraemer HC. Risk factors for childhood overweight: a prospective study from birth to 9.5 years [published correction appears in J Pediatr. 2004 Sep;145(3):424]. *J Pediatr*. 2004;145(1):20-25. doi:10.1016/j.jpeds.2004.03.023

15. Landhuis CE, Poulton R, Welch D, Hancox RJ. Childhood sleep time and long-term risk for obesity: a 32-year prospective birth cohort study. *Pediatrics*. 2008;122(5):955-960. doi:10.1542/peds.2007-3521

16. Van Cauter E, Leproult R, Plat L. Age-related changes in slow wave sleep and REM sleep and relationship with growth hormone and cortisol levels in healthy men. *JAMA*. 2000;284(7):861-868. doi:10.1001/jama.284.7.861

17. Honda Y, Takahashi K, Takahashi S, et al. Growth hormone secretion during nocturnal sleep in normal subjects. *J Clin Endocrinol Metab*. 1969;29(1):20-29. doi:10.1210/jcem-29-1-20

18. Cherniske S. *Caffeine Blues: Wake Up To The Hidden Dangers Of America's # 1 Drug*. New York, NY: Warner Books; 1998.

19. Imaki M, Hatanaka Y, Ogawa Y, Yoshida Y, Tanada S. An epidemiological study on relationship between the hours of sleep and life style factors in Japanese factory workers. *J Physiol Anthropol Appl Human Sci*. 2002;21(2):115-120. doi:10.2114/jpa.21.115

20. Wong YJ, Owen J, Gabana NT, et al. Does gratitude writing improve the mental health of psychotherapy clients? Evidence from a randomized controlled trial. *Psychother Res*. 2018;28(2):192-202. doi:10.1080/10503307.2016.1169332

21. Bailey BW, Allen MD, LeCheminant JD, et al. Objectively measured sleep patterns in young adult women and the relationship to adiposity. *Am J Health Promot*. 2014;29(1):46-54. doi:10.4278/ajhp.121012-QUAN-500

22. Drake C, Roehrs T, Shambroom J, Roth T. Caffeine effects on sleep taken 0, 3, or 6 hours before going to bed. *J Clin Sleep Med*. 2013;9(11):1195-1200. Published 2013 Nov 15. doi:10.5664/jcsm.3170

23. Fujita S, Rasmussen BB, Cadenas JG, Grady JJ, Volpi E. Effect of insulin on human skeletal muscle protein synthesis is modulated by insulin-induced changes in muscle blood flow and amino acid availability. *Am J Physiol Endocrinol Metab*. 2006;291(4):E745-E754. doi:10.1152/ajpendo.00271.2005

24. Fernstrom JD, Larin F, Wurtman RJ. Daily variations in the concentrations of individual amino acids in rat plasma. *Life Sci I*. 1971;10(14):813-819. doi:10.1016/0024-3205(71)90036-1

25. Fernstrom JD, Faller DV. Neutral amino acids in the brain: changes in response to food ingestion. *J Neurochem*. 1978;30(6):1531-1538. doi:10.1111/j.1471-4159.1978.tb10489.x

26. Ober C, Sinatra ST, Zucker M. *Earthing: The Most Important Health Discovery Ever!* Laguna Beach, CA: Basic Health Publications, Inc.; 2014.

27. Harvard Health Publications. Medications That Can Affect Sleep. 2010. www.harvard.edu/newsletters/Harvard-Womens-Health-Watch/2010/July/medications-that-can-affect-sleep. Published July 1, 2010.

28. Whitaker R. *Anatomy of an Epidemic*. New York, NY: Broadway Books; 2010.

29. Goldman E. A new approach to promoting healthy sleep. http://holisticprimarycare.net/topics/topics-o-z/vitamins-a-supplements/1249-a-new-approach-to-promoting-healthy-sleep. Published December 8, 2011.

30. Pagel JF, Zafralotfi S, Zammit G. How to prescribe a good night's sleep. *Patient Care*. 1997;31(4):87-97.

31. Kryger MH, Roth T, Dement WC. *Principles and Practices of Sleep Medicine (2nd ed)*. Philadelphia, PA: W.B. Saunders; 1994.

Chapter 20: Environmental Toxins, Obesogens, and Weight Gain

1. Thomas P. The Big Fat Fix. *Ecologist*. 2006;36(9):33-43.

2. Desvergne B, Feige JN, Casals-Casas C. PPAR-mediated activity of phthalates: A link to the obesity epidemic? *Mol Cell Endocrinol*. 2009;304(1-2):43-48. doi:10.1016/j.mce.2009.02.017

3. Newbold RR, Padilla-Banks E, Jefferson WN, Heindel JJ. Effects of endocrine disruptors on obesity. *Int J Androl*. 2008;31(2):201-208. doi:10.1111/j.1365-2605.2007.00858.x

4. Brucker-Davis F. Effects of environmental synthetic chemicals on thyroid function. *Thyroid*. 1998;8(9):827-856. doi:10.1089/thy.1998.8.827

5. Wetervelt A. Pthalates are everywhere, and the health risks are worrying. How bad are they really? *The Guardian*. Published February 10, 2015.

6. Sathyanarayana S, Alcedo G, Saelens BE, et al. Unexpected results in a randomized dietary trial to reduce phthalate and bisphenol A exposures. *J Expo Sci Environ Epidemiol*. 2013;23(4):378-384. doi:10.1038/jes.2013.9

7. Toxic-Free Future. What are bisphenols? https://toxicfreefuture.org/toxic-chemicals/bisphenols/. Accessed February 24, 2024.

8. Cooper K, Marshall M, Vanderlinden L, Ursitti F. Early Exposures to Hazardous Chemicals/Pollution and Association with Chronic Disease: A Scoping Review. Canadian Environmental Law Association, the Ontario College of Family Physicians and the Environmental Health Institute of Canada. June 2011.

9. Grün F, Blumberg B. Environmental obesogens: organotins and endocrine disruption via nuclear receptor signaling. *Endocrinology*. 2006;147(6 Suppl):S50-S55. doi:10.1210/en.2005-1129

10. Stahlhut RW, van Wijngaarden E, Dye TD, Cook S, Swan SH. Concentrations of urinary phthalate metabolites are associated with increased waist circumference and insulin resistance in adult U.S. males [published correction appears in *Environ Health Perspect*. 2007 Sep;115(9):A443]. *Environ Health Perspect*. 2007;115(6):876-882. doi:10.1289/ehp.9882

11. Lee DH, Lee IK, Song K, et al. A strong dose-response relation between serum concentrations of persistent organic pollutants and diabetes: results from the National Health and Examination Survey 1999-2002. *Diabetes Care*. 2006;29(7):1638-1644. doi:10.2337/dc06-0543

12. Gladen BC, Ragan NB, Rogan WJ. Pubertal growth and development and prenatal and lactational exposure to polychlorinated biphenyls and dichlorodiphenyl dichloroethene. *J Pediatr.* 2000;136(4):490-496. doi:10.1016/s0022-3476(00)90012-x

13. Environmental Working Group (EWG) Science Team. EWG's 2023 Shopper's Guide to Pesticides in Produce. www.ewg.org/foodnews/summary.php. Accessed Nov 2023.

14. Séralini GE, Cellier D, de Vendomois JS. New analysis of a rat feeding study with a genetically modified maize reveals signs of hepatorenal toxicity. *Arch Environ Contam Toxicol.* 2007;52(4):596-602. doi:10.1007/s00244-006-0149-5

Chapter 21: Psycho-Emotional Factors: Discarding Old Programs

No References

Chapter 22: Food Addiction, Mindfulness, and Self-Care: What's Eating You?

1. Holder JM. American College of Addictionology and Compulsive Disorders, Certified Addiction Professional (CAP) Training Program, Module 1.

2. Blum K, Kozlowski GP. Ethanol and Neuromodulator Interactions: A Cascade Model of Reward. (In: Ollat H, Parvez S, Parvez H, Eds. *Alcohol and Behavior.* Utrecht, Netherlands: VSP Press; 1990:131-149.

3. Blum K, Braverman ER, Holder JM, et al. Reward deficiency syndrome: a biogenetic model for the diagnosis and treatment of impulsive, addictive, and compulsive behaviors. *J Psychoactive Drugs.* 2000;32 Suppl:i-112. doi:10.1080/02791072.2000.10736099

4. Holder, JM. Beating Addiction: From Bondage to Freedom. *Alternative Medicine.* May 1999:38-40.

5. Miller M, Miller D. *Staying Clean and Sober.* Orem, UT: Woodland Publishing; 2005.

6. Rao P, Rodriguez RL, Shoemaker SP. Addressing the sugar, salt, and fat issue the science of food way. *NPJ Sci Food.* 2018;2:12. Published 2018 Jul 16. doi:10.1038/s41538-018-0020-x

7. Onaolapo AY, Onaolapo OJ. Food additives, food and the concept of 'food addiction': Is stimulation of the brain reward circuit by food sufficient to trigger addiction? *Pathophysiology.* 2018;25(4):263-276. doi:10.1016/j.pathophys.2018.04.002

8. Holder JM, Duncan RC, Gissen M, Miller M, Blum K. Increasing retention rates among the chemically dependent in residential treatment: auriculotherapy and subluxation-based chiropractic care. *Molecular Psychiatry.* 2001;6(Suppl1):S8.

Chapter 23: Body Image and Emotional Care

No References

Chapter 24: Keys to Successful Lifestyle Change

No References

RESOURCES AND SUPPORT

To reinforce your commitment to the Weightless program, I share the following resources. They will enhance your success and support you on your journey.

BOOKS

1. *Whole*, by T. Colin Campbell, PhD
2. *The China Study*, by T. Colin Campbell, PhD, and Thomas M. Campbell II, MD
3. *Becoming Vegan*, by Brenda Davis, RD
4. *Comfortably Unaware*, by Richard Oppenlander
5. *Food is Climate*, by Glen Merzer
6. *The Pleasure Trap*, by Alan Goldhamer, DC, and Doug Lisle, PhD
7. *Fast Food Genocide*, by Joel Fuhrman, MD
8. *Your Body in Balance*, by Neal Barnard, MD
9. *Rewind Your Body Clock*, by Jayney Goddard
10. *Straight Up Food*, by Cathy Fisher

VIDEOS

1. *What the Health*
2. *Forks Over Knives*

3. *The Game Changers*

4. *Seaspiracy*

5. *Dominion*

6. *Cowspiracy*

7. *A Prayer for Compassion*

8. *Land of Ahimsa, Land of Cruelty*

9. *Eating Our Way to Extinction*

WEBSITES and ONLINE PROGRAMS

1. The National Health Association (healthscience.org)

2. DrFrankSabatino.com online weight-loss program, *Lean for Life*

3. Physicians Committee for Responsible Medicine (PCRM.org)

4. Main Street Vegan (mainstreetvegan.com)

5. Climate Healers (Climate Healers.com)

6. The Complementary Medical Association (the-cma.org.uk)

7. JayneyGoddard.org

ABOUT THE AUTHOR

Dr. Frank Sabatino has been a plant-exclusive physician for over 45 years. He is the past health director of the Shangri-La Natural Hygiene Institute in Bonita Springs, Florida, the Regency Health Resort and Spa in Hallandale, Florida, and the Ocean Jade Health Center in Lauderdale-by-the-Sea, Florida, where for over 30 years he lectured, cared for, and inspired thousands of people to adopt the benefits of a vegan, plant-exclusive lifestyle. He is currently the director of the Balance for Life Health Retreat (BalanceForLifeFlorida.com) in the beautiful city of Deerfield Beach, Florida. Balance for Life is a vegan-lifestyle education center specializing in SOS-free, whole plant-exclusive nutrition, weight regulation, health rejuvenation, stress management, therapeutic fasting, and detoxification.

Dr. Sabatino is a chiropractic physician who also has a Ph.D. in cell biology and neuroendocrinology from the Emory University School of Medicine. The book of his original research on the effects of brain peptides on the regulation of reproductive hormones was published in 1988. While a professor at the University of Texas School of Medicine, he did extensive landmark research on calorie restriction, stress, and aging, and has published a number of major scientific papers in some of the most well-respected peer-reviewed journals in the fields of cell biology, endocrinology, and neuroscience.

He also has written numerous articles for lay magazines and journals in the areas of water-only fasting, clinical plant-based nutrition, healthy weight loss, women's hormones, stress management, addiction, and healthy aging.

He has been featured in a variety of books, news articles, on CNN, and on other cable TV programs. Dr. Sabatino is a past member of the prestigious Brookdale Fellowship in Gerontology and Aging. As a member of the International Association of Hygienic Physicians, he also is widely recognized as an expert in water-only fasting. Dr. Sabatino is certified in the study and care of addictions from the American College of Addictionology and Compulsive Disorders. He is currently the Director of Health Education for the National Health Association (NHA), the oldest hygienic, whole-plant-food lifestyle education organization in the world, and the host of the Health Science Podcast sponsored by the NHA. Dr. Sabatino also serves as a consultant for the TrueNorth Health Center fasting research program and is on the medical advisory board of the T. Colin Campbell Center for Nutritional Studies. He is also the Science and Research Director for The Complementary Medical Association located in the U.K., an organization that promotes coursework and global standards for complementary and integrative healthcare. His online program, *Lean for Life*, promotes the most comprehensive plant-exclusive solution and lifestyle strategies for solving the pandemic of obesity. He is also a proponent of Oriental energy arts and a longtime teacher and student of tai chi and qi gong.

Previous works by the author

1. The role of Neuropeptide Y in the regulation of luteinizing hormone-releasing hormone secretion from the hypothalamus in vitro. Published dissertation manuscript. Emory University School of Medicine, Department of Anatomy and Cell Biology, 1988.

2. *Be Truly Well: It's a SNAP.* 8-part CD series, 1999.

3. *Weightless: Compassionate weight loss for life.* DVD series, 2011.

4. *Lean for Life* online program (DrFrankSabatino.com), 2019.

5. *Lean and Healthy for Life.* 2022, ebook.

6. *Plant-Based Guide to Eating Out in the Real World.* 2023, ebook.

INDEX

Printed in Great Britain
by Amazon